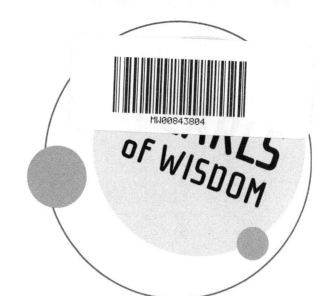

Gastroenterology and Hepatology

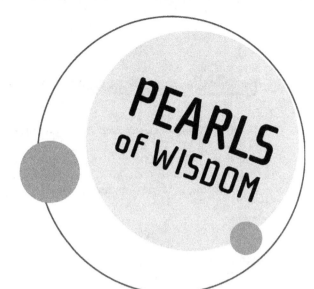

Gastroenterology and Hepatology
BOARD REVIEW
Third Edition

John K. DiBaise, MD
Professor of Medicine
Division of Gastroenterology
Mayo Clinic
Scottsdale, Arizona

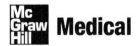 **Medical**

New York Chicago San Francisco Lisbon London Madrid Mexico City Milan
New Delhi San Juan Seoul Singapore Sydney Toronto

Pearls of Wisdom: Gastroenterology and Hepatology Board Review, Third Edition

1 2 3 4 5 6 7 8 9 0   QDB/QDB   17 16 15 14 13 12

ISBN 978-0-07-176166-6
MHID 0-07-176166-7

Notice

Medicine is an ever-changing science. As new research and clinical experience broaden our knowledge, changes in treatment and drug therapy are required. The authors and the publisher of this work have checked with sources believed to be reliable in their efforts to provide information that is complete and generally in accord with the standards accepted at the time of publication. However, in view of the possibility of human error or changes in medical sciences, neither the authors nor the publisher nor any other party who has been involved in the preparation or publication of this work warrants that the information contained herein is in every respect accurate or complete, and they disclaim all responsibility for any errors or omissions or for the results obtained from use of the information contained in this work. Readers are encouraged to confirm the information contained herein with other sources. For example and in particular, readers are advised to check the product information sheet included in the package of each drug they plan to administer to be certain that the information contained in this work is accurate and that changes have not been made in the recommended dose or in the contraindications for administration. This recommendation is of particular importance in connection with new or infrequently used drugs.

This book was set in Garamond by Cenveo Publisher Services.
The editors were Kirsten Funk and Christina M. Thomas.
The production supervisor was Sherri Souffrance.
Project management provided by Rohini Deb, Cenveo Publisher Services.
Quad/Graphics was printer and binder.

This book is printed on acid-free paper.

Library of Congress Cataloging-in-Publication Data

Gastroenterology and hepatology board review/[edited by] John K. DiBaise.—3rd ed.
      p. ; cm.—(Pearls of wisdom)
  Includes bibliographical references.
  ISBN 978-0-07-176166-6 (pbk. : alk. paper)—ISBN 0-07-176166-7
  I. DiBaise, John K.   II. Series: Pearls of wisdom.
  [DNLM: 1. Gastrointestinal Diseases—Examination Questions.   2. Liver Diseases—
Examination Questions. WI 18.2]
  616.3'30076 dc23   2011048191

Tranquilla, confidentiam et claritate ex cogitatione

CONTENTS

GASTROENTEROLOGY

ESOPHAGUS

STOMACH

SMALL INTESTINE

LARGE INTESTINE

GALLBLADDER, BILE DUCTS, AND PANCREAS

NUTRITION

HEPATOLOGY

MISCELLANEOUS TOPICS

CONTRIBUTORS

Bhupinder S. Anand, MD
Professor of Medicine
Baylor College of Medicine
Staff Physician
Michael DeBakey Veterans Association Medical Center
Houston, Texas
Cirrhosis and Its Complications

Jamie S. Barkin, MD, MACP, MACG
Professor of Medicine
University of Miami
Miller School of Medicine
Chief, Division of Gastroenterology
Mt. Sinai Medical Center
Miami, Florida
Acute and Chronic Pancreatitis

Erika S. Boroff, MD
Consultant, Primary Care Internal Medicine
Community Internal Medicine
Mayo Clinic
Scottsdale, Arizona
Gastrointestinal and Hepatobiliary Disorders in Pregnancy

Randall E. Brand, MD
Professor of Medicine
University of Pittsburgh
University of Pittsburgh Medical Center
Pittsburgh, Pennsylvania
Gallbladder and Bile Duct Tumors
Pancreatic Tumors

Thomas J. Byrne, MD, MSCR
Assistant Professor of Medicine
Mayo Medical School
Phoenix, Arizona
Consultant, Divisions of Hepatology and
    Gastroenterology
Mayo Clinic
Scottsdale, Arizona
Autoimmune and Cholestatic Conditions and
    Overlap Syndromes

Elizabeth J. Carey, MD
Assistant Professor of Medicine
Consultant, Divisions of Hepatology and
    Gastroenterology
Mayo Clinic
Phoenix, Arizona
Gastrointestinal and Hepatobiliary Disorders in Pregnancy

Darwin L. Conwell, MD, MS
Associate Professor of Medicine
Harvard Medical School
Associate Physician
Division of Gastroenterology, Hepatology and
    Endoscopy
Brigham and Women's Hospital
Boston, Massachusetts
Gallbladder, Bile Duct and Pancreatic Congenital and
    Structural Abnormalities

Michael D. Crowell, PhD, FACG, AGAF
Professor of Medicine
Consultant, Division of Gastroenterology
Co-Director, Gastrointestinal Physiology and Motility
Mayo Clinic
Phoenix, Arizona
Esophageal Motility Disorders

Joseph J. Cullen, MD
Professor of Surgery
University of Iowa
Carver College of Medicine
Chief, Surgical Services
Veterans Affairs Medical Center
Iowa City, Iowa
Surgical Aspects of Peptic Ulcer Disease

Nora Decher, MS, RD, CNSC
Nutrition Support Specialist
University of Virginia Health System
Digestive Health Center of Excellence
Charlottesville, Virginia
Short Bowel Syndrome

Parakkal Deepak, MD
Lifetract Clinical Research Fellow, Gastroenterology
NorthShore University Health System
Evanston, Illinois
*Gastrointestinal and Hepatobiliary Manifestations of
   HIV and AIDS*
Maldigestion and Malabsorption

Chirag S. Desai, MD
Assistant Professor of Surgery
Division of Transplantation
University of Arizona
Tucson, Arizona
*Congenital and Structural Abnormalities and Pediatric
   Diseases of the Liver*

John K. DiBaise, MD
Professor of Medicine
Division of Gastroenterology
Mayo Clinic
Scottsdale, Arizona
Esophageal Miscellaneous Inflammatory Diseases
Gastric Motility Disorders
Gastrointestinal Bleeding

Michelle O. DiBaise, MPAS, PA-C, DFAAPA
Associate Clinical Professor
Northern Arizona University
Physician Assistant Program
Phoenix, Arizona
Gastrointestinal and Liver Dermatoses

Ivana Dzeletovic, MD
Fellow, Gastroenterology and Hepatology
Division of Gastroenterology
Mayo Clinic
Scottsdale, Arizona
Gastrointestinal and Pancreaticobiliary Endoscopy

Eli D. Ehrenpreis, MD
Chief, Gastroenterology and Endoscopy
Highland Park Hospital
Clinical Associate Professor of Medicine
University of Chicago
Director, Center for the Study of Complex Diseases
NorthShore University Health System
Evanston, Illinois
*Gastrointestinal and Hepatobiliary Manifestations of
   HIV and AIDS*
Maldigestion and Malabsorption

Atilla Ertan, MD, AGAF, MACG
Professor
The University of Texas
Medical School at Houston
Houston, Texas
Medical Aspects of Cholelithiasis

Douglas O. Faigel, MD, FACG, FASGE, AGAF
Professor of Medicine
Division of Gastroenterology and Hepatology
Mayo Clinic College of Medicine
Scottsdale, Arizona
Gastric Tumors

Ronnie Fass, MD
Professor of Medicine
University of Arizona
Chief, Gastroenterology
Neuroenteric Clinical Research Group
Southern Arizona Veterans Administration Health
   Care System
Tucson, Arizona
*Esophageal Congenital and Structural
   Abnormalities*

Nicholas Ferrentino, MD
Associate Professor of Medicine
Fellowship Program Director
Division of Gastroenterology and Hepatology
University of Vermont
College of Medicine
Burlington, Vermont
Hepatic Infectious Disorders
Hepatic Vascular Disorders

M. Isabel Fiel, MD
Professor of Pathology
Department of Pathology
Mount Sinai School of Medicine
New York, New York
Hepatic Tumors and Cysts

Ryan M. Ford, MD
Assistant Professor of Transplant Hepatology and
   Digestive Diseases
Emory University
Atlanta, Georgia
*Alcoholic Liver Disease and Nonalcoholic
   Steatohepatitis*

Temitope Foster, MD, MSCR
Assistant Professor of Medicine
Division of Digestive Diseases
Emory University School of Medicine
Atlanta, Georgia
*Alcoholic Liver Disease and Nonalcoholic
    Steatohepatitis*

David J. Frantz, MD, MS
Fellow, Division of Gastroenterology
Department of Medicine
The University of North Carolina at Chapel Hill
Chapel Hill, North Carolina
Obesity and Eating Disorders

Juan F. Gallegos-Orozco, MD
Assistant Professor of Medicine
College of Medicine
Fellow, Transplant Hepatology
Division of Hepatology
Mayo Clinic
Phoenix, Arizona
*Drug-Induced, Granulomatous, and Other
    Inflammatory Hepatic Diseases*

Eric B. Goosenberg, MD
Senior Gastroenterologist
Abington Memorial Hospital
Abington, Pennsylvania
Attending Gastroenterologist
Holy Redeemer Hospital
Meadowbrook, Pennsylvania
Esophageal Infectious Disorders
Esophageal Tumors

Kunal Gupta, MD, MBA
Clinical Instructor of Medicine
Fellow, Division of Gastroenterology and
    Hepatology
University of Vermont
College of Medicine
Burlington, Vermont
Hepatic Vascular Disorders

Suryakanth R. Gurudu, MD, FACG, FASGE
Assistant Professor of Medicine
Mayo Medical School
Mayo Clinic
Division of Gastroenterology
Scottsdale, Arizona
Small Intestinal Tumors

Stephanie L. Hansel, MD, MS
Assistant Professor
Division of Gastroenterology and Hepatology
Mayo Clinic
Rochester, Minnesota
Gallbladder and Biliary Motility Disorders

Andrew D. Hardie, MD
Assistant Professor of Radiology
Department of Radiology and Radiological Sciences
Medical University of South Carolina
Charleston, South Carolina
Gastrointestinal and Liver Radiology

Jana G. Hashash, MD
Fellow, Division of Gastroenterology, Hepatology, and
    Nutrition
University of Pittsburgh
Pittsburgh, Pennsylvania
Gallbladder and Bile Duct Tumors
Pancreatic Tumors

Rejy Joseph, MD, MRCP
Resident, Department of Medicine
Pennsylvania Hospital
University of Pennsylvania Health System
Philadelphia, Pennsylvania
Small Intestinal Motility Disorders

Doron D. Kahana, MD, FAAP, CPNS
Assistant Clinical Professor of Pediatrics
Department of Pediatrics
Harbor-University of Califronia, Los Angeles
The David Geffen School of Medicine
Torrance, California
*Congenital and Structural Abnormalities and Pediatric
    Diseases of the Liver*

Khalid M. Khan, MBChB, MRCP
Associate Professor
Department of Surgery
University of Arizona
Tucson, Arizona
*Congenital and Structural Abnormalities and Pediatric
    Diseases of the Liver*

Reena Khanna, MD, FRCPC
Division of Gastroenterology
McMaster University
Hamilton, Ontario, Canada
Large Intestinal Miscellaneous Inflammatory Diseases

David G. Koch, MD, MSCR
Assistant Professor
Department of Medicine
Division of Gastroenterology and Hepatology
Medical University of South Carolina
Charleston, South Carolina
Gastrointestinal and Liver Radiology

Joseph Krenitsky, MS, RD
Nutrition Support Specialist
Division of Gastroenterology and Hepatology
University of Virginia Health System
Charlottesville, Virginia
*Clinical Nutrition, Enteral, and Parenteral
    Nutrition Support*

Brian E. Lacy, PhD, MD
Associate Professor of Medicine
Dartmouth Medical School
Director, Gastrointestinal Motility Lab
Dartmouth-Hitchcock Medical Center
Lebanon, New Hampshire
Esophageal Motility Disorders

Linda S. Lee, MD
Assistant Professor of Medicine
Harvard Medical School
Director, Women's Health in Gastroenterology and
    Endoscopic Education
Brigham and Women's Hospital
Boston, Massachusetts
*Gallbladder, Bile Duct, and Pancreatic Congenital and
    Structural Abnormalities*

Elizabeth Lyden, MS
Statistical Coordinator
College of Public Health
University of Nebraska Medical Center
Omaha, Nebraska
Biostatistics for the Gastroenterologist

James A. Madura, II, MD, FACS
Assistant Professor of Surgery
Director, Bariatric Surgery Program
Mayo Clinic
Phoenix, Arizona
*Abdominal Cavity: Congenital Abnormalities, Abscesses,
    and Fistulae*

John K. Marshall, MD, MSc, FRCPC, AGAF
Division of Gastroenterology
McMaster University
Hamilton, Ontario, Canada
Large Intestinal Miscellaneous Inflammatory Diseases

Timothy M. McCashland, MD
Professor of Medicine
Department of Gastroenterology and Hepatology
University of Nebraska Medical Center
Omaha, Nebraska
Acute Liver Failure and Liver Transplantation

Denise McCormack, MD
Resident, Department of Surgery
Danbury Hospital
Danbury, Connecticut
*Gallbladder, Bile Duct, and Pancreatic Infectious Disorders
Pancreas Miscellaneous Inflammatory Diseases*

David W. McFadden, MD, MBA
Professor and Chair
Department of Surgery
University of Vermont
Associate Dean for Regional Academic Affairs
Burlington, Vermont
*Gallbladder, Bile Duct, and Pancreatic Infectious Disorders
Pancreatic Miscellaneous Inflammatory Diseases*

Ibraheem Mizyed, MD
Gastrointestinal Fellow, Division of Gastroenterology
The University of Arizona College of Medicine
Tucson, Arizona
Surgical Aspects of Cholelithiasis

Enrique G. Molina, MD
Senior Fellow
University of Miami
Miller School of Medicine
Mt. Sinai Medical Center
Miami, Florida
Acute and Chronic Pancreatitis

Sandeep Mukherjee, MD
Associate Professor of Medicine
Department of Internal Medicine
Section of Gastroenterology and Hepatology
University of Nebraska Medical Center
Omaha, Nebraska
Viral Hepatitis

Marco A. Olivera-Martínez, MD
Assistant Professor of Medicine
Department of Internal Medicine
Section of Gastroenterology and Hepatology
University of Nebraska Medical Center
Omaha, Nebraska
Viral Hepatitis

Rahul Pannala, MD, MPH
Assistant Professor
Senior Associate Consultant
Division of Gastroenterology
Mayo Clinic
Scottsdale, Arizona
Gastrointestinal and Pancreaticobiliary Endoscopy

Samir Parekh, MD
Assistant Professor of Medicine
Division of Digestive Diseases and The Emory
    Transplant Center
Emory University School of Medicine
Atlanta, Georgia
Metabolic Liver Disorders

Carol Rees Parrish, MS, RD
Nutrition Support Specialist
University of Virginia Health System
Digestive Health Center of Excellence
Charlottesville, Virginia
*Clinical Nutrition, Enteral, and Parenteral
    Nutrition Support*
Short Bowel Syndrome

Shabana F. Pasha, MD
Assistant Professor of Medicine
Vice Chair, Research
Director, Small Bowel Disorders Clinic
Division of Gastroenterology
Mayo Clinic
Scottsdale, Arizona
*Radiation and Ischemic Injury and Vascular
    Abnormalities*

Amir Patel, MD
Department of Medicine
NorthShore University HealthSystems
Teaching Affiliate of The University of Chicago
Evanston, Illinois
Large Intestinal Tumors

Isaac Raijman, MD
Clinical Associate Professor
Baylor College of Medicine and University of Texas
    Health Science Center
Digestive Associates of Houston
Houston, Texas
*Gallbladder and Bile Duct Miscellaneous Inflammatory
    Diseases*

Francisco C. Ramirez, MD
Professor of Medicine
Mayo Clinic College of Medicine
Mayo Clinic
Scottsdale, Arizona
Peptic Ulcer Disease and Its Complications

Yehuda Ringel, MD
Associate Professor of Medicine
Division of Gastroenterology and Hepatology
The University of North Carolina School of
    Medicine
Chapel Hill, North Carolina
Disorders of the Pelvic Floor and Anorectum

Tamar Ringel-Kulka, MD, MPH
Assistant Professor of Maternal and
    Child Health
Gillings School of Global Public Health
The University of North Carolina at Chapel Hill
Chapel Hill, North Carolina
Obesity and Eating Disorders

Rene Rivera, MD
Clinical Instructor
Department of Gastroenterology and Hepatology
University of Rochester Medical Center
Rochester, New York
Gastric Congenital and Structural Abnormalities

Cory A. Roberts, MD
Clinical Associate Professor
University of Texas Southwestern Medical Center
Director, Gastrointestinal and Hepatic Pathology
President, Chairman and Medical Director - ProPath
Dallas, Texas
Gastrointestinal Pathology
Hepatobiliary Pathology

Robin D. Rothstein, MD
Associate Professor of Medicine
Department of Medicine
Pennsylvania Hospital
University of Pennsylvania Health System
Philadelphia, Pennsylvania
Small Intestinal Motility Disorders

Hemant K. Roy, MD
Director, Research and Vice Chair
Section of Gastroenterology
NorthShore Univertsity HealthSystems
Clinical Associate Professor of Medicine
University of Chicago Pritzker School of Medicine
Evanston, Illionis
Large Intestinal Tumors

Kevin C. Ruff, MD
Division of Gastroenterology and Hepatology
Department of Internal Medicine
Mayo Clinic
Scottsdale, Arizona
Gastric Infectious Disorders
Small Intestinal Infectious Disorders

Claudia P. Sanmiguel, MD
Fellow, Gastroenterology
University of California
Los Angeles, California
Large Intestinal Motility Disorders

Neeraj K. Sardana, MD
Clinical Instructor of Medicine
Fellow, Division of Gastroenterology and Hepatology
University of Vermont
College of Medicine
Burlington, Vermont
Hepatic Infectious Disorders

Thomas D. Schiano, MD
Professor of Medicine
Division of Liver Diseases Mount Sinai Medical Center
New York, New York
Hepatic Tumors and Cysts

Kendra K. Schmid, PhD
Department of Biostatistics
College of Public Health
Universty of Nebraska Medical Center
Omaha, Nebraska
Biostatistics for the Gastroenterologist

Ashok N. Shah, MD, MS, FRCP, MACG, AGAF
Professor of Medicine
Department of Gastroenterology and Hepatology
University of Rochester Medical Center
Rochester, New York
Gastric Congenital and Structural Abnormalities
Large Intestinal Congenital and Structural Abnormalities
Small Intestinal Congenital and Structural Abnormalities

Rajiv Sharma, MD
Clinical Instructor
Department of Gastroenterology and Hepatology
University of Rochester Medical Center
Rochester, New York
Small Intestinal Congenital and Structural Abnormalities
Large Intestinal Congenital and Structural Abnormalities

Humberto Sifuentes, MD
Section of Gastroenterology and Hepatology
Georgia Health Sciences University
Augusta, Georgia
Gastrointestinal and Hepatobiliary Manifestations of
*   HIV and AIDS*

Jessica K. Smith, MD
Assistant Professor of Surgery
Division of Gastrointestinal, Minimally Invasive and
   Bariatric Surgery
University of Iowa Hospitals and Clinics
Staff Surgeon, Iowa City Veterans Medical Center
Iowa City, Iowa
Surgical Aspects of Peptic Ulcer Disease

Edy E. Soffer, MD
Gastrointestinal Motility Program
Cedars-Sinai Medical Center
Los Angeles, California
Large Intestinal Motility Disorders

Matthew L. Stephenson, MD
Chief Resident, Department of Radiology
Medical University of South Carolina
Charleston, South Carolina
Gastrointestinal and Liver Radiology

Eugene A. Trowers, MD, MPH, FACP
Clinical Professor of Medicine, Gastroenterology
Department of Medicine
The University of Arizona College of Medicine
Tucson, Arizona
Surgical Aspects of Cholelithiasis

Jon A. Vanderhoof, MD
Executive Medical Advisor
Children's Hospital Boston
Harvard Medical School
Boston, Massachusetts
Pediatric Gastrointestinal Diseases

Hugo E. Vargas, MD
Chair, Division of Hepatology
Professor of Medicine
College of Medicine
Mayo Clinic
Phoenix, Arizona
*Drug-Induced, Granulomatous, and Other
    Inflammatory Hepatic Diseases*

Rajeev Vasudeva, MD, FACG
Clinical Professor
University of South Carolina School of Medicine
Consultant in Gastroenterology
Director of Endoscopy
Palmetto Health Richland
Columbia, South Carolina
Foreign Bodies and Caustic Injury
Gastroesophageal Reflux Disease

Holenarasipur R. Vikram, MD, FACP, FIDSA
Assistant Professor of Medicine
Consultant, Division of Infectious Diseases
Mayo Clinic
Phoenix, Arizona
Large Intestinal Infectious Disorders

Abinash Virk, MD, DTM&H
Associate Professor of Medicine
Mayo Clinic College of Medicine
Rochester, Minnesota
Travel Matters in Gastroenterology

David S. Wolf, MD
Assistant Professor
The University of Texas
Medical School at Houston
Houston, Texas
Medical Aspects of Cholelithiasis

Richard A. Wright, MD
Professor of Medicine
Arthur M. Schoen, MD Chair in Gastroenterology
Division of Gastroenterology, Hepatology and
    Nutrition
University of Louisville
Louisville, Kentucky
Gastric Motility Disorders

Renee L. Young, MD
Associate Professor
Division of Gastroenterology and Hepatology
Department of Internal Medicine
University of Nebraska Medical Center
Omaha, Nebraska
Inflammatory Bowel Disease

PREFACE

Gastroenterology and Hepatology Board Review: Pearls of Wisdom is designed to help you learn about gastrointestinal and liver diseases and prepare you for the In-Service and Board Examination in Gastroenterology and Hepatology. The third edition brings with it many exciting upgrades. Every chapter has been extensively revised by a nationwide team of experts in their field. Several new chapters have been included, such as Gastrointestinal and Liver Radiology. Most notable is the increased use of images in this edition to test you on visual diagnosis. The incorporation of black and white photos directly into each chapter is supplemented with a separate gallery of full color images. Finally, each chapter ends with a list of up-to-date suggested readings for further remediation on the topic.

Before you get started, a few words are appropriate discussing the intent, format, limitations, and proper use of this book. *Gastroenterology and Hepatology Board Review* is primarily intended as a study aid structured in a question and answer format. Most of the questions are short with brief answers. This is to facilitate moving through a large body of information. Such a format, while unlike that in the actual Boards, is useful to enable you to assess your strengths and weaknesses in a particular area. This then allows you to concentrate further studies on areas of interest or weakness. Emphasis has been placed on distilling key facts that are easily overlooked, quickly forgotten, and that somehow seem to occur frequently on in-service and board examinations.

It must be emphasized that any question and answer book is most useful as a learning tool when *used in conjunction* with a subject-specific textbook. Truly assimilating these facts into a framework of knowledge absolutely requires further reading on the surrounding concepts. The more active the learning process, the better the understanding. **Use this book with your preferred source texts handy and open.** When you encounter a question that you cannot recall the answer or that you find of particular interest, you are strongly encouraged to review the pertinent area in the textbook at hand or refer to the recommended reading at the end of each chapter.

The chapters are organized to include all aspects of gastroenterology and hepatology. Some areas are covered more thoroughly than others. The questions within each chapter are randomly arranged to simulate board examinations and the way questions arise in real life. There are areas of redundancy. This is intentional—redundancy is a good thing when preparing for board examinations.

While great effort has been made to verify that the questions and answers are accurate, discrepancies and inaccuracies sometimes occur. Most often this is attributable to variance between original sources. We have tried to verify in several references the most accurate information. Keep in mind that some answers may not be the answers you would prefer. New research and practice occasionally deviates from that, which likely represents the correct answer for test purposes. In addition, this book risks accuracy by aggressively pruning complex concepts down to the simplest level; the dynamic knowledge base and clinical practice of medicine is not like that. **Remember, this book is designed to maximize your score in a test.** Refer to your most current sources of information and mentors for direction in clinical practice.

We welcome your comments, suggestions, and criticism. Please make us aware of any errors you find. We hope to make continuous improvements and would greatly appreciate any input with regard to format, organization, content, presentation, or about specific questions.

Study hard and good luck for the Boards!

John K. DiBaise, MD

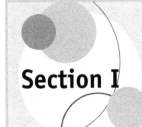

Section I

GASTROENTEROLOGY

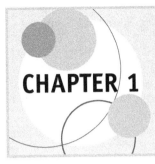

CHAPTER 1

Gastrointestinal Bleeding

John K. DiBaise, MD

○ **What major clinical features help predict which patients who present with gastrointestinal bleeding can be managed without admission to the hospital?**

Absence of hypotension, melena, or hematemesis and age less than 60 years.

○ **A 37-year-old man with a history of alcohol abuse is transferred to your hospital with a history of hematemesis and melena the day before. He has numerous spider telangiectasias on his upper body and mild asterixis. What lesion is being demonstrated on upper endoscopy?**

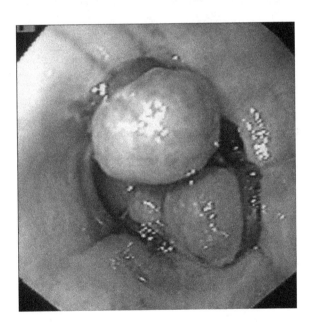

Figure 1-1

Esophageal varices in the distal esophagus that have undergone band ligation.

○ **What is the advantage, if any, of esophageal variceal band ligation compared with sclerotherapy?**

Fewer complications with banding.

○ **What is the presently accepted efficacy rate (of stopping hemorrhage) for sclerotherapy or banding of esophageal varices?**

85%–90%.

○ **Approximately what percentage of patients with esophageal varices that have never bled will experience a variceal hemorrhage in the 1 to 2 years following their diagnosis?**

Approximately one-third.

○ **What endoscopic features of esophageal varices predict a high probability of hemorrhage?**

Large size (ie, grade 3 and 4) and red wale markings.

○ **What is the hepatic wedge pressure gradient below which bleeding from esophageal varices rarely occurs?**

12 mmHg.

○ **True/False: An arteriovenous malformation (angiodysplasia) in a patient who shows no evidence of gastrointestinal blood loss should be cauterized to prevent bleeding.**

False. The vast majority of angiodysplasia discovered at endoscopy are incidental findings and require no treatment.

○ **When considering all the diagnoses found in a large number of patients who present with upper gastrointestinal hemorrhage, approximately what percentage has some form of acid-peptic disease?**

85%.

○ **The national mortality rate from gastrointestinal bleeding has remained stable since 1945 and is approximately what percentage?**

10%.

○ **True/False: Oral iron therapy produces a false positive fecal occult blood test.**

False. It may, however, cause visual interpretation errors.

○ **What is the average amount of blood/day lost in the stool of a healthy individual on no medication as determined by the chromate-tagged red cell test?**

0.5 to 1.5 mL/day.

○ **In experimental animals (and presumably in humans), at what rate must blood be lost into the gut lumen before arteriography is capable of demonstrating a bleeding site?**

0.5 to 1.5 mL/min. The corresponding rate for a nuclear medicine red blood cell scan is 0.1 to 0.4 mL/min.

○ **Approximately what percentage of patients with a gastrointestinal hemorrhage will have no identifiable source despite careful evaluation including small bowel enteroscopy?**

10%.

○ **True/False: Intense inhibition of acid secretion slows or stops acute upper gastrointestinal bleeding.**

False. However, intense inhibition of acid secretion may prevent early rebleeding from peptic ulcer disease.

○ **A 35-year-old man presents with massive hematemesis and anemia following an episode of protracted retching. What does the figure show?**

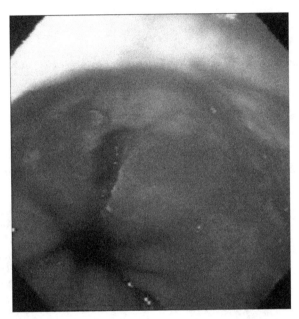

Figure 1-2 See also color plate.

Mallory–Weiss tear.

○ **What percentage of acute hemorrhages due to Mallory–Weiss tears stop spontaneously?**

80%–90%.

○ **Considering all nonvariceal causes of upper gastrointestinal hemorrhage, what is the rebleeding rate (with or without endoscopy)?**

20%.

○ **What is the therapeutic efficacy (range) of a Sengstaken–Blakemore tube in controlling bleeding from esophageal varices?**

65%–85%.

○ **True/False: Varices may return after eradication.**

True. By 2 years, there appears to be a return of varices in 40% of patients.

○   **What are the two major complications of the Sengstaken–Blakemore tube for tamponade of bleeding esophageal varices?**

Aspiration pneumonia and perforation of the esophagus by erroneously inflating the gastric balloon in the esophagus.

○   **What is the primary indication for angiographic infusion of vasopressors or embolization in the treatment of bleeding peptic ulcer disease?**

Failure of therapeutic endoscopy to control bleeding or rebleeding not controlled by a second therapeutic endoscopy in a patient who is of poor operative risk.

○   **True/False: It is accepted as true that cure of *Helicobacter pylori* infection in a patient with a bleeding ulcer will prevent future bleeding episodes.**

True—although not in everyone. The nonsteroidal anti-inflammatory drug (NSAID)-status of the patient and location of the ulcer (ie, gastric or duodenal) may play a role in those cases of recurrent ulcer bleeding.

○   **In a patient with melena but a normal hematocrit, the lesion below was found on upper endoscopy. Based on its appearance, what is the approximate risk of rebleeding from this lesion?**

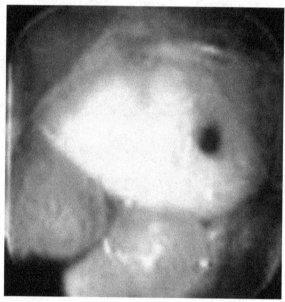

Figure 1-3 See also color plate.

The risk of rebleeding in an ulcer with a flat pigmented spot is about 10%.

○   **True/False: It is the national standard of care that endoscopy be repeated in order to prove healing of a duodenal ulcer that has previously bled.**

False. In contrast, it is generally advised that endoscopy be repeated for gastric ulcers given the risk of neoplasm.

○   **In a patient with a third episode of bleeding from proven duodenal ulcer disease in the second portion of the duodenum, what diagnosis must be considered?**

Zollinger–Ellison syndrome (gastrinoma).

○   **What is the single most common risk factor for ulcer formation in patients who use NSAIDs regularly?**

Age greater than 65 or 70 years.

○   **Upper gastrointestinal hemorrhage is an important clinical problem in critically ill patients and after extensive surgery, especially neurosurgery and cardiac procedures. What, if anything, can be done to reduce the frequency of such bleeding episodes?**

Intravenous or oral acid suppression. Sucralfate may also be useful in this setting.

○   **A 63-year-old "vasculopath" presents with massive GI bleeding about 6 weeks after another episode of bleeding during which an esophagogastroduodenoscopy (EGD) and colonoscopy were normal. An emergent CT scan is obtained. What is the diagnosis?**

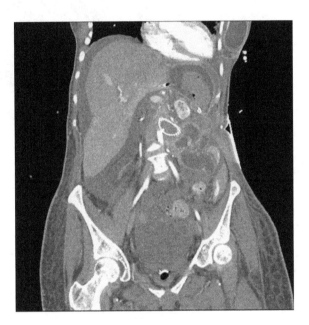

Figure 1-4

An aorto-enteric fistula. The so-called "herald bleeding episode," in which significant bleeding that spontaneously ceases occurs, is characteristic of this condition. Although CT scan is more sensitive than endoscopy to diagnose this condition, the sensitivity of CT is still relatively low. This diagnosis, therefore, requires a high index of clinical suspicion. Endoscopy is often necessary to exclude a peptic process as a cause of the bleed but should be done in conjunction with surgery.

○   **What is the eventual outcome of ischemic colitis in the vast majority of patients?**

Spontaneous cessation of bleeding, usually without requiring blood transfusion and with no complications. Acute perforation (within 3 days) and late stricture formation are uncommon.

○ **A 58-year-old woman with multiple medical problems presents with the sudden onset of severe lower abdominal cramping, an urge to defecate, and passage of a fairly normal stool followed shortly by passage of gross blood. Flexible sigmoidoscopy reveals the following finding. What is the most likely diagnosis?**

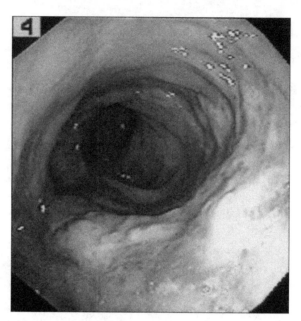

Figure 1-5 See also color plate.

Ischemic colitis.

○ **True/False: Colonic biopsy can differentiate ischemic colitis from *Clostridium difficile* colitis.**
False.

○ **True/False: Diverticular hemorrhage can be controlled by endoscopic means.**
True. If the bleeding site can be identified (uncommonly), injection around the orifice of the diverticulum or the endoscopic placement of clips may be helpful.

○ **What is the most common cause of significant upper gastrointestinal bleeding in patients of child-bearing age?**
Duodenal ulcer disease.

○ **If a patient with bleeding esophageal varices continues to bleed following two attempts at variceal banding or sclerotherapy, what is the recommended next therapeutic maneuver?**
Emergency portosystemic shunt, usually by surgery or by transjugular intrahepatic portosystemic shunt (TIPS), depending on the cause of portal hypertension, severity of the liver disease, and availability. A Sengstaken–Blakemore tube may be necessary in the interim.

○ **True/False: Endotracheal intubation should be considered before endoscopy in patients presenting with hematemesis and hemodynamic instability.**
True.

○ A previously healthy, asymptomatic patient over the age of 60 years presents with the sudden passage of voluminous gross blood with little or no abdominal discomfort. Colonoscopy is performed. What is the most likely diagnosis?

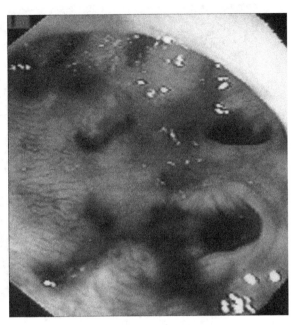

Figure 1-6 See also color plate.

Diverticular bleeding from the colon.

○ What is the most common complication of upper gastrointestinal endoscopy in a patient with active upper gastrointestinal hemorrhage?

Aspiration pneumonia.

○ In an acutely bleeding patient, what is the first step in management?

Support the intravascular volume (ie, fluid resuscitation). Once hemodynamically stable, further evaluation can safely be performed.

○ In a patient who is vigorously bleeding from esophageal varices despite pharmacotherapy and banding of varices and who is waiting for a surgical suite to become available for portosystemic shunt, what therapeutic maneuver is available that may control the hemorrhage?

Sengstaken–Blakemore or Minnesota tube for tamponade.

○ A 26-year-old man presents with hematemesis, fever, and severe pleuritic left chest pain a few hours after a severe vomiting episode. What is the most likely diagnosis?

Boerhaave's syndrome.

○   A 38-year-old man with a history of chronic pancreatitis complicated by pseudocysts in the past presents with a history of hematemesis the evening before. The following picture of the stomach was obtained on upper endoscopy. What is being demonstrated?

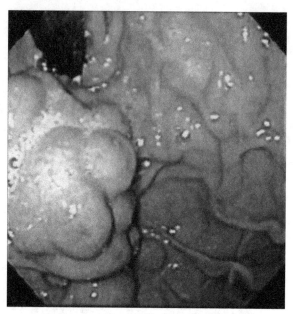

Figure 1-7 See also color plate.

Gastric varices.

○   In the previous case, the patient was found to have isolated gastric varices. What is the most likely underlying cause of the varices?

Splenic vein thrombosis.

○   True/False: Use of intravenous erythromycin prior to endoscopy in patients presenting with hematemesis may be beneficial in reducing the need for a second-look endoscopy.

True. Randomized controlled studies have suggested that a single dose of intravenous erythromycin given 20 to 120 minutes before endoscopy can significantly improve visibility, shorten endoscopy time, and reduce the need for a second-look endoscopy.

○   True/False: Melena can only occur as a result of upper gastrointestinal hemorrhage.

False. It may also occur due to a colonic lesion with slow transit.

○   True/False: Bleeding from gastric cancer is difficult to control.

True. In general, bleeding from tumors of any type is difficult to manage nonsurgically.

○   True/False: The incidence of recurrent ulcer hemorrhage is markedly reduced if *Helicobacter pylori* is eradicated.

True.

○ A 53-year-old woman presents with intermittent painless hematochezia, always following defecation of a normal colored stool, and often with several drops of blood dripping into the commode. There is usually blood on the toilet tissue after defecation. What is the lesion shown below?

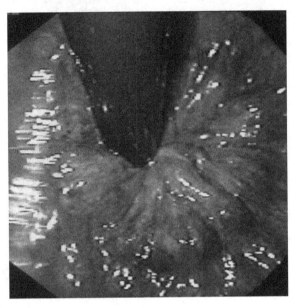

Figure 1-8 See also color plate.

Internal hemorrhoids. An anal fissure should be considered in those who present with hematochezia and painful defecation.

○ **True/False: A clean ulcer base has a very low incidence of rebleeding and requires no endoscopic therapy.**

True. The incidence of rebleeding is less than 5%.

○ **What are some clinical predictors of ulcer rebleeding?**

Shock (hemodynamic instability), anemia, hematemesis, and persistent bloody lavage.

○ **What information can be obtained from a bloody nasogastric aspirate associated with hematochezia?**

The patient is bleeding rapidly from the stomach or duodenum and has an increased risk of morbidity and mortality.

○ **True/False: A negative nasogastric aspirate implies that a patient could not have bled from the stomach or duodenum.**

False. It is possible that a gastric or duodenal ulcer may not have bled for some time and there is no longer blood in the stomach.

○ **True/False: Older patients have increased morbidity and mortality related to ulcer hemorrhage.**

True. This is generally due to the presence of comorbidities. Comorbid illnesses increase the risk of death from ulcer hemorrhage and also increase the risk of rebleeding.

○   **A 55-year-old woman presents with massive hematemesis. Shown below is the endoscopic view. What is your diagnosis and given the finding, what is the likelihood that she will bleed again within the next few days?**

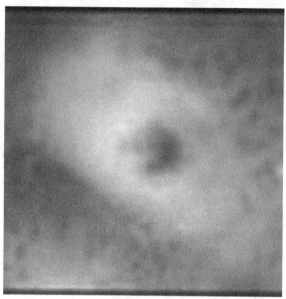

Figure 1-9 See also color plate.

Gastric ulcer in an NSAID user. With a visible vessel, the likelihood of rebleeding within the next 72 hours is 40%–60%.

○   **A 55-year-old man with long-standing untreated gastroesophageal reflux disease (GERD) presents with hematemesis and a normal hematocrit. Upper endoscopy is performed. What is the lesion in the esophagus?**

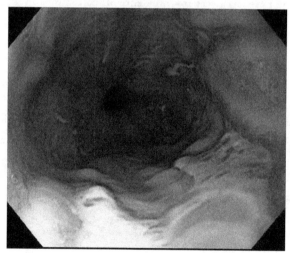

Figure 1-10 See also color plate.

Severe reflux esophagitis.

○   A 60-year-old man presents with scant hematemesis, iron deficiency anemia, and a 15-pound weight loss. An endoscopic view just below the cardioesophageal junction is shown below. What is the most likely diagnosis?

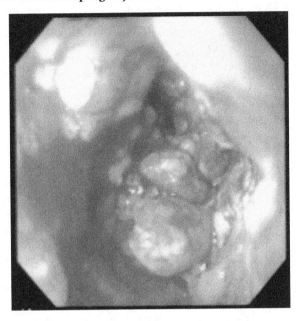

Figure 1-11

Adenocarcinoma of the stomach.

○   A 45-year-old man presents with massive hematemesis. Shown below is the endoscopic view of the gastric fundus. What is your diagnosis?

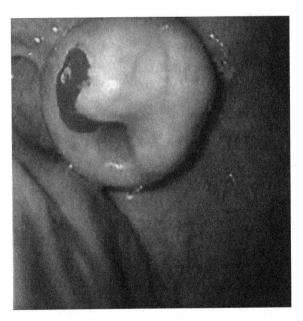

Figure 1-12

Gastrointestinal stromal tumor (GIST).

○ A hemodynamically stable 50-year-old, otherwise healthy, woman with melena was initially treated with nasogastric suction, blood transfusion, and an intravenous proton pump inhibitor. The following day, upper endoscopy was performed and showed the lesions below. What is your diagnosis?

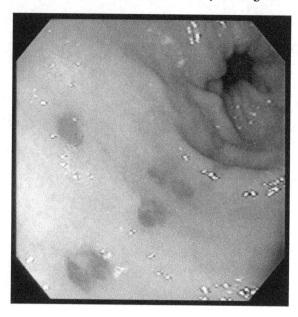

Figure 1-13

Suction trauma due to constant nasogastric suction. Clearly, this was not the cause of the melena.

○ **Which ulcer sites are at higher risk of rebleeding?**

Ulcers located high on the lesser curvature and posteriorly in the duodenal bulb are at higher risk due to their proximity to large arteries (left gastric, pancreatico-duodenal).

○ **What size vessel can be coagulated by monopolar electrocautery?**

Electrocautery can obliterate vessels up to 1 mm in diameter. Coaptive coagulation is needed for vessels larger than 1 mm and can be used for vessels up to 2 mm.

○ **How is blood flow related to the size of the artery?**

The blood flow is related to the fourth power of the radius of the vessel.

○ **Describe the mechanism whereby arteries bleed in ulcer-related hemorrhage.**

There is fibrinoid necrosis of the vessel wall. The vessel bleeds from both sides and does not contract because it is not completely severed.

○ **True/False: Endoscopic therapy should be utilized whenever a nonbleeding visible vessel is found.**

True. The high risk of rebleeding in this situation mandates endoscopic treatment.

○ **What specific causes of gastrointestinal bleeding are associated with increased mortality?**

Esophageal varices and gastric cancer.

○ **A 71-year-old man presents with recurrent hematemesis of uncertain etiology despite several prior upper endoscopies. Another EGD is performed. A retroflexed view in the stomach is shown. What is the most likely cause of the bleeding?**

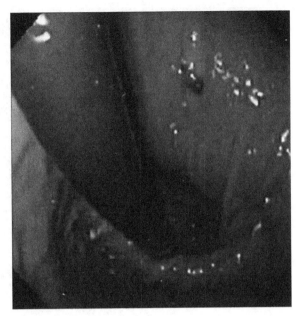

Figure 1-14 See also color plate.

A Dieulafoy lesion, which is a 'caliber-persistent' artery that protrudes from the mucosa with little or no surrounding ulceration. This lesion is usually treated with combination therapy using injection plus thermal therapy. Endoscopic band ligation and clipping may also be effective.

○ **What is the overall rate of rebleeding for ulcers?**

About 15%–20%.

○ **What is the rate of rebleeding after endoscopic treatment of an ulcer?**

About 10%–30%.

○ **True/False: According to a consensus statement from the National Institutes of Health, heater probe, bipolar electrocautery, injection therapy, and clipping are about equal in the ability to control ulcer hemorrhage.**

True—in experienced hands.

○ **A 42-year-old man presents with melena. On examination, he is found to have pigmented spots on the buccal mucosa. What syndrome may he have?**

Peutz–Jegher's syndrome.

○ **A 47-year-old woman presents with melena and is found to have increased lunulae (Terry's nails). What may be the cause of her bleeding?**

Variceal hemorrhage or severe portal hypertensive gastropathy due to chronic liver disease.

○   **A 70-year-old woman presents with hematemesis. At endoscopy, erythematous linear streaks are noted in the antrum giving a watermelon appearance. What are the most likely diagnosis and treatment of choice?**

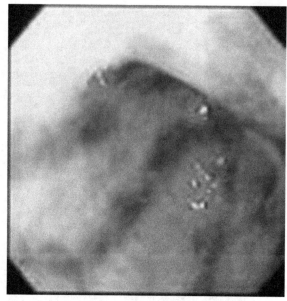

Figure 1-15 See also color plate.

Gastric antral vascular ectasia (GAVE), which is most commonly treated using thermal ablative techniques. Successful treatment using band ligation has also been described in small case series.

○   **A 23-year-old woman presents with right lower quadrant pain and hematochezia. Upper and lower gastrointestinal endoscopy are negative and the bleeding seems to have stopped. Which nuclear medicine scan might be useful at this point?**

The patient could be bleeding from a Meckel diverticulum, which could be identified by such a scan.

○   **What methods are available for the prevention of a first esophageal variceal hemorrhage?**

Therapy with nonselective beta blockers and long-acting nitrates has been shown to be effective. Prophylactic band ligation has also been shown to be effective.

○   **A patient presents with melena and is noted to have telangiectatic lesions on the lips, oral cavity, and nailbeds. What diagnosis should be considered?**

Osler–Weber–Rendu syndrome (ie, hereditary hemorrhagic telangiectasia syndrome).

○   **Why does angiodysplasia occur mainly in the right colon?**

The increased wall tension of the right colon is due to the larger diameter. The veins become partially obstructed and over years become dilated and tortuous forming the angiodysplasia.

○   **How common are angiodysplasia?**

More than 25% of asymptomatic individuals over age 60 have been found to have angiodysplasia.

○ A 40-year-old man, who receives hemodialysis for renal failure, bleeds intermittently but significantly. On colonoscopy, the following lesion is seen. What is it? How is it treated?

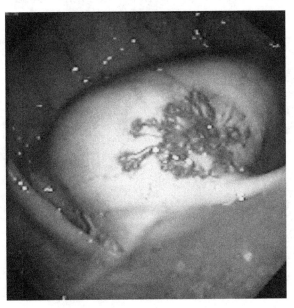

Figure 1-16 See also color plate.

Cecal angiodysplasia, commonly called arteriovenous malformation (AVM). Several endoscopic, angiographic, and surgical methods are available to obliterate these lesions. Noncontact treatments such as argon plasma coagulation seem to be the most popular method currently.

○ True/False: Angiodysplasia can present as occult intestinal bleeding.

True.

○ Where in the colon is the most common site of diverticular hemorrhage?

The left side of the colon. Diverticula in the proximal half of the colon are more likely to bleed; however, diverticula isolated to the left side of the colon are far more common.

○ True/False: If a patient on home fecal occult blood testing has one of six fecal occult blood test windows positive, this is a significant finding requiring colonoscopy.

True.

○ A 31-year-old man presents with abdominal distention and hematemesis. Upper endoscopy reveals blood coming from beyond the second portion of the duodenum. What is the most likely diagnosis?

A jejunal volvulus with partial obstruction and ischemic necrosis.

○ A 51-year-old man presents with fever, right upper quadrant pain, and hematemesis. Endoscopy reveals blood in the second part of the duodenum without any lesion noted. What is one possible cause of this scenario?

Acute cholecystitis with a cystic artery aneurysm that has bled into the bile duct.

○   **A 31-year-old man presents with a 3-month history of progressively worsening bloody diarrhea, abdominal cramping, and tenesmus. He also describes painful erythematous nodules on his lower legs. Flexible sigmoidoscopy reveals the finding below. What is the most likely diagnosis?**

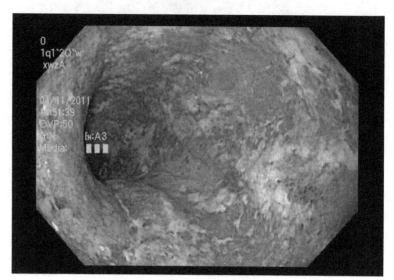

Figure 1-17 See also color plate.

Ulcerative colitis.

○   **An 81-year-old man presents with chronic unexplained iron-deficiency anemia. Colonoscopy is normal and upper endoscopy demonstrates a large hiatal hernia as shown below. What is the most likely cause of the iron-deficiency anemia?**

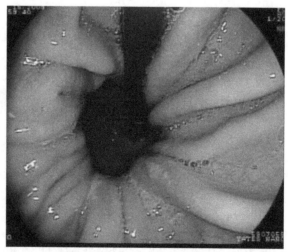

Figure 1-18 See also color plate.

Chronic occult bleeding from Cameron erosions at the diaphragmatic hiatus.

○   A 63-year-old man appears in the emergency room stating that he passed "a lot" of gross blood the day before without any other symptoms. His hematocrit is 22%. Following a bowel preparation, colonoscopy is performed. No blood is seen and the only abnormality identified is shown in the figure below. Is it the source of his bleeding?

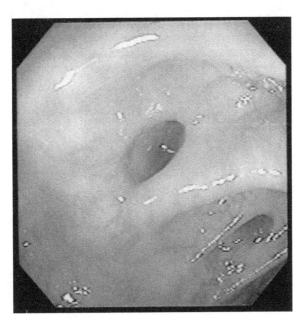

Figure 1-19

In the absence of any other demonstrable lesions, diverticulosis must be assumed to be the cause of the hemorrhage.

○   **What is the role of enteroscopy in the evaluation and management of occult gastrointestinal intestinal bleeding?**

Enteroscopy may be useful after a negative colonoscopy and upper endosocopy. If a telangiectasia is found, it can be coagulated using thermal techniques.

● ● ● SUGGESTED READINGS ● ● ●

Barkun AN, Bardou M, Kuipers EJ, et al; International Consensus Upper Gastrointestinal Bleeding Conference Group. International consensus recommendations on the management of patients with nonvariceal upper gastrointestinal bleeding. *Ann Intern Med.* 2010;152(2):101.

Davila RE, Rajan E, Adler DG, et al. Standards of Practice Committee. ASGE Guideline: the role of endoscopy in the patient with lower-GI bleeding. *Gastrointest Endosc.* 2005;62(5):656.

Garcia-Tsao G, Sanyal AJ, Grace ND, Carey W; Practice Guidelines Committee of the American Association for the Study of Liver Diseases; Practice Parameters Committee of the American College of Gastroenterology. Prevention and management of gastroesophageal varices and variceal hemorrhage in cirrhosis. *Hepatology.* 2007;46(3):922.

Raju GS, Gerson L, Das A, Lewis B; American Gastroenterological Association. American Gastroenterological Association (AGA) Institute medical position statement on obscure gastrointestinal bleeding. *Gastroenterology.* 2007;133(5):1694.

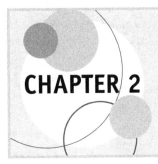

CHAPTER 2

Gastrointestinal Pathology

Cory A. Roberts, MD

○ **Where in the esophagus are you most likely to find heterotopic gastric mucosa (inlet patch)?**

The cervical region is the most common location.

○ **What is the underlying pathophysiology of achalasia?**

It is characterized, in part, by nearly complete absence of the myenteric plexus within the esophagus.

○ **What infectious agent and disease present a nearly identical clinical and pathologic scenario as idiopathic achalasia?**

Infection with *Trypanosoma cruzi* causes Chagas' disease which results in findings similar to achalasia.

○ **In a patient with achalasia, what type of esophageal tumor occurs at an increased rate compared to the general population?**

Squamous cell carcinoma.

○ **True/False: An esophageal biopsy report says there are 23 eosinophils per high-power field. This person has eosinophilic esophagitis.**

It depends on where in the esophagus the biopsies were obtained. EoE is a clinicopathologic diagnosis whereby there are 15 or more eosinophils per high-power field and an absence of pathologic reflux by pH studies and/or lack of response to high-dose proton pump inhibitors. Biopsies taken from the mid- and proximal esophagus are more specific for EoE. Furthermore, while the pathologist can suggest EoE as a diagnosis, they will typically not have all of the clinical data to make the diagnosis with certainty.

○ **What is the most common type of esophagitis in biopsy specimens and what are the histologic features?**

Reflux esophagitis is the most common type and is characterized by epithelial hyperplasia, elongation of the papillae, basal hyperplasia, spongiosis, vascular ectasia within the papillae, and epithelial infiltration by neutrophils and eosinophils. The histology can be identical to eosinophilic esophagitis, hence the reason that EoE is a clinicopathologic diagnosis.

○ **List some risk factors for development of squamous cell carcinoma of the esophagus.**

Smoking, alcohol, history of lye stricture, achalasia, previous radiation, Plummer–Vinson's syndrome, and tylosis.

○   **A 47-year-old man with frequent, long-standing classical reflux symptoms undergoes endoscopy. A 7-cm circumferential segment of columnar appearing mucosa proximal to the gastric folds is seen. A representative biopsy is shown below. What is the diagnosis?**

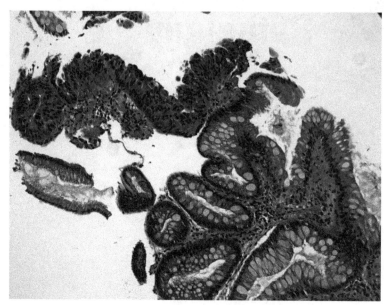

Figure 2-1 See also color plate.

Barrett's esophagus with high-grade dysplasia. Note the goblet cells on the right and high-grade dysplasia on the left.

○   **In a biopsy of Barrett's esophagus, at what pH should one use an alcian blue stain to demonstrate the specific mucin seen in the specialized intestinal metaplastic cells?**

The alcian blue stain should be at an acidic pH of 2.5.

○   **True/False: In progressive systemic sclerosis (scleroderma), the esophagus is commonly involved.**

True. About 80% of patients have some esophageal abnormality. Most of these will also have Raynaud's phenomenon.

○   **What are the typical histological findings in the esophagus of a patient with progressive systemic sclerosis?**

Smooth muscle atrophy, fibrosis, and hyaline thickening with luminal narrowing of small arterioles.

○   **What benign tumor of the esophagus is characterized by bland, granular appearing cells in the subepithelial tissue that are S100 positive by immunohistochemistry?**

Granular cell tumor.

○   **What is the most common type of tissue heterotopia in the stomach?**

Pancreatic tissue is most common and is usually present in the submucosa of the distal stomach or pylorus.

○ **A 34-year-old male patient with recurrent solid dysphagia but no reflux symptoms undergoes upper endoscopy that demonstrates multiple concentric rings. Biopsies from the mid-esophagus are shown below. What is the diagnosis?**

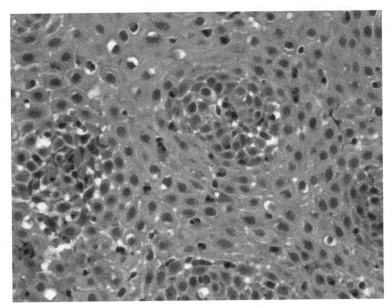

Figure 2-2 See also color plate.

This is the classic description of eosinophilic esophagitis. Typical histologic findings include 15 or more eosinophils per high-power field, spongiotic change (intraepithelial edema), degranulation of eosinophils, and possibly eosinophilic microabscesses and/or a luminal predominance of eosinophils.

○ **What microbial organism is associated with development of extra-nodal marginal zone lymphoma also known as lymphoma of gastric mucosa-associated lymphoid tissue (MALT)?**

Helicobacter pylori.

○ **What stain(s) would you use to highlight *Helicobacter pylori* in a gastric biopsy tissue section?**

A number of stains can be used. Commonly used, inexpensive, and easily performed stains are Giemsa and Diff-Quik. Silver-based stains also work well but are more technically challenging and slightly more expensive. At present, most laboratories use an immunohistochemical stain directed toward the organism as this is the only stain that will typically detect the organism in the lamina propria, will still react with treated organisms that may have an altered morphology (coccus rather than the bacillus), and will also react with *Helicobacter heilmannii.*

○ **What three forms of hypertrophic gastropathy are characterized by enlarged rugal folds?**

Menetrier's disease, hypertrophic-hypersecretory gastropathy, and gastric gland hyperplasia in Zollinger–Ellison syndrome.

○ **Describe the usual histologic appearance of Menetrier's disease.**

Gastric glandular atrophy with pronounced hyperplasia of the overlying superficial mucus-producing cells.

○ **On upper endoscopy, a yellowish, sessile polypoid lesion is seen in the stomach. The biopsy is shown below. What is the diagnosis?**

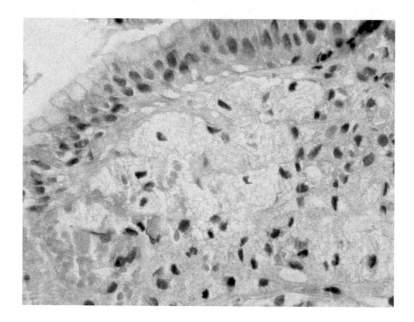

Figure 2-3

Xanthoma or xanthelasma. This benign incidental lesion is characterized by an accumulation of foamy histiocytes within the lamina propria.

○ **True/False: In Menetrier's disease, the antrum is typically spared and the transition to the other involved areas is abrupt.**

True.

○ **What demographic characteristics and clinical presentation are typically seen in Menetrier's disease?**

It is three times as common in men as women, typically ranges in age from the fourth to sixth decade of life, and presents with weight loss, abdominal, pain and occasionally peripheral edema (due to protein-losing enteropathy).

○ **Where in the stomach would you be most likely to find an adenomatous gastric polyp?**

The antrum.

○ **True/False: Gastric polyps are frequently a component of familial adenomatous polyposis and Gardener's syndrome.**

True. Gastric polyps of some type (adenomatous, fundic gland, or hyperplastic/regenerative) are present in more than half of the patients. Most commonly, the polyps are of the fundic gland type which may harbor low-grade dysplasia.

○ **Where are gastrinomas typically found in patients with Zollinger–Ellison syndrome?**

The majority are in the pancreas or duodenum.

○ **Describe the typical histologic features of "chemical" gastritis.**

In "chemical gastritis" or reactive gastropathy, the foveolae are hyperplastic with increased luminal serrations, the antral glands are atrophic, the lamina propria is fibrotic with splayed smooth muscle fibers, and there is an increased number of congested and somewhat ectatic superficial capillaries.

○ **What is the most common site of origin of primary lymphoma in the gastrointestinal tract?**

The stomach is the site of origin in about 50% of the cases—usually of the extra-nodal marginal zone type (ie, MALT lymphoma).

○ **What is the most common segment of the gut affected by GISTs?**

The stomach accounts for about half of all cases.

○ **What is the typical histology of a Meckel's diverticulum?**

This is a congenital anomaly that results from persistence of the proximal vitelline duct and is usually found within 90 cm of the ileocecal valve on the antimesenteric border. It is usually lined by small intestinal mucosa; however, gastric, duodenal, colonic, or pancreatic mucosa may also be found.

○ **How does a fundic gland polyp differ histologically from a hyperplastic polyp?**

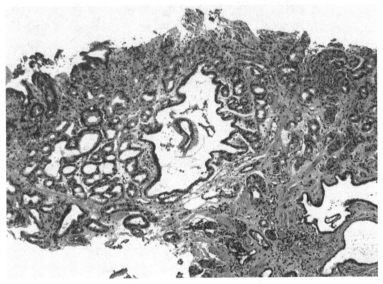

Figure 2-4 See also color plate.

As shown here, fundic gland polyps have fundic epithelial-lined microcysts and shortened foveolae. Proton pump inhibitors can also cause dilatation of gastric pits. In this case, there is surface low-grade dysplasia and this patient had a history of familial adenomatous polyposis.

○ **What is the "rule of two's" as it refers to Meckel's diverticulum?**

Meckel's diverticulum is typically found within two feet of the ileocecal valve, is two inches long, causes symptoms in 2% of cases, and is found in 2% of the population.

○   **True/False: Hirschsprung's disease is more common in males than females.**

True. Hirschsprung's disease is characterized by a loss of both the submucosal (Meissner's) and myenteric (Auerbach's) plexuses with resultant nerve trunk hyperplasia. The gender incidence varies—males are four times more likely to have a short segment of affected colon, while patients with long segments are more frequently female. In addition, 10% of Hirschsprung's disease is found in patients with trisomy 21 (Down's syndrome).

○   **A 57-year-old woman with known autoimmune gastritis undergoes upper endoscopy demonstrating several small proximal gastric polyps. A biopsy is shown below. What is the diagnosis?**

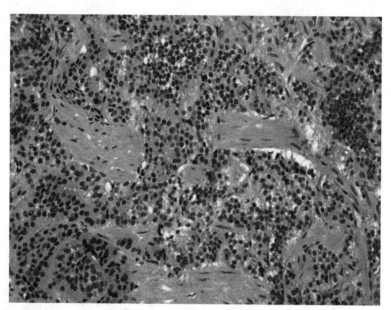

Figure 2-5 See also color plate.

Carcinoid. These patients develop predominantly hyperplastic gastric polyps; however, about 10% will show foci of dysplasia. They also tend to develop low-grade neuroendocrine tumors (carcinoids) and adenocarcinoma. The adenocarcinoma is typically of the intestinal type and appears to arise from the intestinal metaplasia that is the hallmark of atrophic gastritis histology.

○   **What is the main histologic finding in patients with gluten-sensitive enteropathy?**

Blunted small bowel villi with an increased number of intraepithelial lymphocytes and lamina propria plasma cells associated with crypt hyperplasia. The Marsh criteria stratify differing degrees of histologic involvement in celiac disease.

○   **What would you expect to see histologically in the small bowel from a patient with disaccharidase deficiency?**

Normal mucosa.

○   **Where would you look in a small bowel biopsy for the causative agent of Whipple's disease?**

The *Tropheryma whippelii* organisms reside in macrophages that are "stuffed" with organisms amidst an expanded lamina propria. These organisms can be confused with mycobacterial organisms. An acid fast stain is useful to differentiate between the two (*T. whippelii* is acid fast negative); however, an immunohistochemical stain is also available.

○ The spindle cell tumor shown below had a thin pedicle attaching it to the gastric muscle wall. Histologic evaluation showed the tumor to be positive for immunohistochemical stains for c-kit (CD117) and DOG1. What is the diagnosis?

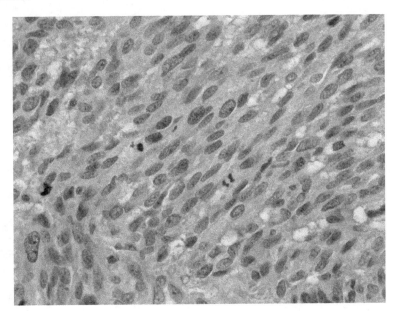

Figure 2-6

Gastrointestinal stromal tumor (GIST). Note the abundant mitotic figures in the image.

○ A 67-year-old man on chronic hemodialysis presents for further evaluation of chronic diarrhea. A small bowel biopsy contains glassy eosinophilic material which stains positively with a Congo red stain. What is the diagnosis?

Gastrointestinal amyloidosis. Thioflavin-T is another stain for amyloid.

○ What diagnostic technique is necessary to diagnose microvillus inclusion disease on a biopsy specimen?

Electron microscopy. This autosomal recessive condition is characterized by the absence of surface villi and, ultrastructurally, microvillus inclusions are found within the cytoplasm of the enterocytes. Unfortunately, death prior to the age of two is common unless small bowel transplantation occurs.

○ What is the inheritance pattern of abetalipoproteinemia?

Autosomal recessive.

○ What condition of the large intestine typically occurs in premature infants, can be associated with umbilical artery catheterization, and results in abdominal distention, loss of bowel sounds, bloody stools, and the presence of pneumatosis intestinalis?

Neonatal necrotizing enterocolitis.

○ In what segment of the small bowel do primary small bowel adenocarcinoma most commonly occur?

The duodenum.

○   **A 27-year-old man presents with a 6-week history of bloody diarrhea, tenesmus, and abdominal cramping. He is otherwise healthy but has noticed a painful, erythematous rash on his shins. Colon biopsies are shown below. What is the most likely diagnosis?**

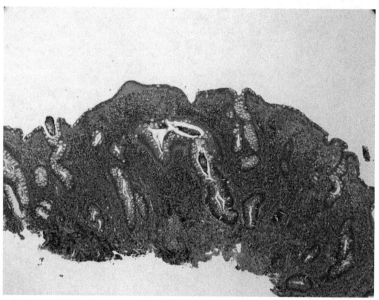

Figure 2-7 See also color plate.

Ulcerative colitis. Note the marked architectural distortion, increased inflammation, and diminished goblet cells.

○   **A 72-year-old woman presents with chronic watery diarrhea. Stool tests and a colonoscopy were normal. Random colonic biopsies revealed the findings demonstrated in the figure. What is the most likely diagnosis?**

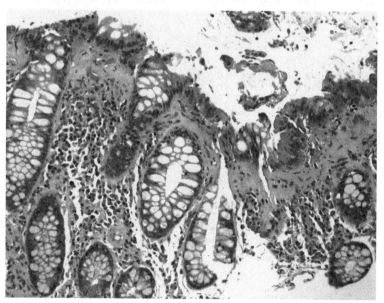

Figure 2-8 See also color plate.

Collagenous colitis. Note the markedly thickened subepithelial collagen table. This condition is much more common in elderly women.

○   **What arbitrary thickness must the subepithelial collagen band reach or exceed to qualify for the diagnosis of collagenous colitis?**

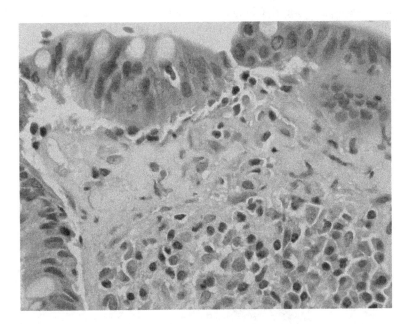

Figure 2-9

The normal subepithelial collagen band measures up to 7 microns and, in collagenous colitis, it reaches 10 microns or greater.

○   **What is major abnormality demonstrated in this colon biopsy specimen taken from a 73-year-old woman with watery diarrhea?**

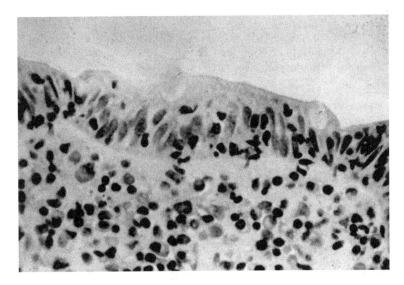

Figure 2-10

Increased intraepithelial lymphocytes. She was subsequently diagnosed with lymphocytic colitis.

○   **What specific race and disease might you expect to find in a patient with an endocrine tumor of the duodenum which is of the delta-cell type?**

African-American patients with von Recklinghausen's disease have an increased incidence of delta-cell type endocrine tumors of the duodenum. Delta cells produce somatostatin.

○   **An 80-year-old male presents with bloody diarrhea and severe left-sided abdominal pain. On sigmoidoscopy, patchy areas of ulceration and inflammation extending from the splenic flexure to about 15 cm distally are noted. A representative biopsy specimen is shown below. What is the diagnosis?**

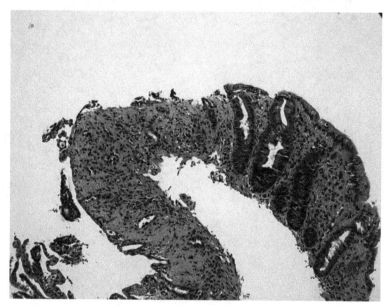

Figure 2-11 See also color plate.

This is a classic presentation and histology of ischemic colitis. The histology is characterized by abrupt transition of normal mucosa to inflamed, ulcerated mucosa with hyalinization of the lamina propria, surface epithelial degeneration/sloughing with more preservation of the basal aspect of the crypts, and rare fibrin thrombi.

○   **A tumor is resected from the ileum and your friendly pathologist tells you that, grossly, the tumor is well circumscribed, nodular, and has a distinctly yellow cut surface. What type of tumor do you suspect this is?**

This is the classic appearance of a carcinoid tumor.

○   **What autosomal dominant condition is found in people of Mennonite descent in Canada, is associated with diarrhea and dehydration in childhood, and can be deadly?**

Torkelson syndrome. These patients sometimes show evidence of common variable immunodeficiency. Histologically, the changes are nonspecific and include blunting of the villi, edema, and focal acute inflammation.

○   **What is acrodermatitis enteropathica?**

This is an autosomal recessive condition that is found in children, usually responds to administration of zinc sulfate, and shows ultrastructural rodlike fibrillar inclusions within Paneth cells.

COLOR INSERT

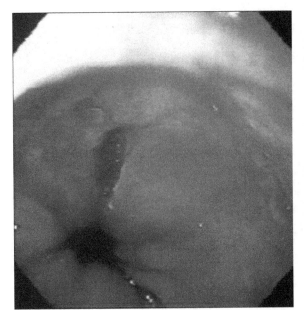

Figure 1-2

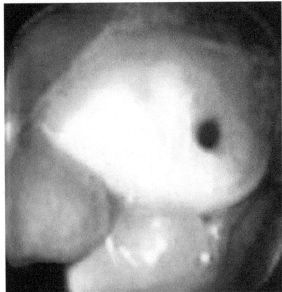

Figure 1-3

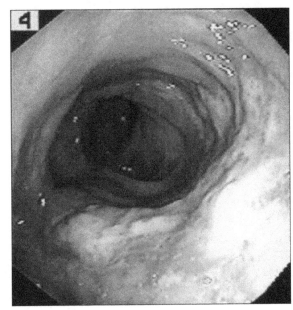

Figure 1-5

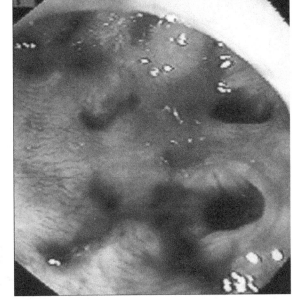

Figure 1-6

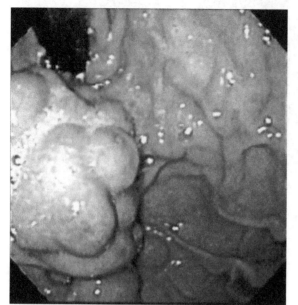

Figure 1-7

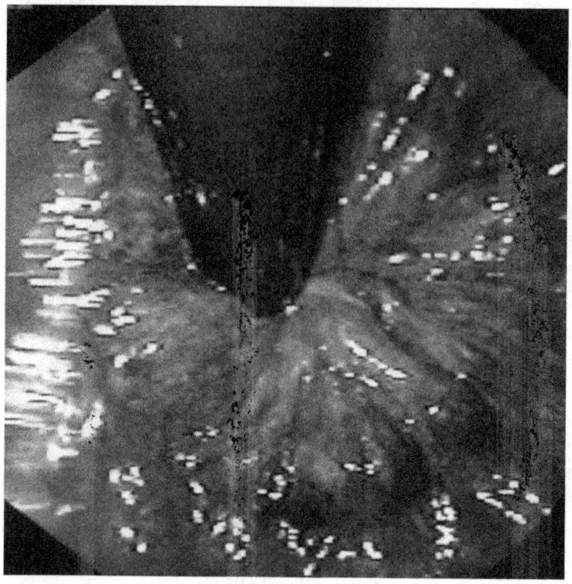

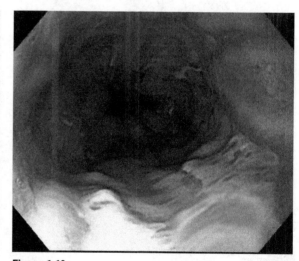

Figure 1-8

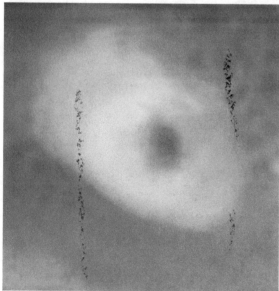

Figure 1-9

Figure 1-10

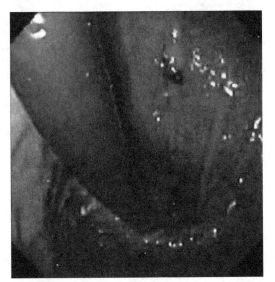

Figure 1-14

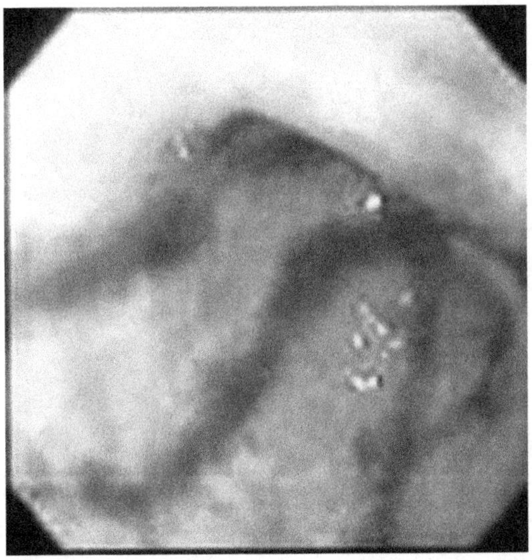

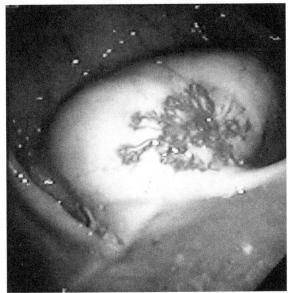

Figure 1-15

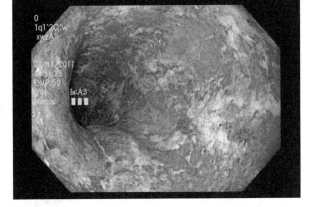

Figure 1-16

Figure 1-17

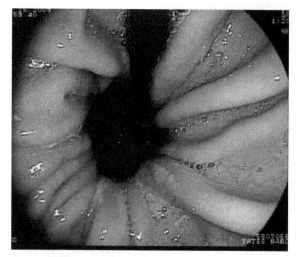

Figure 1-18

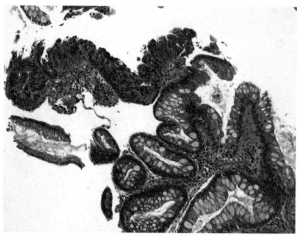

Figure 2-1

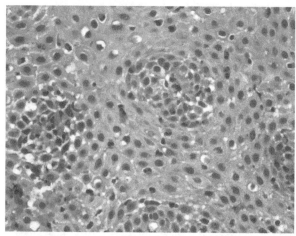

Figure 2-2

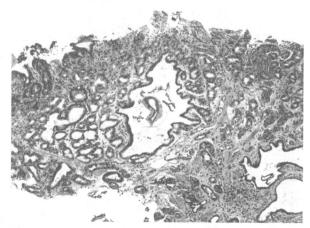

Figure 2-4

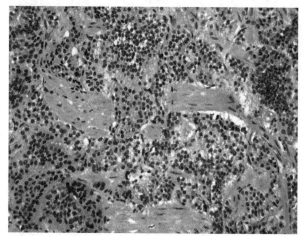

Figure 2-5

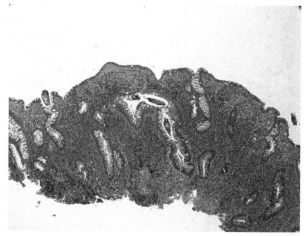

Figure 2-7

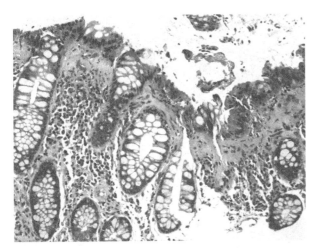

Figure 2-8

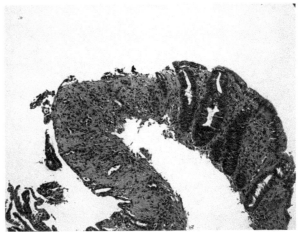

Figure 2-11

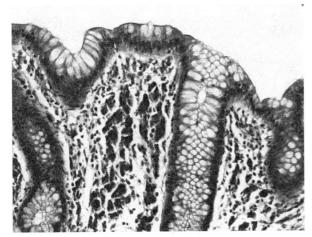

Figure 2-13

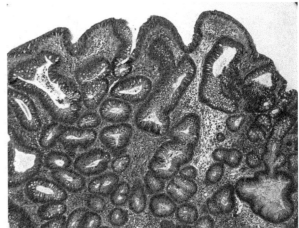

Figure 2-14

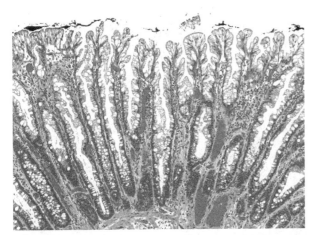

Figure 2-15

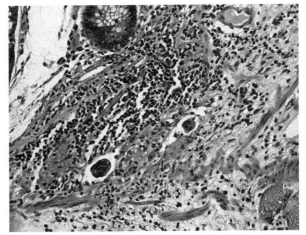

Figure 2-16

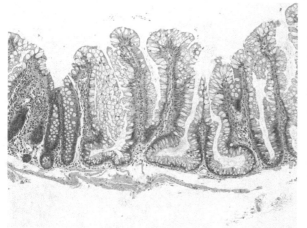

Figure 2-17

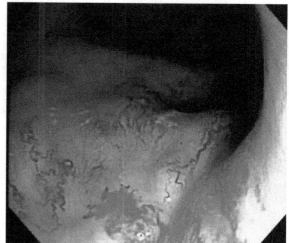

Figure 6-1

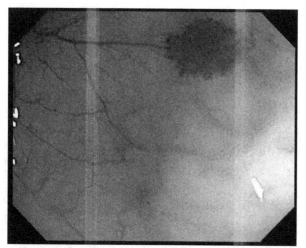

Figure 6-2

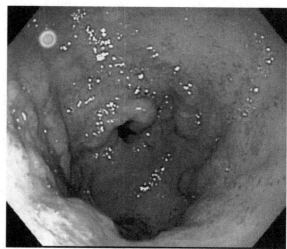

Figure 6-3

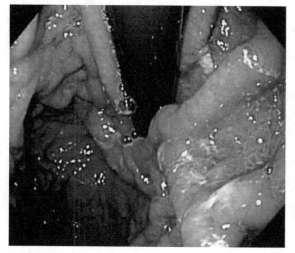

Figure 6-4

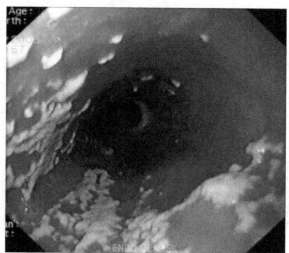

Figure 9-1

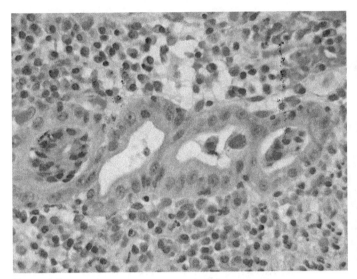

Figure 9-2

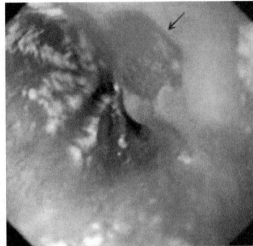

Figure 9-3

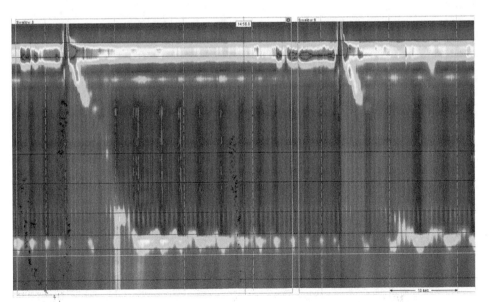

Figure 10-1

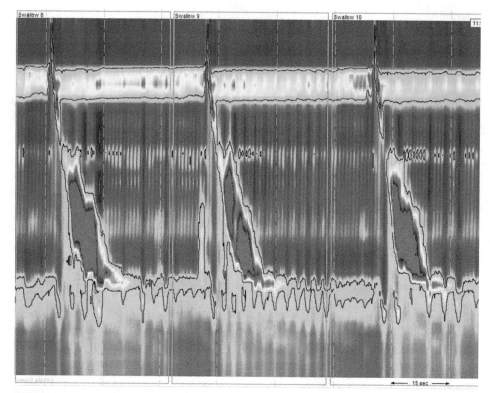

Figure 10-2

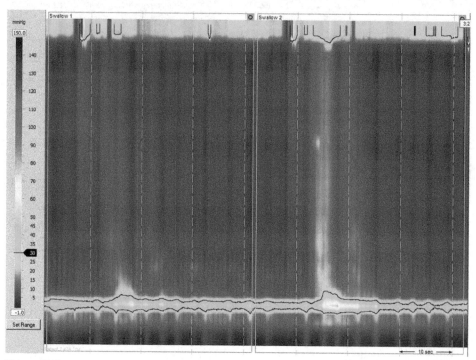

Figure 10-3

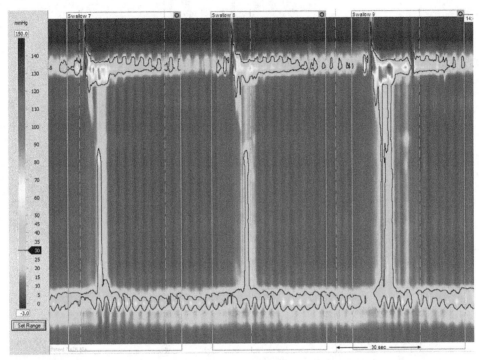

Figure 10-4

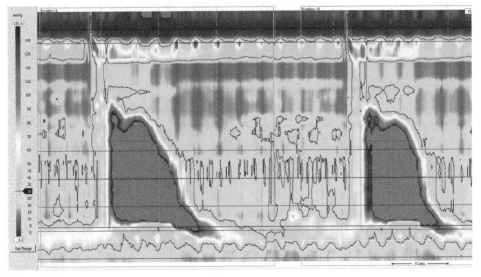

Figure 10-5

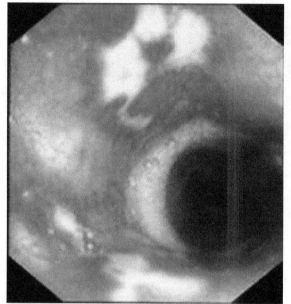

Figure 11-1

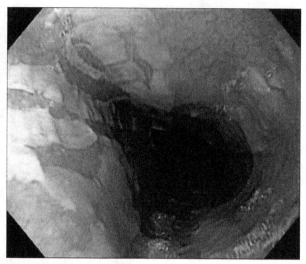

Figure 11-2

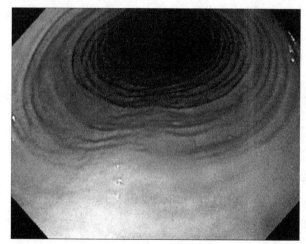

Figure 11-3

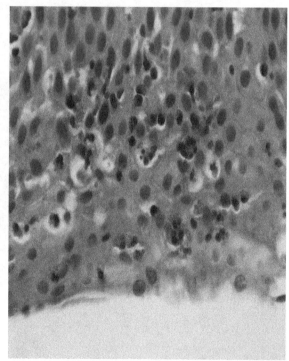

Figure 11-4

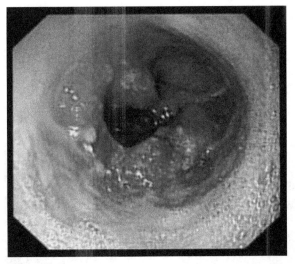

Figure 12-1

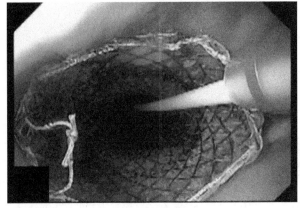

Figure 12-2

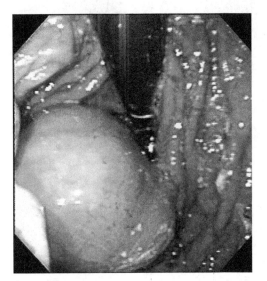

Figure 17-4

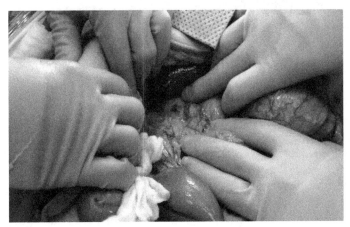

Figure 19-2

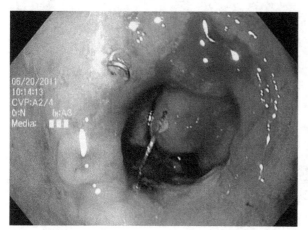

Figure 19-3

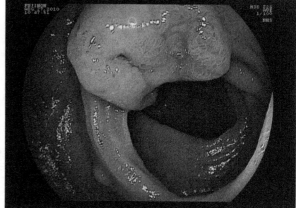

Figure 23-1

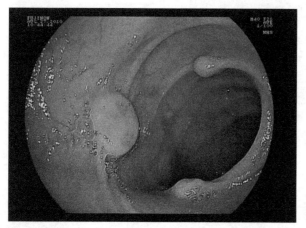

Figure 23-2

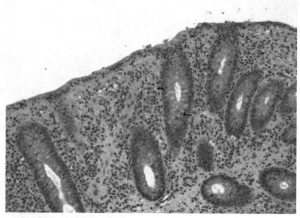

Figure 27-1A (Figure used with permission of Dr J. Radhi, McMaster University, Hamilton, ON, Canada.)

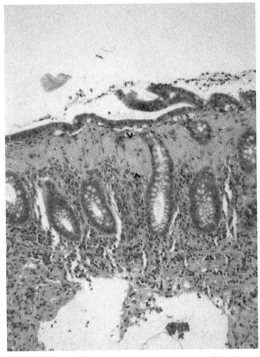

Figure 27-1B (Figure used with permission of Dr J. Radhi, McMaster University, Hamilton, ON, Canada.)

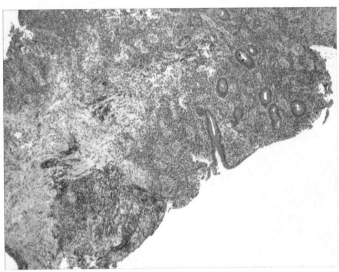

Figure 27-2 (Figure used with permission of Dr J. Radhi, McMaster University, Hamilton, ON, Canada.)

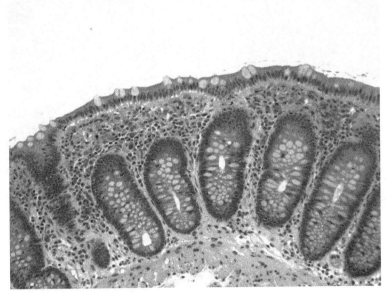

Figure 27-3 (Figure used with permission of Dr J. Radhi, McMaster University, Hamilton ON, Canada.)

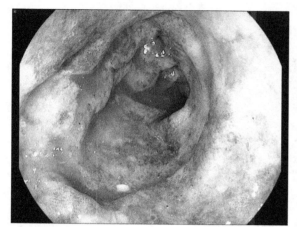

Figure 27-4

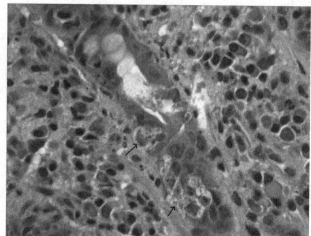

Figure 27-5 (Figure used with permission of Dr J. Radhi, McMaster University, Hamilton ON, Canada.)

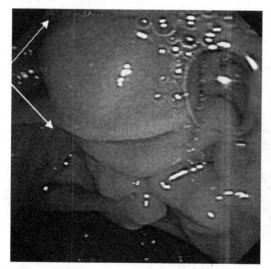

Figure 31-1C

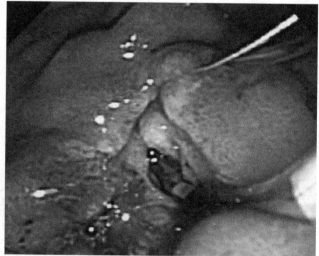

Figure 31-1D

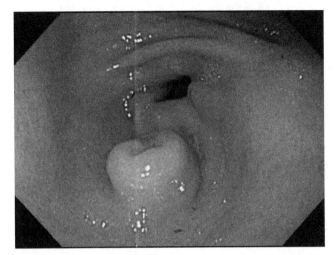

Figure 31-4

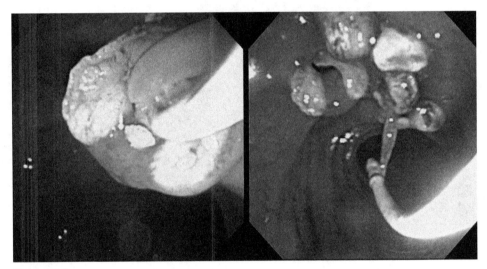

Figure 39-3

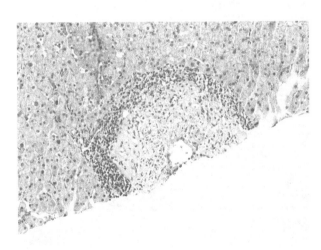

Figure 51-6

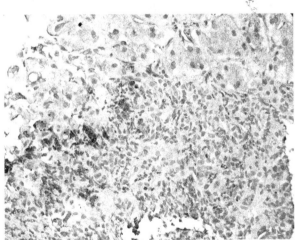

Figure 51-14

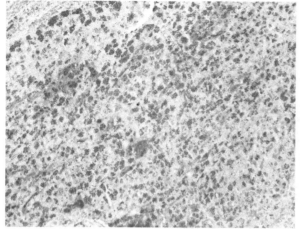

Figure 51-15

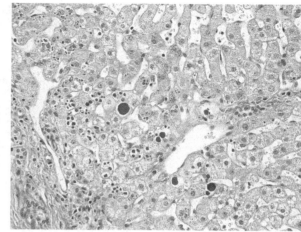

Figure 51-16

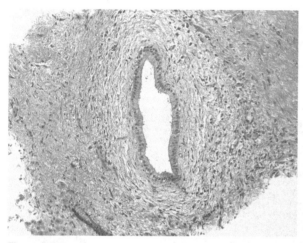

Figure 51-17

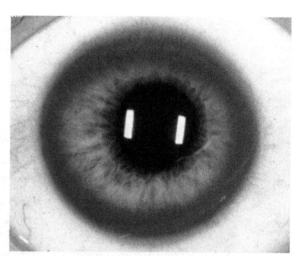

Figure 53-1

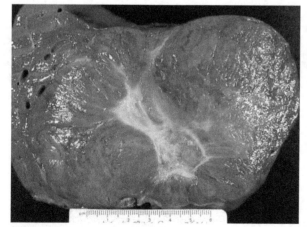

Figure 54-2

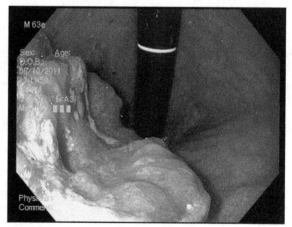

Figure 62-5A

○   A recently hospitalized man presents to your office complaining of persistent, voluminous, nonbloody diarrhea. Colonoscopy is normal. A representative random colon biopsy is shown in the figure. What is your diagnosis?

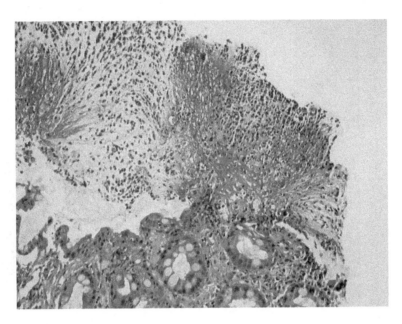

Figure 2-12

This is the classic low-power appearance of pseudomembranous colitis. The biopsy shows the characteristic eosinophilic fibrinous surface debris with a "mushroom" or volcanic eruption appearance. Interestingly, stool tests were negative in this patient.

○   **What pinworm would you expect to find either as an incidental finding in the appendix or, less commonly, associated with acute appendicitis?**

Enterobius vermicularis. This organism is found in about 3% of appendectomy specimens in the United States.

○   **A patient undergoes appendectomy for acute appendicitis. Histologic sections of the appendix show multinucleated giant cells which are called Warthin–Finkeldey cells. What viral illness do you suspect?**

Warthin–Finkeldey cells occur in the prodromal stage of measles infection in the appendix. The patient will likely develop a typical measles rash in the near future.

○   **What is the difference between acquired and congenital diverticula?**

Either acquired (pseudo-)diverticula lack a muscularis propria or they are greatly attenuated, whereas congenital diverticula, such as a Meckel's diverticulum, are true diverticula as they contain all three layers of the intestinal wall.

○   **What is the term given to describe the presence of numerous submucosal gas-filled cysts which create polypoid projections in the mucosa of the bowel?**

Pneumatosis cystoides intestinalis. In children, it is associated with necrotizing enterocolitis and in adults, there is usually an associated gastrointestinal disorder or chronic obstructive pulmonary disease.

○ **What is diagnosis in this biopsy from a 60-year-old woman with diarrhea? Colonoscopy was notable for a subtle brownish discoloration mainly to the right side of the colon. The pigmented material in the biopsy is iron stain negative.**

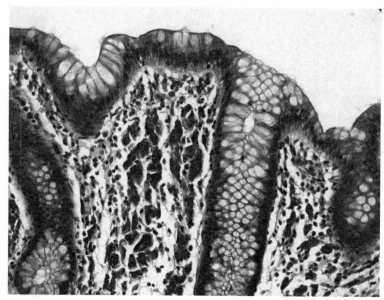

Figure 2-13 See also color plate.

Melanosis coli.

○ **What is the general descriptive term under which the specific diagnoses lymphocytic and collagenous colitis reside?**

Microscopic colitis.

○ **Describe the microscopic features you would expect to see in a biopsy of solitary rectal ulcer syndrome (mucosal prolapse syndrome).**

In spite of the name "solitary," about one out of ten cases is not solitary at all but rather is multiple. The crypts are dilated with irregular branching which can impart a villiform appearance. The goblet cells are often mucin depleted and the lamina propria exhibits fibrosis, vascular congestion and there is often vertical streaking of smooth muscle bundles in the superficial lamina propria.

○ **Behcet's syndrome in the colon is characterized by what histologic/endoscopic findings?**

It is characterized by ulcers occurring in various parts of the large intestine with an associated "lymphocytic vasculitis" of the submucosal veins. This can result in a colitis which may mimic Crohn's disease.

○ **What is the most common polyp in children?**

Juvenile or retention polyp; however, in spite of the name "juvenile," more than 30% of cases are diagnosed in adults. The most common site of occurrence is in the rectum.

○ **True/False: Arteriovenous malformations in the large intestine are most commonly found in the rectum.**

False. The vast majority are in the cecum and ascending colon.

○ **What type of polyp is depicted below?**

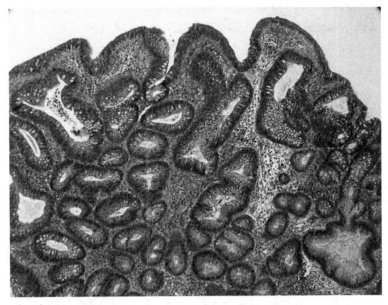

Figure 2-14 See also color plate.

This is a tubular adenoma characterized by hyperchromatic epithelium due to goblet cell depletion, nuclear enlargement, and nuclear pseudostratification. There is mild architectural disarray but no villous component.

○ **What is the risk of malignant transformation in the rectal polyp shown in the photomicrograph below?**

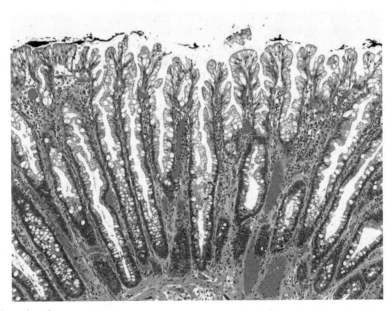

Figure 2-15 See also color plate.

None. This is a benign, nonneoplastic hyperplastic polyp as evidenced by the surface and crypt epithelium with serrated glandular lumina, abundant mucin, crypts without basal flattening or branching, and lack of crypt dilatation or hyperserration.

○   **Name three histologic features that help determine the presence of so-called pseudoinvasion of the stalk in an adenomatous polyp as opposed to true malignant invasion?**

   1. The glands are surrounded by a loose lamina propria stroma not a desmoplastic tissue response.
   2. There are associated hemosiderin-laden macrophages.
   3. The glands in the stalk are identical to those that are more superficially located.

○   **A polypectomy of a 1.5-cm pedunculated polyp demonstrates adenomatous changes with evidence of adenocarcinoma. Your pathologist tells you that there is lymphatic space invasion by the tumor (as shown below). What other features do you need to know about in order to arrive at an appropriate decision regarding the need for further therapy and/or surveillance for this patient?**

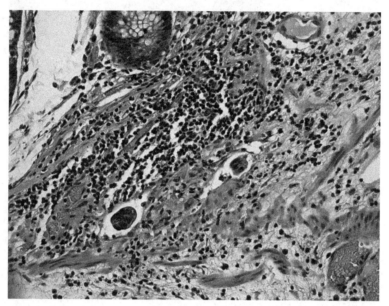

Figure 2-16 See also color plate.

The presence of lymphatic invasion, distance to the margin (need at least 1 mm), and grade (high-grade worse prognosis) of the tumor are the three factors one must know in order to decide if there is need for a resection or if the polypectomy is curative.

○   **Describe the inheritance pattern in Peutz–Jeghers syndrome.**

Autosomal dominant. It is characterized by multiple hamartomatous polyps of the gastrointestinal tract and abnormal pigmentation of mucosa and skin.

○   **What is the malignant potential of the hamartomatous gastrointestinal polyps seen in Peutz–Jeghers syndrome?**

While these patients face a higher risk for development of a carcinoma, it is not related to the polyps but to an increased rate of malignancy in other organs such as the breast or pancreas.

○   **What is the name of the syndrome characterized by the combination of adenomatous polyposis of the colon and associated tumors of the central nervous system, typically gliomas?**

Turcot's syndrome.

○   This polyp was found in the proximal ascending colon of a 63-year-old man and measured 1.1 cm. The endoscopist was initially not sure if it was a polyp or just a prominent fold. What is the diagnosis?

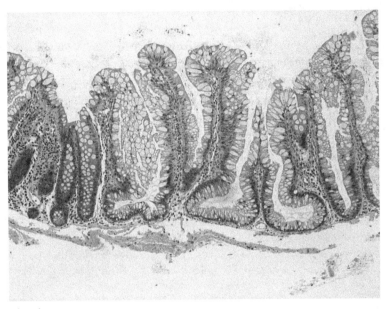

Figure 2-17 See also color plate.

Sessile serrated adenoma referred to by some as sessile serrated polyp. Note the preservation of goblet cells even at the base of the crypts and the prominent flattening or splaying of the base of the crypts. This example also demonstrates herniation through the muscularis mucosae which is sometimes seen in these polyps.

○   **What is the name of the syndrome composed of colorectal carcinoma with multiple sebaceous tumors and keratoacanthomas?**

The Muir–Torre syndrome.

○   **What are the components and inheritance of Cowden's syndrome?**

It is characterized by the presence of oral mucosal papillomas, trichilemmomas of the face, and acral hyperkeratosis. Approximately one-third of the patients have intestinal polyposis. Inheritance is autosomal dominant.

○   **What is the Cronkhite–Canada syndrome?**

This syndrome is characterized by the presence of numerous gastrointestinal polyps and abnormalities of the nails termed onychodystrophy.

○   **Where is the allele called DCC (deleted in colon cancer) located?**

On chromosome 18q where it encodes for a molecule in the cell adhesion molecule family. The expression of this protein is absent or markedly reduced in almost 75% of colon cancers.

○   **In some patients with a genetic predisposition to development of adenocarcinoma of the colon, there is an abnormality of the DNA on chromosome 2. What is the abnormality?**

Microsatellite instability.

○ **What are the four proteins that immunohistochemical stains can and should be used to evaluate for in a mismatch repair positive tumor?**

MLH1, MSH2, MSH6, and PMS2.

○ **According to recent recommendations, which patients with colorectal carcinomas should be screened for microsatellite instability or mismatch repair gene status?**

Recently, recommendations have changed and suggest that all patients under age 70 with a new colorectal carcinoma diagnosis should be screened regardless of family history, tumor location, or histology as studies have shown a significant number of hereditary nonpolyposis colorectal cancer (HNPCC) patients will be missed if only traditional screening tools are used.

○ **What does it mean if a tumor is found to be positive for all four mismatch repair immunohistochemical stains (MLH1, MSH2, MSH6, and PMS2)?**

It means there is no evidence of a replication error positive tumor (also known as a mismatch repair positive tumor) and, therefore, no evidence of HNPCC (aka Lynch) syndrome. Positive stain results are normal. The absence of staining means there is a defect in that particular gene as evidenced by the lack of expression of that protein and indicates there is evidence of a mismatch repair positive tumor, thus a need to further investigate and determine if the cause is Lynch syndrome or a sporadic error that is not inherited or heritable.

○ **If a tumor is found to be MLH1 negative, what is a logical next step?**

Evaluate the tumor for BRAF1 to determine if the loss of MLH1 is a sporadic event or a sign of HNPCC.

○ **Where in the colon do most carcinomas in the Lynch syndrome occur?**

They are typically right sided.

○ **How does the prognosis of Lynch syndrome colonic carcinomas compare to traditional colorectal tumors?**

It is better.

○ **Describe the typical clinical features of sessile serrated adenomas.**

They are typically right sided but can occur anywhere in the colon. They tend to be larger, leading some authorities to say that any polyp with serrated architecture that is larger than 5 mm and located to the right of the splenic flexure should be considered a sessile serrated adenoma (SSA). They are often ill defined endoscopically, sometimes appearing simply as prominent folds and making determination of the precise size and extent difficult.

○ **Describe the typical histologic features of sessile serrated adenomas.**

They have serrated gland lumina (often hyperserrated), dilatation of the involved crypts, persistence of goblet cells at the bottom of the crypts, and flattening of the crypts at the base along the muscularis mucosae creating the image of an upside down letter T or an L or backward L. Additionally, they often have increased superficial mitoses and so-called dysplastic goblet cells.

○ **What is the name of the carcinogenic pathway that sessile serrated adenomas follow?**

The serrated pathway. They have the ability to progress to malignancy more quickly than the traditional adenoma to carcinoma sequence of classic or traditional colorectal carcinoma.

○ **What is a dysplasia-associated lesion or mass (DALM)?**

This is an endoscopically visible area of histologically confirmed dysplasia in a patient with chronic inflammatory bowel disease. One cannot reliably distinguish DALM from a sporadic adenoma not related to inflammatory bowel disease histologically. The same histologic appearance, if submitted as part of surveillance in a setting where there was no visible lesion, would be called flat low-grade dysplasia. The endoscopic appearance is critical in all dysplastic lesions in chronic inflammatory bowel disease.

○ **What is the predominant histologic finding indicative of acute graft versus host disease in mucosal biopsies of the gastrointestinal tract?**

Apoptosis of individual crypt cells. Apoptosis refers to individual cell necrosis characterized by dark fragments of what was the nucleus (so-called "nuclear dust"). There is typically not a significant mononuclear cell infiltrate accompanying this, so close microscopic examination is necessary.

● ● ● **SUGGESTED READINGS** ● ● ●

Odze RD, Goldblum JR, eds. *Surgical Pathology of the GI Tract, Liver, Biliary Tract, and Pancreas.* 2nd ed. Philadelphia: Saunders Elsevier; 2009.

Fenoglio-Preiser CM, Noffsinger AE, Stemmermann GN, Lantz PE, Isaacson PG. *Gastrointestinal Pathology: An Atlas and Text.* Wolters Kluwer Health/Lippincott Williams & Wilkins; 2007.

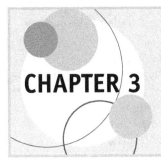

CHAPTER 3

Abdominal Cavity: Congenital Abnormalities, Abscesses, and Fistulae

James A. Madura, II, MD, FACS

○ **What are the two main anatomic features of intestinal malrotation that lead to clinical symptoms?**

1. Ladd bands, which cross the duodenum, can cause duodenal obstruction.
2. Narrow mesenteric base/pedicle, which results in excessive small bowel mobility, can lead to volvulus and bowel ischemia.

○ **True/False: Intestinal rotational anomalies are always associated with other congenital gut anomalies.**

False. While intestinal malrotation and nonrotation are often associated with other gut anomalies, particularly those in which the intestines are located outside the peritoneal cavity (eg, congenital diaphragmatic hernia or abdominal wall defects), they can also occur in children and adults who have no associated anomalies.

○ **True/False: Intestinal nonrotation is not as dangerous as malrotation because the base of the mesentery is usually wider than in malrotation and the risk of volvulus is less.**

True.

○ **True/False: Intestinal malrotation is a disorder of infancy and does not occur in adults.**

False. Although intestinal malrotation has been considered primarily a disease of infancy with infrequent occurrence beyond the first year of life, more recent reports suggest it is not uncommonly first detected in adults.

○ **True/False: Intestinal malrotation in adults usually presents as an abdominal catastrophe (eg, volvulus with bowel ischemia).**

False. Intestinal malrotation in adults is often detected incidentally as part of an evaluation of chronic nonspecific gastrointestinal symptoms. Volvulus and other complications of malrotation appear to occur less commonly in adults.

○ **True/False: The cornerstone of the surgical treatment of intestinal malrotation is to restore the normal configuration of the bowel.**

False. The restoration of normal bowel configuration is not possible. The objective of the Ladd procedure is to minimize the risk of future volvulus by widening the base of the mesentery and placing the bowel in a position of nonrotation (ie, small bowel on the right and colon on the left). Division of Ladd bands, if present, and an appendectomy is also done.

○ **True/False: Adults with asymptomatic or incidentally discovered malrotation should undergo the Ladd procedure.**

This remains controversial with proponents on both sides and so there is no clear right or wrong answer. Because it is not clear that the risk of volvulus decreases with age and it is difficult to determine with imaging studies whether a patient with a rotational anomaly has a narrow-based mesentery, many surgeons recommend surgery regardless of the patient's age or the presence of symptoms characteristic of malrotation. One approach that has been advocated is the use of diagnostic laparoscopy to assess the mobility of the colon and the width of the mesentery. In patients with narrow mesenteric attachment and potential colonic mobility, definitive laparoscopic correction can then be undertaken.

○ **How and where is particulate material in the peritoneal cavity normally cleared from the cavity?**

Through modified lymphatics located along the diaphragm undersurface, stomas of which open when the diaphragm relaxes creating negative intra-abdominal pressure. Diaphragmatic muscle contractions then force lymph cephalad, aided by one-way valves.

○ **The presence of rebound or percussive tenderness and guarding helps to diagnose peritonitis in what way?**

They indicate extension to and irritation of the abdominal wall peritoneal surface, whereas localized inflammatory processes between visceral surfaces produce nonspecific, dull aching pain that may be difficult to localize.

○ **What is the desired timing for initiating antibiotics to treat peritoneal contamination?**

The estimated "grace period" is 4 to 6 hours after contamination, the earlier the better. Antibiotics should always be started before percutaneous or surgical intervention.

○ **Clinically significant *Candida* peritonitis, usually responsive to low-dose amphotericin B or fluconazole, is most likely to be found in what situations?**

In patients on long-term antibiotics, after gastric perforations in acid suppressed patients and in immunocompromised individuals.

○ **True/False: The process of abscess formation and maturation is deterrent but not cidal to contained bacteria.**

True. While abscess formation and maturation initially retards bacterial escape and septicemia and decreases bacterial access to oxygen and glucose, it also creates a barrier to penetrating phagocytes and systemic antibiotics. Therefore, bacteria can persist as vegetative forms and can rejuvenate in a changed environment; ergo, the surgical principle that abscesses must be drained.

○ **What are the most common aerobic and anaerobic organisms recovered from intra-abdominal abscesses?**

Aerobic: *Eschericia coli*
Anaerobic: *Bacteroides fragilis*

○ **Although the overall incidence of intra-abdominal abscess has progressively declined, what is the most common cause?**

While formerly perforated appendicitis, colonic diverticulitis is now the most common cause as a result of more rapid diagnosis and treatment of appendicitis.

○ **When searching for an intra-abdominal abscess, a high-resolution CT scan is the procedure of choice with three limitations. Name the limitations.**

 1. Interloop abscesses.

 2. Inability to differentiate sterile from contaminated fluid collections.

 3. The post abdominal surgery patient.

○ **Percutaneous drainage of abscesses after CT scan identification should be avoided in what situations?**

 • Noninfected peripancreatic phlegmon.
 • Infected organized hematomas.
 • Abscess with enteric fistulae.
 • Fungal infections.
 • Abscess within necrotic tumors.

○ **How often are abdominal x-ray findings of pneumoperitoneum in an unoperated patient associated with a perforated hollow viscus?**

 90%. These cases require urgent surgical intervention.

○ **Aside from iatrogenic causes of nonsurgical pneumoperitoneum, the second most common source of gas/air in the abdominal cavity is from where?**

 Above the diaphragm. Ruptured alveoli can lead to pneumomediastinum which can: 1) rupture into the pleural space and then into the abdomen directly through the diaphragmatic hiatus or fenestrations, or 2) dissect into the retroperitoneum and then rupture through the mesentery.

○ **Name three other causes of noniatrogenic, spontaneous pneumoperitoneum.**

 1. Introduction of air through the female genital tract during sexual activity.

 2. Pneumatosis cystoides intestinalis.

 3. Cocaine use.

○ **True/False: In patients with significant abdominal distension who develop oliguria unresponsive to hemodynamic changes or corrections, increased intra-abdominal pressure (IAP or "compartment syndrome") should be considered.**

 True. Following the diagnosis of IAP (intra-abdominal pressure above 20 mmHg) measured with a bladder catheter and manometer, appropriate efforts, including surgical exploration, directed at intra-abdominal decompression should be followed with diuresis expected afterward.

○ **An adolescent of Iranian or Jordanian ancestry develops episodic, nonradiating, diffuse abdominal pain with associated fever and without any postepisode sequelae. What inherited disorder may he have?**

 Familial Mediterranean Fever.

○ **A 25-year-old woman describes the acute onset of severe localized right lower quadrant pain. A CT scan is performed revealing epiploic appendagitis. What is the most appropriate treatment?**

 Pain is addressed with analgesia and should resolve in a week's time. No surgical or other medical treatment is required. Epiploic appendagitis is a self-limiting condition resulting from torsion or venous thrombosis of a fatty projection (epiploic appendage) from usually the ascending colon.

○ **Aerophagia may cause sudden localized or diffuse abdominal distention with normal bowel sounds and localized tympany and pain. Most often, the air collects in what two places?**

Stomach and splenic flexure of the colon.

○ **Although the specific risk of postoperative abdominal adhesive complications may vary according to the acute need and location of the initial surgical procedure, what is the approximate overall risk of hospital readmission later for these complications?**

Studied over a 10-year follow-up interval, 4% of 30,000 initial procedures and 5.5% of hospital readmissions were directly attributable to postoperative adhesions.

○ **A rectal shelf of Blumer is often associated with metastatic gastric or breast cancer. How is this distinguished from a rectal stricture?**

The Blumer shelf is an extrarectal mass indenting the anterior wall of the rectum and is distinguished from a stricture by the fact that: 1) it does not encircle the circumference and 2) often the mucosa can be made to move over the shelf.

○ **Carnett's test is a physical examination means of differentiating an abdominal wall mass from an intra-abdominal mass (and abdominal wall pain from intra-abdominal pain). How is this test performed?**

The supine patient is asked to extend his legs and lift his/her feet up from the bed or table, thereby tensing the abdominal musculature. Alternatively, the patient can raise his/her head. An intraperitoneal mass will nearly disappear when the abdominal muscles tighten, whereas an abdominal wall mass will persist. Likewise, pain from an intra-abdominal source will usually lessen, whereas abdominal wall pain will not.

○ **Abdominal wall crepitance surrounding an early postoperative incision but without wound discharge, pain, odor, or skin discoloration has what significance?**

It is innocuous. Termed "pseudo-gas gangrene," it occurs because air is entrapped in the subcutaneous tissue. It will soon be absorbed. This is especially common after laparoscopic procedures. If there is any doubt, prompt surgical intervention in the form of wound exploration should be undertaken to rule out early clostridial soft tissue infection.

○ **Acute development of a tender lump in the right lower quadrant after spasmodic coughing, about half-way between the umbilicus and pubic tubercle, may likely be due to what?**

Rectus muscle rupture or torn inferior epigastric artery. This may be differentiated from a strangulated Spigellian hernia by the absence of vomiting. Patients that are pregnant or on anticoagulant therapy are at increased risk for this problem.

○ **What four structures may remain patent rather than obliterate in the umbilicus at birth?**

1. Umbilical vein.
2. Omphalo-mesenteric duct (fecal).
3. Hypogastric arteries.
4. Bladder-urachal fistula (urine).

○ **What is a likely cause of a sudden appearance of feculent discharge from the umbilicus in a middle-aged, unoperated patient?**

Colonic diverticulitis or colon carcinoma.

○ **Acute mesenteric lymphadenitis is as common as acute appendicitis and can mimic this disease in children. After what age does the incidence drop and become exceedingly unlikely?**

Fifteen years of age.

○ **Acute extra-abdominal conditions that are common and may mimic acute inflammatory intra-abdominal disease in adults number at least three. Name them.**

1. Coronary occlusion/myocardial infarction.

2. Diaphragmatic pleurisy.

3. Herpes zoster.

○ **A psychogenic disease, usually occurring in females, in which acute abdominal symptoms are out of proportion to physical findings and in which there are often several surgical scars on the abdomen is suggestive of what diagnosis?**

Münchausen's syndrome.

○ **What type of bowel fistulae frequently spontaneously close if surrounding active bacterial peritonitis is cleared?**

Lateral bowel fistulae, which permit normal progression of some intestinal contents beyond the fistula through normal bowel.

○ **If a colonic fistula is present, whether cutaneous or internal, what is the problem with treatment by proximal loop colostomy or cecostomy?**

Neither procedure is totally diverting and thereby may cause persistent contamination.

○ **The six major physical deterrents to spontaneous closure of an enterocutaneous fistula are**

Remember the mnemonic FRIEND:

1. **F**oreign body

2. **R**adiation

3. **I**nflammation/Infection/Inflammatory bowel disease (Crohn's)

4. **E**pithelialization (gastrointestinal mucosa has fused with the skin)

5. **N**eoplasia

6. **D**istal obstruction

○ **The two potential benefits of parenteral nutritional support for bowel fistula closure are**

1. Increased proportion close without surgical intervention.

2. Reduced average time for closure.

○ **True/False: All enterocutaneous fistula treatment is aided by the use of somatostatin or octreotide. What are theoretical reasons for use of these agents?**

False. Theoretical reasons for use include: 1) more rapid closure interval of high output fistulae by reducing the volume of pancreatic enzyme secretion, and 2) reduced duration of parenteral nutrition and its inherent morbidity because of more rapid closure rate. The ultimate closure of low volume fistulae is not enhanced by use of these peptides.

○   **A defect in what lining or layer through which any abdominal wall hernia—be it umbilical, hiatal, inguinal, or incisional—must extrude is called?**

The "endoabdominal fascia." This is a continuous lining of the abdominal cavity that is given other names when it lies over various muscles, such as transversalis (muscle) fascia, psoas (muscle) fascia, and so on.

○   **How does gastroschisis in newborns differ from omphalocele?**

- Gastroschisis is a defect of the abdominal wall lateral to the umbilicus that results when the abdominal wall has failed to close, whereas omphalocele is a defect in closure of the umbilical ring.
- No sac is found over the protruded intestines in gastroschisis, whereas an amniotic sac usually lies over the intestines in omphalocele.
- Omphalocele is associated with other birth defects, gastroschisis is not.
- Bowel loss is more likely in gastroschisis due to amniotic fluid peritonitis and bowel torsion/infarction.

○   **Persons with cystic remnants or fibrous bands at the umbilical end of the omphalomesenteric duct are at risk for what problems?**

Acute volvulus and intestinal obstruction. Occasionally, an acute abdomen due to cyst infection may occur.

○   **What is the persistence of the intestinal end of the omphalomesenteric duct called?**

Meckel's diverticulum. This is a true intestinal diverticulum with all intestinal wall layers represented.

○   **Congenital abdominal hernias that are caused by abnormal rotation of the intestine and create obstructive symptoms in adults (usually) have what two anatomic descriptions.**

1. "Right mesocolic" with entrapment of proximal small bowel in mesentery under the right colon.
2. "Left mesocolic" with entrapment of rotated small bowel under the left/sigmoid colon.

○   **One month after an uncomplicated aortic aneurysm repair, a 65-year-old man presents with a painless, gradually distended abdomen. Shifting dullness and a fluid wave are noted on examination. Paracentesis returns a milky white fluid rich in triglycerides. What is the diagnosis and initial treatment?**

Chylous ascites from surgically disrupted lymphatics. Post surgical chylous ascites usually resolves with supportive therapy. Paracentesis is reserved for diagnosis and symptoms. A diet eliminating long chain triglycerides should be instituted. Octreotide (100 mcg subcutaneously three times per day) can be tried in refractory cases. Prolonged bowel rest with parenteral nutrition support should be considered for more refractory cases. Rarely, surgical ligation of the lymphatics is necessary.

● ● ● SUGGESTED READINGS ● ● ●

Nehra D, Goldstein AM. Intestinal malrotation: varied clinical presentation from infancy through adulthood. *Surgery.* 2011;149(3): 386-393.

Schecter WP, Hirshberg A, Chang DS, et al. Enteric fistulas: principles of management. *J Am Coll Surg.* 2009;209(4):484-491.

Mazuski JE, Solomkin JS. Intra-abdominal infections. *Surg Clin North Am.* 2009;89(2):421-437.

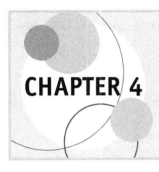

CHAPTER 4

Foreign Bodies and Caustic Injury

Rajeev Vasudeva, MD, FACG

○ **Where in the gastrointestinal tract is the most common site of foreign body impaction?**

The esophagus is the most common site, especially at the level of the hypopharynx. Other common places are areas of physiologic narrowing and include the pylorus, retroperitoneal duodenum, ileocecal valve, and the anus. The ileocecal region is the most frequent site of perforation beyond the esophagus.

○ **Where in the esophagus are objects likely to become lodged?**

Objects may become lodged at any of the areas of physiologic narrowing (cricopharyngeus, aortic arch, the left main stem bronchus, immediately above the esophagogastric junction) or any other area of structural abnormality (stricture).

○ **True/False: Most foreign body ingestions occur in children between the ages of 5 and 8 years.**

False. Most foreign body ingestions occur between the ages of 6 months to 3 years.

○ **Which adults are at an increased risk for swallowing foreign bodies?**

Adults at increased risk include those who wear dentures, those who are mentally retarded, those with psychiatric illnesses, and prisoners.

○ **What is the most common symptom in patients presenting with an esophageal foreign body?**

Dysphagia is the most common symptom followed by odynophagia, chest pain, choking, and drooling. The presence of respiratory distress and inability to swallow oral secretions suggests a need for urgent intervention.

○ **What are the most common symptoms of complete esophageal obstruction due to a foreign body?**

Ptyalism (drooling), regurgitation, and choking.

○ **True/False: Most ingested foreign bodies that become lodged in the esophagus pass spontaneously.**

True. Seventy percent of ingested foreign bodies pass spontaneously and <1% result in perforation.

○ **What is the most common physical finding in patients presenting with an ingested foreign body?**

Usually the physical examination is normal; however, signs of crepitation should always be sought.

○   **A chest x-ray reveals an ingested foreign body aligning itself in the sagittal plane. Is the object more likely to be located in the esophagus or trachea?**

Trachea. Tracheal foreign bodies align themselves sagittally and are best seen on lateral projections.

○   **What is the best study for identifying a radiopaque foreign body in the esophagus?**

Frontal view chest x-ray. Objects in the esophagus align themselves in an anteroposterior projection.

○   **True/False: Contrast studies of the esophagus may be useful in determining the type and location of an ingested foreign body.**

False. Contrast studies should be avoided due to their increased risk of aspiration and interference with subsequent endoscopic visualization.

○   **What is the best imaging study to identify and localize a nonradiopaque foreign body in the esophagus?**

CT scan can localize and identify the foreign body in >80% of cases.

○   **How often do pointed sharp objects perforate the intestinal tract and how are they best removed?**

Fortunately, up to 90% of objects pass spontaneously without complication and rarely perforate. Pointed objects should be removed with the pointed end trailing in order to avoid mucosal injury. Under these circumstances, an overtube or a hood attached to the tip of the endoscope should be used.

○   **True/False: Enzyme preparations such as papain should be tried prior to endoscopy in all cases of meat impaction.**

False. Besides being ineffective, it is important to avoid papain and other enzyme preparations because of an increased risk of perforation.

○   **Prior to endoscopic removal of an ingested safety pin, what should be done by the endoscopist to increase the success rate?**

Rehearsal of the retrieval process (dry run) should always be performed in order to facilitate removal of an object.

○   **True/False: Blindly pushing a foreign body into the stomach followed by endoscopic retrieval is routinely advocated.**

False. This technique should be avoided unless the lumen beyond the obstructing foreign body is adequately visualized and patent. In general, once the foreign body has passed into the stomach, it does not need to be retrieved as it will usually pass through the gastrointestinal tract without any problem.

○   **A 72-year-old woman is brought to the emergency room 72 hours after swallowing a pointed object. What is the best management at this point?**

Endoscopic removal should be attempted in this patient if it can be localized and is retrievable. Indications for prompt removal of ingested foreign bodies include the presence of complete esophageal obstruction and ingestion of sharp, pointed, or toxic objects (disc [button] batteries) lodged in the esophagus.

◯   **True/False: A 23-year-old man presents with fever, chills, neck pain, and obvious subcutaneous emphysema 2 hours after accidentally swallowing a fish bone. Endoscopic removal by an experienced gastroenterologist is the most appropriate management for this patient.**

False. This patient has evidence of possible esophageal perforation. Therefore, surgical evaluation is the treatment of choice.

◯   **What is the most appropriate management for a patient who is found to have an ingested foreign body that is embedded in the esophageal wall?**

Surgery. If it appears to be removable endoscopically, after consultation with a surgeon, endoscopic removal could be considered.

◯   **True/False: Immediate endoscopic removal is the best approach for management of ingested latex packets of cocaine.**

False. Endoscopic removal of such drug packets is unwise because of the potential for rupture upon manipulation. If packets fail to progress or if there are signs suggesting leakage, urgent surgical intervention is indicated.

◯   **What is the appropriate management of ingested elemental mercury in the intestine?**

Observation and possibly cathartics to hasten its elimination as long as there is no evidence of perforation or leakage outside the digestive tract.

◯   **What is the best approach to take when an esophageal stricture is found once the foreign body has been removed or pushed into the stomach?**

Dilatation of the stricture. If there is local mucosal trauma or bleeding or the patient is not cooperative or visualization of the field is suboptimal, the stricture is best dilated at a later time.

◯   **True/False: The location of the perceived discomfort is predictive of the most likely site of a foreign body lodged in the esophagus.**

False. As with dysphagia in general, the location of the perceived discomfort does not usually correlate with the anatomic location of the obstructing foreign body.

◯   **What size objects should be considered for endoscopic removal?**

Long objects >6 cm in children and >10 cm in adults should be removed. Rounded objects <2.5 cm usually pass through the pylorus in adults and can be managed conservatively.

◯   **When should endoscopy be utilized in the management of an ingested disc (button) battery?**

Endoscopy should be performed promptly if the disc battery is lodged in the esophagus. If it has passed into the stomach, conservative measures may be employed and the patient observed. If the battery has remained in the stomach for more than 48 hours, is >1.5 cm, and has mercury, it should be promptly removed.

◯   **How long should you wait before contemplating endoscopic or surgical removal of a foreign body?**

Blunt objects such as coins, if located in the esophagus, should be removed urgently. Asymptomatic blunt objects that fail to leave the stomach after 2 weeks should be removed endoscopically. Surgical removal of blunt objects beyond the stomach that fail to advance after 7 to 10 days (sharp objects >3 days) should be considered. Surgical intervention is otherwise indicated if fever, vomiting, overt bleeding, or abdominal pain develops.

○ **True/False: Adults are more likely than children to ingest caustic substances?**

False. It is estimated that 17,000 children, half of whom are under 4 years of age, accidentally ingest caustic substances each year. Although relatively uncommon in adults, it predominantly involves adults who are inebriated, mentally retarded, psychotic, or suicidal.

○ **What factors are implicated in the pathogenesis of caustic injury to the gut?**

The nature, concentration, and physical state of the agent, the amount ingested, the time of exposure ("dwell time"), as well as the amount of re-exposure secondary to vomiting or reflux are important factors.

○ **Where are common caustic agents implicated in accidental or intentional ingestion found?**

The individual's home. Many household products contain strong alkaline caustic agents. These include drain cleaners, oven cleaners, swimming pool–cleaning products, dishwasher detergents, hair relaxers, bleaches, and lye soaps.

○ **How do alkaline agents cause injury?**

Alkaline agents cause liquefaction (saponification) necrosis, which dissolves superficial mucosa, and rapidly diffuse into deeper tissues. Blood vessel thrombosis causes further cellular necrosis potentially resulting in full-thickness burns.

○ **How do acidic agents cause injury?**

Acidic agents produce a coagulation necrosis of the surface epithelium and tend to produce less penetration.

○ **What region of the gastrointestinal tract is more commonly affected by acidic agent ingestion?**

Acidic agents usually cause extensive damage to the stomach. The esophagus is relatively spared due to a combination of factors including rapid transit through the esophagus, greater resistance of esophageal squamous epithelium to acid, and the protection afforded by superficial coagulation necrosis preventing deeper injury. Nevertheless, 20%–50% of patients may have significant esophageal burns from ingestion of highly concentrated sulfuric or hydrochloric acid.

○ **True/False: There is good correlation between oral/pharyngeal burns and esophageal or gastric injury.**

False. The lack of oral or pharyngeal burns does not preclude the possibility of extensive esophageal or gastric injury.

○ **True/False: Gastric lavage with water or administration of emetics plays an important role in the management of caustic ingestions.**

False. Gastric lavage is contraindicated in both alkaline and acid ingestions due to increased risk of perforation and aspiration. Emetics should always be avoided due to re-exposure to the caustic agent.

○ **True/False: Administration of acid neutralizers is helpful immediately after caustic ingestion.**

False. The heat produced in the neutralization reaction may actually increase tissue injury. Additionally, since most alkali injuries occur very rapidly, acid neutralization is ineffective.

○ **When should endoscopic examination be carried out in patients with suspected caustic ingestion?**

Although there are differing opinions, most experts agree on the need to document extent of damage by performing endoscopy within 12 to 24 hours.

○ **How often does endoscopic injury occur in patients with caustic ingestion?**

<50%.

○ **What is the most sensitive imaging study to detect a suspected early perforation following caustic ingestion?**

CT scan of the chest and abdomen with oral contrast.

○ **What are the 'Grades' of injury caused by caustic ingestion?**

The extent of injury can be divided into three degrees of injury. First-degree injury is characterized by mild friability, erythema, and edema only. Second-degree injury extends into the wall, occasionally to the muscularis propria. Ulceration, necrosis, and exudate may be seen. Third-degree injury involves the full thickness of the wall. A dark exudate with sloughing of the mucosa, hemorrhage, ulceration, and necrosis are typically seen.

○ **True/False: Endoscopic findings accurately predict the pathological depth of tissue injury.**

False. Grades of injury on endoscopy are not as precise as the pathologic degree of burn.

○ **What is the management and prognosis of patients based on the Grade of endoscopic injury?**

Patients with first-degree injury have an excellent prognosis and can be started on a liquid diet, which can be advanced in 1–2 days as tolerated. Patients with second-degree injury develop strictures in >70% of cases, usually within 2–4 weeks, requiring endoscopic or surgical intervention. Patients with third-degree injury have a high mortality and may require urgent surgical intervention.

○ **What is the role of antibiotics and corticosteroids in the management of caustic ingestions?**

The lack of controlled trials precludes definitive arguments in support of any therapeutic modality. The use of antibiotics and corticosteroids is fraught with controversy in the literature. However, corticosteroids may be considered if symptoms of laryngeal edema are present. Antibiotics are recommended in proven or suspected infection and in patients with second- and third-degree injury.

○ **When do strictures usually develop following caustic ingestion?**

Most strictures (80%) present within the first 8 weeks after injury. However, they can occur insidiously over months to years after the initial event.

○ **What are the usual sites of stricture development in the esophagus and stomach following caustic ingestion?**

Strictures tend to develop at sites of pooling such as the cricopharyngeus, aortic arch, bifurcation of the trachea, and lower esophageal sphincter in the esophagus and the antrum of fasting patients and the mid-body in patients who have food present in the stomach at the time of caustic ingestion.

○ **What is another long-term complication of caustic ingestion?**

The development of squamous cell carcinoma of the esophagus. The latency period varies from 12 to 41 years and is shorter for injuries occurring after childhood. Specific surveillance protocols have not been defined.

● ● ● SUGGESTED READINGS ● ● ●

Eisen GM, Baron TH, Dominitz JA, et al. American Society for Gastrointestinal Endoscopy. Guideline for the management of ingested foreign bodies. *Gastrointest Endosc.* 2002;55:802-806.

Weiland ST, Schurr MJ. Conservative treatment of ingested foreign bodies. *J Gastrointest Surg.* 2002;6:496-500.

Smith MT, Wong RKH. Esophageal foreign bodies: types and techniques for removal. *Curr Treat Op Gastroenterol.* 2006;9:75-84.

Poley JW, Steyerberg EW, Kuipers EJ, et al. Ingestion of acid and alkaline agents: outcome and prognostic value of early upper endoscopy. *Gastrointest Endosc.* 2004;60:372-377.

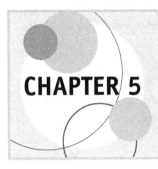

CHAPTER 5

Pediatric Gastrointestinal Diseases

Jon A. Vanderhoof, MD

○ **Formula-fed and human milk-fed infants have different patterns of gut microbiota colonization. The stools of breast-fed infants have a predominance of which bacterial genus?**

Bifidobacterium.

○ **What is the coefficient of fat absorption in a normal individual?**

In a normal individual, 93% of fat is absorbed. In newborn infants, the number drops to a level of 90% and even less in premature infants. Nevertheless, its caloric density (9 kcal/g) makes it an excellent source of calories, even in premature infants.

○ **Absent responses to which gastrointestinal hormones occur in gluten-sensitive enteropathy prior to treatment?**

Cholecystokinin, secretin, and glucose-dependent insulin trophic peptide.

○ **In the medical evaluation of anorexia nervosa, laboratory studies to screen for pregnancy, inflammatory bowel disease, thyroid disease, central nervous system disorders, drug abuse, celiac disease, and metabolic disorders are routinely done. What additional serum study may be useful in this scenario?**

Serum carotene. It is often elevated in anorexia nervosa.

○ **What disorder should be suspected in a patient with a history of caustic ingestion who develops a late onset or worsening of dysphagia?**

Esophageal carcinoma.

○ **What percentage of school-age children have chronic abdominal pain to the extent that it interferes with normal daily activity?**

10%.

○ **What is the most useful diagnostic tool to identify the cause of chronic recurrent abdominal pain of childhood?**

Careful history and physical examination.

○ **Chronic, nonspecific diarrhea or 'toddler diarrhea,' the most common cause of chronic diarrhea in this age group, is best treated utilizing what dietary maneuvers?**

High-fat, low-carbohydrate diet.

○ **Constipation in school-age children has been identified as a possible consequence of intolerance to what dietary component?**

Cow's milk protein.

○ **Why is cow's milk allergy so common in infants?**

The infant's gut is more permeable to macromolecules in the first month of life permitting greater antigen exposure. Since cow's milk is the only antigen utilized in infants under a month of age, allergy to this protein is more common than other dietary protein allergies.

○ **An 8-month-old infant develops diarrhea and gas production every time he is given cow's milk. Both mother and father have been diagnosed with lactose intolerance. The family physician has recommended the child undergo a lactose breath hydrogen test. Could this be done in an 8-month-old infant?**

Yes. Breath hydrogen testing can be performed in infants and is useful in the investigation of bacterial overgrowth, specific carbohydrate malabsorption, and measuring intestinal transit. Lactose intolerance at this age is almost always secondary and is usually due to cow's mild allergy.

○ **True/False: Cow's milk protein allergy results in life-long lactose intolerance.**

False. Most children outgrow the allergy by 3 to 5 years of age. As a consequence, when suspected, allergy testing is rarely necessary and a trial of cow's milk protein exclusion should be recommended.

○ **What is the most common cause of acute abdomen in the infant age group?**

Intussusception.

○ **What is the most common cause of painless, lower gastrointestinal bleeding in school-age children?**

Colonic polyp, usually of the juvenile type.

○ **Infantile failure to thrive is a serious condition requiring early identification and treatment. What is responsible for nearly all the mortality in this condition?**

Abused or seriously neglected infants.

○ **What is the most common malignant tumor of the gastrointestinal tract in children, and occurs most frequently in the distal ileum?**

Lymphoma.

○ **What is the drug of choice if sedation is required for esophageal manometry?**

Chloral hydrate, 50 mg/kg. It does not affect lower esophageal sphincter pressure or the amplitude of esophageal contractions.

○ **What is the most common type of tracheoesophageal fistula?**

Proximal esophageal atresia with a fistula between the trachea and the distal esophagus accounts for 85%.

○ **What is the major value of an upper gastrointestinal x-ray in an infant with frequent emesis?**

An upper gastrointestinal barium-contrast x-ray excludes anatomical lesions, gastric outlet obstruction, and proximal small bowel anomalies. It does not reliably diagnose or exclude gastroesophageal reflux.

○ **What is the most common cause of idiopathic portal hypertension in a child without liver disease?**

Portal vein thrombosis. Further history may reveal that a venous umbilical catheter was placed during the newborn period.

○ **True/False: Newborn infants are achlorhydric.**

False. Newborn infants have high serum gastrin levels and normal stimulated gastric acid production has been demonstrated in the first few days of life.

○ **How long does an infant need to receive nothing by mouth after a pyloromyotomy for pyloric stenosis?**

They can eat as soon as they wake up.

○ **What is the most common cause of erosive gastritis associated with eosinophilic infiltrates on biopsy in a 6-week-old infant?**

Cows' milk protein allergy. Eosinophilia, more common in small bowel and rectal biopsies, may be seen in esophageal and gastric biopsies as well.

○ **An institutionalized child with Down's syndrome presents with abdominal pain and is found to have an iron-deficiency anemia. What is the most likely cause?**

The child needs an upper gastrointestinal endoscopy as children with Down's syndrome have a high incidence of celiac disease. It should also be kept in mind that institutionalized children also have a higher incidence of symptomatic *Helicobacter pylori* disease.

○ **When should gut malrotation be surgically repaired?**

Only if symptomatic; however, it is often difficult to determine if the symptoms, such as abdominal pain, are directly related to the malrotation.

○ **How do you differentiate between gastroschisis and omphalocele?**

An omphalocele involves the umbilicus but a gastroschisis does not. An omphalocele is also covered by peritoneal membrane, which may or may not be apparent, but a gastroschisis is not covered by this membrane.

○ **What is a common cause of lactase deficiency in infants less than 6 months of age?**

Infection or enteropathy due to cow's milk protein intolerance. Primary acquired lactose intolerance does not occur until after the age of 5 years.

○ **Bacterial proliferation in small bowel bacterial overgrowth is diminished by an increase in which macronutrient and concurrent decrease in which macronutrient?**

Increase in fat and a decrease in carbohydrate.

○ **What percentage of children with celiac disease present with chronic diarrhea and failure to thrive?**

This is unknown. However, as the child ages, classic symptoms become less apparent and he/she may present merely with abdominal pain and short stature.

○ **What is the most common, non-IgE-mediated food-related immunologic reaction?**

Milk protein. Although IgE-mediated food allergies occur, they are manifested by gastrointestinal symptoms and, oftentimes, respiratory symptoms and/or skin reactions occurring within 2 hours after food ingestion.

○ **What is the safest, most effective drug therapy for eosinophilic gastroenteritis in a child who does not respond completely to dietary restrictions?**

Oral fluticasone, although a budesonide slurry and oral cromolyn sodium may also be effective. Although systemic corticosteroid therapy is highly efficacious, long-term treatment is often associated with numerous side effects.

○ **What is the definition of short bowel syndrome?**

The presence of malabsorption and malnutrition following massive small bowel resection. It is not based solely on the length of remaining bowel; however, it generally does not become clinically apparent until about three-quarters of the small bowel has been removed.

○ **What is the most common and frequently unrecognized gastrointestinal complication in a child with short bowel syndrome?**

Chronic small bowel bacterial overgrowth.

○ **What type of triglyceride has the most potent effect on enhancement of intestinal adaptation after massive small bowel resection?**

Long-chain triglyceride.

○ **What would characteristically be found on upper endoscopy in a child who presents with stool lymphocytes, lymphopenia, hypoalbuminemia, and hyperlipidemia?**

Scattered milky white spots with a snowflakelike appearance. These represent markedly dilated lymphatics in the lamina propria and/or the submucosa (lymphangiectasia).

○ **Currant jelly stools in an infant with severe irritability and a palpable sausage-shaped abdominal mass is the classic description of what disorder?**

Intussusception. This classic presentation is seen in only about 15%. More commonly, emesis and abdominal pain with various forms of rectal bleeding are seen.

○ **What is the most likely consideration in a pediatric patient carrying the tentative diagnosis of pseudo-obstruction who never demonstrates ileus or air fluid levels?**

Munchausen-by-proxy.

○ **Children presenting with significant abdominal pain may warrant screening by stool microscopy for what particular infectious agents?**

Parasitic infections may present solely with abdominal pain in the absence of other gastrointestinal symptoms.

○ **What is the most common anomaly of an omphalomesenteric duct remnant?**

Meckel's diverticulum.

○ **What are the most common tumors of the lower gastrointestinal tract in children?**

Benign polyps including the juvenile polyp, hamartomatous polyp, inflammatory fibroid polyp, and lymphoid polyp. Malignant adenomas of the colon are usually seen in conjunction with familial polyposis syndromes.

○ **What is the most common cause of abdominal pain in children who present to the Emergency Room?**

Gastroenteritis. The most common error is to diagnose gastroenteritis in a child who actually has a retrocecal appendicitis.

○ **What single most important factor reduces the morbidity and mortality of Hirschsprung's disease in children?**

Enterocolitis is a major cause of mortality in infants with Hirschsprung's disease. Therefore, the recognition and treatment of Hirschsprung's disease before enterocolitis develops is important.

○ **What is the most likely cause of acute diarrhea in school-age children who present with watery stools, vomiting, and a low-grade fever that spontaneously resolves within 24 hours?**

Norovirus.

○ **Continuing oral feedings in patients with acute infectious enteritis is done primarily to avoid what complication?**

Weight loss.

○ **A 6-year-old boy treated with amoxicillin-clavulanic acid for otitis media develops *Clostridium difficile* diarrhea requiring treatment with metronidazole. After successful treatment, he experiences a recurrence of *C. difficile* 3 weeks later. What would be the most beneficial course of action to prevent recurrence again?**

Retreat with metronidazole and initiate and maintain a probiotic such as *Saccharomyces boulardii* for 2 to 3 months.

○ **What fat soluble vitamin is least well absorbed in patients with cholestatic liver disease?**

Vitamin E.

○ **How reliable are IgA antigliadin antibodies in children under 2 years of age in screening for celiac disease?**

The reliability of IgA antigliadin antibodies under 2 years of age deteriorates significantly. Consequently, the test cannot be reliably used as a screening test in this age group.

○ **In IgA-deficient patients, is there a suitable alternative screening test for celiac disease?**

Deaminated antigliadin IgG antibodies may be used in this population.

○ **Persistent mild elevation of serum aminotransferase levels in an 8-year-old overweight boy is most likely suggestive of what disorder?**

Nonalcoholic fatty liver disease (NAFLD) has now become commonplace even in the pediatric age group and carries with it a significant risk of ongoing chronic liver disease and metabolic syndrome.

○ **Anti-tumor necrosis factor (TNF) alpha therapy for inflammatory bowel disease in children is commonly associated with what complication?**

Infection is the most common complication of anti-TNF therapy. There is also a risk of lymphoma, especially associated with a combination of anti-TNF therapy and immunomodulators. The risk of lymphoma appears to be somewhat greater in children and adolescents than in adults, although the complication is still quite rare.

○ **True/False: A 2-month-old infant has been constipated since birth. A barium enema is performed which shows no transition segment. Hirschsprung's disease has been effectively excluded in this infant.**

False. The barium enema is notoriously unreliable in infants as a screening tool for Hirschsprung's disease as a definitive transition zone with dilated proximal bowel usually does not develop this early.

○ **True/False: A 7-year-old girl with a history of unremitting bloody diarrhea for 2 years has continuous, acute, and chronic inflammatory changes on her colonoscopic biopsies throughout the colon, and has responded poorly to high-dose corticosteroids and immunomodulators. She has a normal small bowel x-ray and a normal upper gastrointestinal endoscopy. A decision has been made to refer her for colectomy. It is safe to assume that she has ulcerative colitis.**

False. It is difficult to make a definitive diagnosis of ulcerative colitis in this age range. Video capsule endoscopy has been approved for use in children over 3 years of age and would provide additional reassurance that she does not have small bowel involvement suggestive of Crohn's disease prior to proceeding with colectomy.

○ **True/False: An infant with chronic spitting and regurgitation has been placed on a proton pump inhibitor for suspected gastroesophageal reflux. It is necessary to continue the child on this medication for the next 6 months.**

False. There is no evidence that proton pump inhibitors symptomatically improve infants with uncomplicated gastroesophageal reflux. While this is a common practice, it is probably of little benefit in this setting.

○ **Dysphagia in a 10-year-old child with a normal barium-contrast upper GI series is most likely to be due to what condition?**

Eosinophilic esophagitis. This disorder is becoming quite common in the pediatric age group. In children, the diagnosis may be apparent endoscopically; however, the mucosa may appear normal early in the disease, so biopsies of the distal, middle, and proximal esophagus, preferably at least four at each location, are needed for making the diagnosis. A normal upper GI series would reliably exclude most other organic causes of dysphagia including achalasia and stricture.

○ **What role does food allergy play in eosinophilic esophagitis in children?**

It has been demonstrated that eosinophilic esophagitis can be treated effectively with an elemental diet strongly suggesting that food allergy plays a key pathogenic role. In children, initial therapy should consist of dietary management either by excluding the most common food allergens or by using a diet directed by allergy testing excluding highly reactive foods. Both approaches have been shown to be beneficial. If symptoms remain and histology does not improve, anti-inflammatory medications such as swallowed fluticasone or budesonide may be utilized.

• • • SUGGESTED READINGS • • •

Steele R. Diagnosis and management of coeliac disease in children. *Postgrad Med J.* 2011 Jan;87(1023):19-25.

Ruemmele FM. Pediatric inflammatory bowel diseases: coming of age. *Curr Opin Gastroenterol.* 2010 Jul;26(4):332-336.

du Toit G, Meyer R, Shah N, et al. Identifying and managing cow's milk protein allergy. *Arch Dis Child Educ Pract Ed.* 2010 Oct;95(5):134-144.

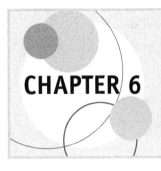

CHAPTER 6

Radiation and Ischemic Injury and Vascular Abnormalities

Shabana F. Pasha, MD

○ **Which cells in the gastrointestinal tract are most prone to be damaged by radiation?**

Crypt cells in the intestine as they have a high turnover rate.

○ **When do acute and chronic radiation injury occur after radiation exposure?**

Acute radiation injury occurs within 6 weeks of radiation exposure. Chronic radiation injury typically occurs 6 months after radiation exposure, but can occur up to 30 years after exposure.

○ **What are the histopathological changes characteristic of acute radiation enteritis?**

Inflammatory cell infiltrate, reduced crypt mitoses, crypt microabscesses, and ulceration.

○ **What are the histopathological changes characteristic of chronic radiation injury?**

Epithelial atrophy, obliterative endarteritis, submucosal fibrosis, mucosal ischemia, and necrosis.

○ **What are the most common symptoms of acute radiation esophagitis?**

Dysphagia, odynophagia, and substernal chest pain, typically occurring 2–3 weeks after initiation of radiation therapy.

○ **How does radiation dosage correlate with esophageal symptoms and signs?**

30 Gy	retrosternal burning and odynophagia
40 Gy	mucosal erythema and edema
50 Gy	incidence and severity of esophagitis increases
60–70 Gy	strictures, perforations, and fistulae

○ **What other factors potentiate radiation-induced esophageal damage?**

The manner of delivery with an accelerated fractionation schedule may result in more injury. Concomitant chemotherapy may also potentiate radiation injury and is particularly common with doxorubicin.

○ **What are late effects of esophageal radiation injury?**

Esophageal stricture and fistula formation.

○ **What patient factors are associated with the development of chronic radiation enteritis?**

Decreased body mass index, chronic co-morbidities (diabetes mellitus, hypertension, inflammatory bowel disease), smoking, and prior intestinal surgery.

○ **What treatment factors are associated with the development of chronic radiation enteritis?**

Radiation dose and fractionation, radiation technique, volume of small bowel irradiated, and concomitant chemotherapy.

○ **What is the most common late manifestation of radiation-induced small bowel injury?**

Partial small bowel obstruction.

○ **What are the radiologic findings of chronic radiation enteritis on barium contrast radiography?**

Mucosal edema, separation of intestinal loops, and flocculation.

○ **What are the most common causes of diarrhea in patients with chronic radiation enteritis?**

Malabsorption (lactose, bile salts, fat), small intestinal bacterial overgrowth, enteroenteric fistula, and gastrointestinal dysmotility.

○ **What are the most common symptoms associated with the condition demonstrated in the figure?**

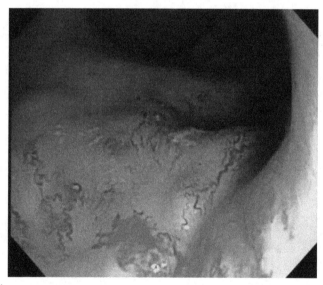

Figure 6-1 See also color plate.

The figure demonstrates the typical endoscopic appearance of chronic radiation proctopathy. Rectal bleeding, tenesmus, and low-volume diarrhea are the most common symptoms.

○ **What is the most serious complication after endoscopic therapy with argon plasma coagulation (APC) for chronic radiation proctopathy? When does this typically occur?**

Rectourethral fistula. It occurs if aggressive APC treatment is performed within 6–24 months after radiation in patients with seed implants.

○ **What is the most common location of radiation-induced rectal ulcers?**
Anterior wall of the rectum, approximately 6–8 cm proximal to the anal verge.

○ **What are the most common vascular abnormalities found in the gastrointestinal tract?**
Angioectasia.

○ **What are the characteristic histopathologic findings in an angioectasia?**
Dilated thin-walled vessel lined with endothelium, with or without smooth muscle fibers.

○ **What is being demonstrated in the figure and where in the colon are these lesions most commonly located?**

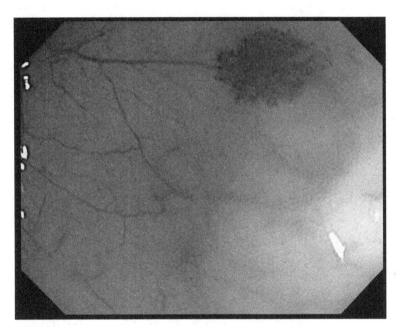

Figure 6-2 See also color plate.

Angioectasia. Cecum and ascending colon.

○ **True/False: Left-sided colonic angioectasia are more likely to bleed than those on the right side of the colon.**
False.

○ **What percent of patients with colonic angioectasia have concomitant small bowel angioectasia?**
10%.

○ **What is the initial test of choice to evaluate the small bowel for angioectasia after a negative esophagogastroduodenoscopy (EGD) and colonoscopy in patients with obscure gastrointestinal bleeding?**
Video capsule endoscopy.

○   **What is Heyde syndrome?**

Gastrointestinal bleeding from angioectasia in patients with aortic stenosis.

○   **What is the proposed mechanism by which aortic stenosis leads to development of angioectasia?**

Disruption of the vonWillebrand multimers during passage through the narrowed aortic valve leads to acquired vonWillebrand disease. It is considered that the increased prevalence of angioectasia in this setting is due to the increased detection rather than a true increased incidence, as the patients with this disease usually present with bleeding.

○   **What are the clinical criteria for the diagnosis of hereditary hemorrhagic telangiectasia (HHT) aka Osler–Weber–Rendu syndrome?**

Epistaxis, telangiectasias (multiple sites including lips, oral cavity, fingers, and nose), visceral vascular malformations (pulmonary, gastrointestinal, cerebral, or spinal), and family history (first-degree relative) of HHT.

○   **At what age do patients with HHT present with gastrointestinal bleeding?**

Fourth decade of life.

○   **What are the histopathological changes typically seen in association with the condition shown in the figure?**

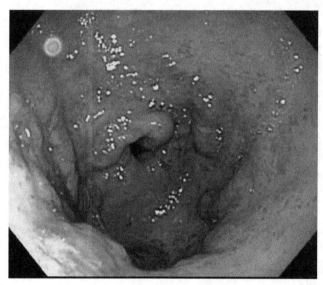

Figure 6-3 See also color plate.

The figure demonstrates the typical appearance of gastric antral vascular ectasia (GAVE, aka "watermelon stomach"). Dilated capillaries with focal thrombosis, dilated and tortuous veins in the submucosa, and fibromuscular hyperplasia of the muscularis mucosa are the usual histological findings.

○   **What conditions are associated with GAVE?**

GAVE is usually seen in middle-aged and older women. It is associated with achlorhydria, atrophic gastritis, cirrhosis, CREST syndrome, and bone marrow transplantation.

○ **What is the treatment of GAVE?**

Supportive treatment with iron therapy and packed red blood cell (PRBC) transfusions, endoscopic ablation (eg, APC), and, rarely, antrectomy for refractory cases.

○ **An endoscopy is performed on a 43-year-old man with long-standing alcoholism and stigmata of chronic liver disease on physical exam. Describe the mucosal changes seen on endoscopy. What is the most likely diagnosis?**

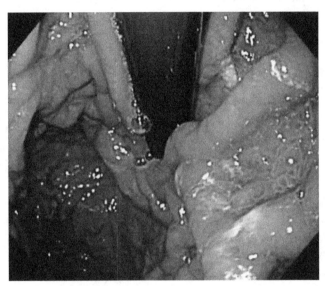

Figure 6-4 See also color plate.

Snake skin or mosaic appearance of the mucosa in the gastric body and fundus is seen. The most likely diagnosis in this case is portal hypertensive gastropathy.

○ **What is the treatment of portal hypertensive gastropathy (PHG)?**

Supportive treatment with iron supplementation, PRBC transfusions, and nonselective beta blockers; transjugular intrahepatic portosystemic shunt (TIPS) for refractory cases.

○ **What is a Dieulafoy lesion?**

It is a dilated aberrant submucosal artery. Focal pressure from the artery can lead to erosion of the overlying mucosa causing severe and often intermittent GI bleeding. Although the most common location is 6 cm distal to the gastroesophageal junction along the lesser curvature, Dieulafoy lesions have been described throughout the GI tract.

○ **What diseases are associated with cutaneous vascular nevi and gastrointestinal bleeding?**

Blue Rubber Bleb Nevus syndrome and Klippel–Trenaunay–Weber syndrome.

○ **What gastrointestinal lesions are seen in Blue Rubber Bleb Nevus syndrome?**

Venous malformations, most commonly located in the small bowel.

○ **What is superior mesenteric artery syndrome?**

Impingement of the superior mesenteric artery on the duodenum, when the angle between the root of the spinal muscular atrophy (SMA) and aorta is narrowed to less than 25 degrees. It usually occurs after rapid weight loss in adults. Symptoms include postprandial epigastric pain, vomiting, and early satiety.

○ **What is celiac artery compression syndrome?**

Celiac artery compression syndrome, also referred to as median arcuate ligament syndrome and Dunbar syndrome, is characterized by postprandial abdominal pain thought to be related to compression of the celiac artery by fibers of the median arcuate ligament.

○ **True/False: The etiology of celiac artery compression syndrome remains a source of controversy.**

True. Indeed, even the existence of this syndrome remains a source of controversy. As a consequence, so do the diagnosis and treatment.

○ **What are the clinical findings in celiac axis compression syndrome?**

Postprandial epigastric pain, diarrhea, weight loss, and presence of an abdominal bruit that increases with expiration. The characteristic radiologic finding is compression of the celiac axis by the median arcuate ligament.

○ **What are the risk factors for acute mesenteric ischemia?**

Advanced age, atherosclerosis, cardiac arrhythmias, low cardiac output states, valvular heart disease, and intra-abdominal malignancy.

○ **What are the causes of acute mesenteric ischemia?**

Superior mesenteric artery embolism (50%), superior mesenteric artery thrombosis, mesenteric venous thrombosis, and nonocclusive ischemia.

○ **What is the classical clinical presentation of acute mesenteric ischemia?**

Severe abdominal pain (periumbilical) out of proportion to the physical examination.

○ **What is the gold standard test in the diagnosis of acute mesenteric ischemia?**

Mesenteric angiography; multidetector CT angiography is a noninvasive alternative.

○ **Intestinal angina, sitophobia, and weight loss are the classical findings of what vascular disorder?**

Chronic mesenteric ischemia. Sitophobia refers to a fear of eating.

○ **True/False: In patients with classic chronic mesenteric ischemia, two of the three mesenteric vessels must typically be occluded or severely stenotic for the patient to experience symptoms of abdominal pain because of the extensive collateral network of the bowel.**

True.

○ **What is the mechanism of injury to the colon in ischemic colitis?**

Hypoxia due to nonocclusive ischemia followed by reperfusion injury with release of oxygen-free radicals and toxins.

○   **True/False: Mesenteric angiography is an important test in the diagnosis of ischemic colitis.**

False, for reasons noted in the preceding question.

○   **What proportion of patients with ischemic colitis develop gangrenous colitis?**

15%.

○   **What are the most common locations where ischemic colitis occurs?**

Splenic flexure and sigmoid colon.

○   **Why is isolated ischemic colitis of the right colon associated with a worse prognosis than other areas of the colon?**

A large proportion of these patients have silent superior mesenteric artery obstructive disease and are at risk for acute mesenteric ischemia of the small intestine.

○   **What is the classical clinical triad seen in Henoch–Schonlein purpura?**

Abdominal pain, arthritis, and palpable purpura.

○   **What are the gastrointestinal manifestations in Behcet's disease?**

Ulcerations in the terminal ileum, cecum, ascending colon, and esophagus that mimic Crohn's disease clinically and endoscopically. Pancreatitis may also occur.

● ● ● SUGGESTED READINGS ● ● ●

Czito BG, Willett CG. Radiation injury. In: Feldman M, Friedman L, Brandt L, eds. *Sleisenger and Fordtran's Gastrointestinal and Liver Disease*. 9th ed. Philadelphia, PA: Saunders Elsevier; 2010:639-651.

Coia AR, Myerson RJ, Tepper JE. Late effects of radiation therapy on the gastrointestinal tract. *Int J Radiation Oncology Biol Phys.* 1995;31:1213-1236.

Brandt LJ, Landis CS. Vascular lesions of the gastrointestinal tract. In: Feldman M, Friedman L, Brandt L, eds. *Sleisenger and Fordtran's Gastrointestinal and Liver Disease*. 9th ed. Philadelphia, PA: Saunders Elsevier; 2010:593-608.

American Gastroenterological Association Medical Position Statement: Guidelines on intestinal ischemia. *Gastroenterology.* 2000;118:951.

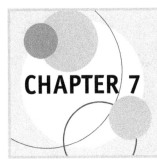

CHAPTER 7

Travel Matters in Gastroenterology

Abinash Virk, MD, DTM&H

○ **Name three clinical syndromes associated with neurologic abnormalities (parathesias, ataxia, hypotension, seizures, and muscle paralysis) that occur following ingestion of toxin-containing fish.**

Puffer fish poisoning (tetrodotoxin), paralytic shellfish poisoning (saxitoxin), and ciguatera poisoning (ciguatoxin).

○ **What is the most common cause of fish poisoning in the United States?**

Ciguatera. This is commonly seen in Florida, Hawaii, and the Caribbean.

○ **What is ciguatera fish poisoning?**

Ciguatera poisoning occurs after consumption of ciguatoxins present in certain fish. Large carnivorous tropical fish such as grouper, amberjack, red snapper, barracuda, and sea bass can harbor a toxin that cannot be detected by odor, taste, or color. The ciguatoxin accumulates in carnivorous fish that have consumed smaller herbivorous fish that feed on dinoflagellates such as *Gambierdiscus taxicus*. Risk is higher at tropical destinations such as the Caribbean and Indo-Pacific Islands.

○ **True/False: Ciguatera poisoning causes both gastrointestinal and neurological symptoms.**

True. Acute gastrointestinal (nausea, vomiting, and cramps) and neurologic symptoms occur within 2–6 hours of ingestion and last for about 1 week. Rarely, the neurologic symptoms of paresthesias and motor weakness can persist for months to years.

○ **Which contaminated fish poisoning may cause flushing, vertigo, and burning sensation and is effectively treated with antihistamines?**

Scromboid.

○ **What is scromboid poisoning?**

Scromboid poisoning presents within 30 minutes of consumption of toxic fish. Scromboid results from improper cooling of fish and resultant bacterial growth that degrades histidine in the fish muscles into histamine and histamine-like products called saurine. The histamine consumption causes flushing, nausea, emesis, and abdominal cramps, and can cause anaphylactoid symptoms within minutes of ingestion of the fish. The fish looks and smells normal but is often reported to have a "peppery" taste. Spoiled tuna, mackerel, and skipjacks are often implicated. If any of these fish has an unpleasant odor or clouded eyes, it should be avoided.

○ **What infectious organisms can a traveler acquire with raw oyster consumption?**

Raw oyster consumption is associated with acquisition of hepatitis A, *Vibrio vulnificus* and *Cryptosporidium parvum*. A single oyster or mollusk can filter >14 liters of water and concentrate pathogens in the gills.

○ **True/False: A causative agent is found in most patients with traveler's diarrhea (TD) suffering from prolonged diarrhea.**

False.

○ **What microorganism is the most common cause of TD?**

Enterotoxigenic *Escherichia coli* is the most common cause of TD when a pathogen is isolated. In approximately 40%–50% patients with TD, no pathogen is isolated in stool cultures suggesting a possible viral etiology.

○ **What is an approach to patients with persistent (TD) in whom a specific pathogen cannot be identified?**

1. Treatment with an antibiotic directed at common bacterial pathogens.
2. Empiric course of antiprotozoal therapy if the above approach does not alleviate symptoms.
3. Endoscopic evaluation if the above fails.

○ **What is the current recommendation for the treatment of TD?**

For mild to moderate diarrhea (fewer than 4 bowel movements per day without blood or fever), either loperamide or bismuth subsalicylate can be used effectively. For more severe diarrhea, an antimicrobial drug should be used, usually a fluoroquinolone or trimethoprim-sulfamethoxazole. Rifaximin is also approved for the treatment of TD. Antimotility agents should not be used when bloody stools or high fever is present.

○ **What are potential infectious causes of bloody diarrhea in a traveler?**

Campylobacter and *Shigella* are the most common causes of bloody diarrhea in a short-term traveler. Other causes of bloody diarrhea include *Salmonella*, *E. coli* O157:H7, and *Entamoeba histolytica*. Acute amebic bloody diarrhea should be considered particularly in those returning after prolonged travel, especially if off the beaten track. *Clostridium difficile* colitis must also be considered in the differential diagnosis in patients on doxycycline for malaria prophylaxis or taking antibiotics for other reasons.

○ **What is the most likely cause of diarrhea after trekking in Nepal during the rainy season?**

Cyclospora should be considered high in the differential diagnosis.

○ **What infection should be considered in a patient with fever, elevated transaminases, and doughnut-shaped granulomas on liver biopsy who recently returned from travels to a New Zealand farm?**

Coxiella burnetii or Q or "Query" fever is a zoonosis that occurs worldwide. Transmission is primarily by inhalation of small droplets of barnyard dust or ingestion of contaminated dairy products; however, tick bites or human-to-human transmission can occur. Symptomatic acute infections may present with nonspecific generalized febrile illness with or without signs or symptoms of pneumonia and/or hepatitis or other organ involvement. Biopsy of the liver shows pathognomonic doughnut-shaped epithelioid granulomas.

○ **What infection needs to be considered in a traveler with diarrhea, right lower quadrant pain, and mesenteric lymphadenitis?**

Yersinia enterocolitica infection can mimic acute appendicitis. This will resolve spontaneously; however, in severe presentations, antibiotic therapy with trimethoprim/sulfamethoxazole, quinolones, or doxycycline is effective.

○ **What condition predisposes to *Yersinia enterocolitica* septicemia?**

Iron overload states such as in hemochromatosis, cirrhosis, and hemolytic processes.

○ **What vaccines are contraindicated in patients receiving immunosuppressive medications including TNF-alpha antagonists?**

Live-attenuated viral or bacterial vaccines such as Varicella–Zoster vaccine, live-attenuated influenza vaccine (LAIV), yellow fever, measles, mumps, and rubella (MMR), oral typhoid vaccine, or oral polio (not available in the United States).

○ **What vaccines are recommended for the short-term healthy traveler to a developing country?**

Hepatitis A and, in some cases, depending on destination risk, typhoid vaccines would be the most commonly recommended vaccines. Both diseases are food and water transmitted. Routine vaccines should be up to date for the age and underlying medical history of the patient. Japanese encephalitis, hepatitis B, and rabies vaccines would be recommended in addition if traveling for several months in South East Asia, while travel to some countries in Africa and South America may require yellow fever vaccine. Meningococcal vaccine is recommended for travel to certain countries in Africa and to Saudi Arabia during Hajj pilgrimage.

○ **What are the adverse effects from yellow fever vaccination?**

Yellow fever vaccine is a live-attenuated vaccine which can cause a multisystemic organ failure (with 50% mortality) in 1 in 250,000 doses in otherwise healthy adults. The risk is higher in adults over 60 years of age and immunocompromised hosts. Affected individuals develop fever, constitutional symptoms, jaundice, hematemesis, hypotension, and shock. Laboratory findings show transaminitis with aspartate aminotransferase being significantly higher than alanine aminotransferase. Yellow fever vaccine also has a neurotropic adverse effect which is lethal but less frequent.

○ **What protozoal conditions are potential causes of constipation, ileus, or intestinal obstruction in travelers or immigrants from developing countries?**

Amebiasis due to *Entamoeba histolytica* from many developing countries and Chagas disease due to *Trypanosoma cruzii* among those returning or immigrating from Central and South American countries.

○ **What are common clinical presentations of trichinosis?**

Trichinosis is acquired by ingestion of raw or undercooked pork, bear, or walrus meat. Initial symptoms include nonspecific diarrhea and abdominal discomfort. However, in the subsequent 1–2 weeks, fever with peri-orbital edema, shortness of breath (diaphragm involvement), and myalgias may occur. A leukemoid reaction with eosinophilia and normal sedimentation rate are unique to trichinosis.

○ **What are adverse gastrointestinal effects of scuba diving?**

Nitrogen gas expansion, related to Boyle's law, may result in expansion of the gases and stretching of the intestines. Rarely, this can result in bowel overdistention and rupture. Barotrauma may also cause an insufficiency of mesenteric blood flow.

○ **Consumption of unpasteurized milk is associated with what infections?**

Brucella melitensis or *abortus*, *Listeria* species, and *Mycobacterium bovis* (presents just like *Mycobacterium tuberculosis*) can be acquired by the consumption of unpasteurized milk or milk products. Populations at risk particularly for *Listeria monocytogenes* include pregnant women and immunosuppressed persons. Meningitis can be a fatal occurrence with this infection.

○   **What infection is associated with raw or improperly stored seafood or food contaminated with seawater?**

Vibrio parahemolyticus.

○   **What is the significance of isolating *Entamoeba hartmanni*, *Endolimax nana*, or *Iodamoeba butschlii* in stool?**

None. These are nonpathogenic protozoa along with *Entamoeba coli*. The presence of these usually indicates consumption of contaminated food and water. No intervention is needed.

○   **Lack of stomach acid (achlorhydria) increases the vulnerability to what infectious diseases?**

Giardiasis, cholera, salmonellosis, tuberculosis, and enterotoxigenic *E. coli*.

○   **What is the most likely infectious organism if a patient calls to report having seen a worm in his stool months after travel to a developing country?**

Ascaris lumbricoides or round worm is large and the most commonly seen worm passed in stool or occasionally from other orifices. It can also migrate into and cause obstruction of the common bile duct.

○   **What are some noninfectious causes of posttravel fatigue, anorexia, nausea, and elevated liver tests?**

The liver dysfunction may be due to "Gordo-lobo yerba tea," which, like germander and comfrey teas, contains pyrrolizidine alkaloids. Hepatic veno-occlusive disease may follow.

○   **What parasite may cause inflammatory colon polyps?**

Schistosomal infection may result in inflammatory colon polyps that appear grossly similar to hyperplastic and adenomatous lesions. Identifying the worm and/or the ova in tissue biopsy or in stool ova and parasite examination can make a definitive diagnosis. Serology is also available.

○   **What are the differences between the enterotoxins produced by *Vibrio cholera* and *Clostridium perfringens*?**

Clostridial enterotoxin has maximal activity in the ileum and minimal activity in the duodenum, just the opposite of cholera toxin.

○   **What is the most common vehicle for *Clostridium perfringens* gastroenteritis?**

Meat or poultry that is cooked, stored, and then reheated. Heat-resistant spores that survive the cooking process germinate within the food during the cooling period. On reheating, sporulation of the cells occurs with subsequent enterotoxin production.

○   **What is the optimal management of patients with cholera?**

The key components of management are aggressive rehydration along with electrolyte replacement, antibiotic therapy (such as doxycycline, azithromycin, or ciprofloxacin), and management of complications such as hypoglycemia or electrolyte imbalance.

○   **What is the most likely diagnosis of persistent fevers, weight loss, diarrhea, shortness of breath, splenomegaly, and pancytopenia in an immunocompromised individual who went spelunking in Mexico 2 months ago?**

Disseminated histoplasmosis from exposure to bat droppings in the caves. *Histoplasma capsulatum* can be identified in the GI tract of 70%–90% of patients with progressive disseminated histoplasmosis, although only 3%–12% have symptoms.

○ **What are gastrointestinal manifestations of chronic Chagas disease?**

Trypanosoma cruzi infection causes destruction of the autonomic and enteric innervation leading to dysfunction of the digestive system especially the esophagus and colon. Mega-esophagus is more frequently seen than megacolon. Symptoms include dysphagia, chest pain, active and passive regurgitation, heartburn, hiccups, cough, ptyalism (drooling), enlargement of the salivary glands—mainly the parotids—and emaciation. Thirty percent will have cardiac problems as well. The risk of acquiring Chagas disease in the course of usual travel itineraries is low. Chronic Chagas disease can be seen in the United States among immigrants from endemic countries in Central and South America.

○ **Mild elevation of transaminases along with fever and rash presenting within 1 week of return from a 1-week trip to Haiti is most likely caused by what infection?**

Dengue fever, transmitted by the *Aedes* sp. mosquitoes, which is present in more than 100 tropical countries. Infected persons usually have fever, chills, frontal headache, characteristic blanching rash, severe myalgias, and malaise. Laboratory tests often show mild neutropenia, thrombocytopenia, and mild elevations of transaminases. Diagnosis is clinical and based on short incubation period of about 7 days. Repeat infection with another strain of dengue virus can result in dengue shock or dengue hemorrhagic syndrome. Insect precautions are advised for travelers to endemic countries.

○ **What parasites do you need to consider in a Chinese immigrant with eosinophilia, low-grade fever, and right upper quadrant pain?**

Liver flukes such as *Clonorchis sinensis* and *Opisthorchis viverrini* infect and reside in the biliary tract. Fascioliasis, contracted from water vegetation, often produces a right upper quadrant "hot sensation," hepatomegaly, and ascending cholangitis. Raw fish ingestion may lead to clonorchiasis that presents as pancreatitis. Cholangiography may detect the characteristic sacculated and dilated biliary tree of opisthorchiasis or brown leaflike fasciola fluke. Diagnosis is often made by finding typical eggs in stool or duodenal aspirates. Cholangiocarcinoma has been associated with chronic *Clonorchis* infection.

○ **What are some adverse effects of transdermal scopolamine patches commonly used for motion sickness prevention?**

A transdermal scopolamine patch is very effective for the prevention of motion sickness but anticholinergic reactions are occasionally seen. Anticholinergic reactions can result in dry mouth, urinary retention, and/or unilateral or bilateral blurred vision (dilation of the pupil [mydriasis] and paralysis of accommodation [cycloplegia]). Removal of the patch results in the resolution of symptoms within 12 hours.

○ **Profuse diarrhea, fatigue, and weight loss in a Guatemalan immigrant unresponsive to metronidazole would most likely be due to which of the following:**

1. *Helicobacter pylori* **infection?**
2. *Necator americanus* **contracted from walking barefoot in the muddy soil?**
3. *Leptospira canicularis* **associated with the domestic dogs?**
4. *Cryptosporidium parvum* **from drinking the well-water?**
5. *Cyclospora cayetanensis?*

Cyclospora cayetanensis is prevalent in developing countries. Outbreaks in the United States have occurred following importation of Guatemalan raspberries, pesto dishes, and mesclun lettuce. Fecal contamination of water and food is often the source.

○   **What is the drug of choice for the treatment of Cyclosporiasis?**

The drug of choice for cyclosporiasis in adults is trimethoprim-sulfamethoxazole (TMP-SMX; one double-strength 160 mg/800 mg tablet orally twice daily) for 7–10 days. Longer duration may be required for an immunocompromised host. Alternatives include ciprofloxacin or nitazoxanide in sulfa allergic patients.

○   **What is Anisakiasis?**

Anisakiasis is an acute infection caused by *Anisakis simplex* or *Pseudoterranova decipiens* larvae (fish roundworms) imbedded in salmon, cod, tuna, pike, herring, or squid. Risk of infection occurs with consumption of raw, undercooked, pickled, or salted fish. Most infections are with a single larva and, uncommonly, by two or more larvae. The larvae try to attach to the gastric mucosa but eventually die. Very few get beyond the stomach but all eventually die since humans are not the final host.

○   **What are the classical symptoms of Anisakiasis? How is it treated?**

Classical symptoms of anisakiasis are acute onset of excruciating abdominal pain, nausea, and emesis associated with sweating beginning a few hours after eating undercooked fish. Extraction by endoscopic forceps provides immediate relief. No antiparasitic medication is available for treatment. Freezing fish to –35°C for 15 hours or cooking the fish will prevent the infection.

○   **What parasite is most frequently found in stool in the United States?**

Giardia lamblia. It is found in 4%–7% of stools tested in US laboratories. The overall rate of detection is 7.4 cases per 100,000 population with a higher incidence in late summer or early fall.

○   **What are the most common symptoms of Giardiasis?**

Diarrhea with foul-smelling stools, malaise, flatulence, and nausea are the most common symptoms. Diarrhea is usually without fever or blood.

○   **What is the best test to diagnose Giardiasis?**

Giardia stool antigen. Due to intermittent shedding, it is best to obtain at least two stools separated by a few days. The enterocapsule "string test" is seldom utilized in present day, but can identify Giardia in the duodenum with a 96% success rate.

○   **What is the optimal treatment for Giardiasis?**

Tinidazole 2 g as a single dose has been shown to be more effective than metronidazole. Alternative treatments include metronidazole 250 mg orally three times a day for 5–7 days or nitazoxanide 500 mg orally twice a day for 3 days. In 2002, nitazoxanide was the first new drug to be FDA-approved for the treatment of Giardia in 40 years.

○   **Which of the following statements below is correct in relation to a 43-year-old woman who presents with malaise, 10-pound weight loss, low-grade fever, mucoid diarrhea with flatulence and right lower quadrant aching and presence of fecal "green-tinted crystals" and hypochromic microcytic anemia following a recent trip to rural Mexico?**

a. **A colonoscopy would aid in the diagnosis.**

b. **The persistent mucoid discharge suggests a right-sided colonic lesion.**

c. **Ameboma, chronic appendiceal abscess, Crohn's ileitis, and tubercular or yersinea infections are all diagnostic considerations.**

d. **A limited trial of medical therapy, while avoiding alcohol, is justified before surgical intervention.**

All are correct. A constricting cecal ameboma associated with colonic ulcerations was visualized on colonoscopy. These regressed on metronidazole and paromomycin therapy with negative biopsies 2 months later. Pineapple crystals display a greenish tinge with long acicular forms and are often mistaken for Charcot–Leyden and fatty acid crystals. The simple use of a flurochrome, calcoflor compound as a wet mount will enhance the detection of not only amebic cysts but filamentous fungi, microsporidia, and *Pneumocystis carinii.*

○ **A 50-year-old Somali male immigrant, who immigrated 6 years ago, presents with low-grade fever, weight loss, intermittent massive hematemesis, and left upper abdominal pain. Evaluation confirms splenomegaly. He is noted to have mild eosinophilia. What is the most likely diagnosis?**

Schistosomiasis is most likely caused by *Schistosoma mansoni* and secondary complications of hepatic cirrhosis and portal hypertension. Diagnosis can be confirmed by stool ova and parasite evaluation, serology, and/or rectal squish biopsy. Chronic complications are irreversible but treatment with praziquantel may decrease progression.

○ **What is the most common infectious cause of chronic nonbloody diarrhea in the United States?**

Cryptosporidium parvum. The testing for *Cryptosporidium* should be specifically requested; otherwise, it can be missed on routine stool ova and parasite examination. The best method for detection is immunofluorescence microscopy followed closely by enzyme immunoassays.

○ **What is the treatment of choice for Cryptosporidium?**

Most infections will be self-limiting and do not require pharmacological treatment; however, if symptoms persist, then treatment is with nitazoxanide 500 mg orally twice a day for 3 days. Alternatives are paromomycin, azithromycin, or a combination of the two. There is no clearly effective regimen in advanced HIV/AIDS patients. Treatment with highly active antiretroviral therapy (HAART) appears to decrease the risk of infection and symptoms.

○ **Massive hepatosplenomegaly with cachexia, pancytopenia, and reversed albumin:gamma-globulin ratio in a soldier returning home from Afghanistan is suggestive of what infectious disease?**

Visceral leishmaniasis is caused by *Leishmania donovani* and other species. It is transmitted by the bite of the female sandfly, *Phlebotomus* sp. Visceral leishmaniasis is endemic in 88 countries with more than 90% of cases occurring in India, Nepal, Bangladesh, Brazil, and Sudan. Diagnosis is mostly by demonstration of the parasite in macrophages in bone marrow specimen or other tissue biopsies.

○ **What food is usually implicated in the vomiting syndrome caused by *Bacillus cereus*?**

Fried rice.

○ **Improperly canned products may contain what potentially lethal infection?**

Clostridium botulinum. Its spores are resistant to heat and its neurotoxin can block acetylcholine at the neuromuscular junction, resulting in fatal respiratory muscle paralysis.

• • • SUGGESTED READINGS • • •

Practice Guidelines for the Management of Infectious Diarrhea. *Clin Infect Dis.* 2001;32(3):331-351.

Drugs for Parasitic Infections. *Treatment Guidelines from the Medical Letter.* 2007;5(suppl):e1-e15.

Rosenblatt JE. Approach to diarrhea in returned travelers. In: Elaine Jong and Christopher Sanford, eds. *The Travel and Tropical Medicine Manual.* 4th ed. Philadelphia, PA: Saunders-Elsevier, 2003:430-447.

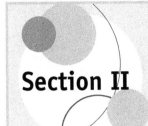

Section II

ESOPHAGUS

CHAPTER 8

Esophageal Congenital and Structural Abnormalities

Ronnie Fass, MD

○ **What type of fistula is the most common embryologic developmental anomaly?**

Tracheoesophageal fistula (85%–90%). In the most common subtype, the upper part of the esophagus ends as a blind sac, while the lower part is connected posteriorly to the trachea.

○ **What is the H-type tracheoesophageal fistula?**

This occurs when the esophagus and the trachea are attached by a short connection, creating an H-type fistula.

○ **What is the most common congenital abnormality associated with esophageal atresia?**

Cardiac abnormality, most commonly patent ductus arteriosus and septal defects.

○ **When considering an operation for congenital tracheoesophageal fistula, what is the most important anatomic information the surgeons need?**

The type of fistula and whether the distance between the upper and lower ends of the esophagus is long (long gap) or closely approximated (short gap).

○ **What is the most common anatomic presentation of esophageal duplication?**

In up to 80% of the cases, it presents as a cyst without luminal connection.

○ **Where in the esophagus are duplication cysts most commonly encountered?**

The most common location is the distal third (60%) followed by the proximal third (23%).

○ **At what age do vascular rings usually become symptomatic?**

Most commonly during infancy and early childhood, although they may present at any age.

○ **What are the most common vascular rings encountered in the pediatric population?**

Double aortic arches and right-sided aortic arch with either patent ductus arteriosus or ligamentum arteriosum.

○   **True/False: Dysphagia lusoria is most commonly associated with an aberrant aortic arch.**

False. Dysphagia lusoria is most commonly associated with an aberrant right subclavian artery. The aberrant artery arises from the left side of the aortic arch and on its course to the right arm compresses the esophagus posteriorly.

○   **How common is an aberrant right subclavian artery in the general population?**

It has been estimated to occur in up to 1% of the population.

○   **True/False: Up to 50% of aberrant right subclavian arteries cause dysphagia.**

False. The vast majority (90%) are asymptomatic.

○   **What are the esophageal A-ring, B-ring, and C-ring?**

These are radiographic terms. The A-ring is usually asymptomatic and involves hypertrophied or hypertonic muscle typically 1.5–2 cm above the squamocolumnar junction. The B-ring is synonymous with Schatzki's ring and involves only mucosa. A C-ring refers to the indentation on the esophagus created by the diaphragmatic crura.

○   **How common is a Schatzki's ring?**

Unknown, because most of Schatzki's rings are asymptomatic. They are found in up to 14% of routine barium esophagrams.

○   **What is the relationship between luminal diameter of Schatzki's ring and dysphagia symptoms?**

Patients with Schatzki's ring and esophageal lumen less than 13 mm will almost always experience dysphagia, between 13 and 20 mm may or may not have dysphagia (about 50%) and greater than 20 mm will rarely have dysphagia.

○   **What "syndrome" has been associated with Schatzki's ring?**

"Steakhouse syndrome," which refers to the occurrence of acute dysphagia due to food impaction.

○   **What pathogenetic mechanisms have been implicated in the formation of Schatzki's ring?**

Pill-induced, gastroesophageal reflux disease, and congenital.

○   **True/False: Endoscopy is the best diagnostic test to detect an esophageal ring.**

False. The barium esophagram is a more sensitive test. The use of a barium tablet or marshmallow may help even further to identify a subtle ring and to estimate its luminal diameter.

○   **How can a muscular ring be differentiated from Schatzki's ring radiographically?**

On barium swallow, the caliber of the muscular ring varies, and the stenosis may disappear with full distension. The Schatzki's ring does not vary in appearance.

○   **What is the usual histology of a Schatzki's ring?**

As the rings are most often located at the gastroesophageal junction, the upper surface usually has squamous epithelium, and the lower surface is covered with columnar cells.

○ **What are typical clinical signs of Schatzki's ring?**

Age greater than 40, intermittent solid dysphagia, and worse when eating is hurried.

○ **What percent of patients with Schatzki's ring remain symptom-free after esophageal dilation at 1-, 2-, and 3-year follow-up?**

68%, 35%, and 11%, respectively. Usually, passage of a large caliber dilator (eg, 16–19 mm) is most helpful.

○ **What endoscopic treatment options may be helpful for Schatzki's rings that have been refractory to esophageal dilatation?**

Four-quadrant biopsies of the ring or four-quadrant incisions of the ring using a needle-knife papillotome.

○ **Where is the most common location of an esophageal web?**

Esophageal webs can appear anywhere in the esophagus but tend to occur most commonly in the proximal part.

○ **What percentage of patients with dysphagia will be found to have an esophageal web?**

5%–15%.

○ **What is the Plummer–Vinson or Paterson–Kelly syndrome?**

Esophageal web that is associated with glossitis, iron-deficiency anemia, and koilonychia.

○ **What types of cancers have been associated with Plummer–Vinson syndrome?**

Pharyngeal and proximal esophageal squamous cell cancers.

○ **True/False: Esophageal webs that are associated with iron deficiency improve with iron supplements.**

False. The esophageal webs do not seem to consistently improve with iron therapy.

○ **What dermatological diseases have been associated with esophageal webs?**

Cicatricial pemphigoid and epidermolysis bullosa. Other associated skin diseases include Stevens–Johnson syndrome and psoriasis.

○ **After allogeneic bone marrow transplantation, what complication has been associated with the development of an esophageal web?**

Graft-versus-host disease.

○ **True/False: Esophageal webs are more common in women.**

True.

○ **What esophageal disorders have been associated with webs?**

Inlet patch, Zenker's diverticulum, and esophageal duplication cyst.

○ **True/False: Zenker's diverticulum is the most common esophageal diverticulum.**

False. Although Zenker's diverticulum is commonly thought of as an esophageal diverticulum, it actually forms in a hypopharyngeal location; in Killian's triangle just proximal to the cricopharyngeus muscle.

○ **What is the estimated prevalence of Zenker's diverticulum in the general population?**

0.01%–0.11%.

○ **At what age does a Zenker's diverticulum commonly present?**

Almost half of the cases will present during the seventh to eighth decade of life.

○ **How commonly does squamous cell carcinoma occur in a Zenker's diverticulum?**

It is seen in approximately 0.4% of patients.

○ **What surgical techniques are used to treat a Zenker's diverticulum?**

Diverticulopexy, diverticulectomy, and cricopharyngeal myotomy.

○ **True/False: Endoscopic approaches have also been described to treat a Zenker's diverticulum.**

True. Endoscopic incision of the septum between the diverticulum and the esophageal lumen is included as a treatment option for the Zenker's diverticulum.

○ **What is the most common cause of midesophageal diverticula?**

Esophageal motor dysfunction resulting in high intraluminal pressure, outpouching, and the formation of pulsion diverticula.

○ **True/False: Most patients with midesophageal diverticula complain of dysphagia.**

False. In most patients, the diverticula are asymptomatic and are incidentally discovered during barium esophagram. In a small percentage of patients, they can cause dysphagia and chest pain.

○ **What is a traction diverticulum?**

Midesophageal diverticula were once considered to arise as a result of traction due to paraesophageal inflammation, most commonly from tuberculosis and fungal diseases.

○ **What is the likely cause of epiphrenic diverticula?**

As with midesophageal diverticula, esophageal motor disorders are believed to be the underlying mechanism for epiphrenic diverticula, which occur just proximal to the lower esophageal sphincter (LES).

○ **What esophageal motility abnormalities have been documented in association with epiphrenic diverticula?**

Achalasia, diffuse esophageal spasm, hypertensive lower esophageal sphincter, and nutcracker esophagus.

○ **What percent of dysphagia cases are due to esophageal diverticula?**

Less than 5%.

○ **What is esophageal intramural pseudodiverticulosis?**

Multiple, small (1–3 mm), flask-shaped outpouching of the esophagus.

○ **What is the pathogenesis of esophageal intramural pseudodiverticulosis?**

Cystic dilations of the esophageal gland ducts.

○ **What infection can be detected in about one half of patients with esophageal intramural pseudodiverticulosis?**

Esophageal candidiasis.

○ **What esophageal lesion is almost always associated with esophageal intramural pseudodiverticulosis?**

Esophageal stricture located in the upper or midesophagus. The pseudodiverticula are often observed distal to the stricture.

○ **What is the incidence of an inlet patch?**

It ranges between 4% and10%.

○ **What type of gastric mucosa can be found in an inlet patch?**

Gastric corpus or fundic mucosa that can include functional parietal and chief cells.

○ **What complications have been described in association with an inlet patch?**

Uncommonly, proximal esophageal stricture, ulcer, and esophageal adenocarcinoma.

○ **What symptom has been suggested to be associated with an inlet patch?**

Globus sensation. Obliteration of the patch may result in symptom resolution.

● ● ● **SUGGESTED READINGS** ● ● ●

Kinottenbelt G, Skinner A, Seefelder C. Tracheo-oesophageal fistula (TOF) and oesophageal atresia (OA). *Best Pract Res Clin Anaesthesiol.* 2010 Sep;24(3):387-401.

Tobin RW. Esophageal rings, webs, and diverticula. *J Clin Gastroenterol.* 1998 Dec;27(4):285-295.

Poyrazoglu OK, Bahcecioglu IH, Dagli AF, Ataseven H, Celebi S, Yalniz M. Heterotopic gastric mucosa (inlet patch): endoscopic prevalence, histopathological, demographical and clinical characteristics. *Int J Clin Pract.* 2009 Feb;63(2):287-291.

Levitt B, Richter JE. Dysphagia lusoria: a comprehensive review. *Dis Esophagus.* 2007;20(6):455-460.

CHAPTER 9

Esophageal Infectious Disorders

Eric B. Goosenberg, MD

○ **Which infectious forms of esophagitis are most common in AIDS patients?**

Candida albicans, *Herpes simplex* virus (HSV), and cytomegalovirus (CMV).

○ **A 47-year-old man with chronic obstructive pulmonary disease (COPD) on inhaled steroids complains of a 3-week history of dysphagia without weight loss or other systems. An endoscopy is performed with the finding demonstrated in the figure. What is the most likely diagnosis?**

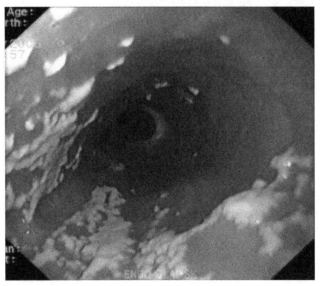

Figure 9-1 See also color plate.

Candida esophagitis.

○ **What are the most common risk factors for *Candida albicans* esophagitis?**

Immunosuppression, most commonly due to corticosteroid use (particularly when inhaled), AIDS or cancer chemotherapy, or suppression of normal oropharyngeal flora by antibiotic use.

○ **Which AIDS patients are at greatest risk of contracting *Candida* esophagitis?**

Those with a CD4 cell count less than 100/mm³, those not taking antiretroviral therapy (ART, formerly referred to as HAART for highly active antiretroviral therapy), and those who have failed to restore immunocompetence while receiving treatment for HIV.

○ **True/False: The most common cause of odynophagia in an AIDS patient is *Candida* esophagitis.**

False. This symptom, particularly in the absence of dysphagia and oral thrush, is more often due to ulcerative esophagitis, such as that occurs in *Herpes simplex* or CMV infection, idiopathic ulcers of advanced HIV infection, pill-induced esophagitis, or severe reflux esophagitis.

○ **What underlying medical conditions increase the risk of developing *Candida* esophagitis?**

Gastric hypochlorhydria, diabetes mellitus, adrenal dysfunction, alcoholism, and conditions associated with impaired esophageal peristalsis/transit such as achalasia, benign strictures, esophageal cancer, and scleroderma.

○ **True/False: Failure of an AIDS patient with dysphagia to respond to a course of fluconazole is strongly suggestive of a resistant strain of *Candida*.**

False. It is more likely that the patient has some other form of esophagitis.

○ **True/False: Infectious esophagitis in patients having undergone bone marrow or solid organ transplant is most commonly due to Candidiasis.**

False. HSV and CMV are the most common pathogens in this setting, as well as during acute rejection after transplantation.

○ **How should an immunocompetent patient who recently received a course of antibiotic therapy and now has *Candida* esophagitis be treated?**

A nonabsorbable oral agent such as nystatin is usually adequate and less expensive than systemic alternatives.

○ **How should an AIDS patient with *Candida* esophagitis be treated?**

A systemically absorbable antifungal agent such as fluconazole should be given as a loading dose of 400 mg once, followed by 200–400 mg daily (orally or intravenously) for a total of 14 to 21 days. Voriconazole or posaconazole could be used alternatively but are usually reserved for cases refractory to fluconazole. Caspofungin (and related echinocandins, micafungin, and anidulafungin) are given intravenously but are also usually reserved for fluconazole failures in patients requiring hospitalization because of severe dysphagia. Amphotericin B is effective but can only be given intravenously and has the greatest toxicity. As a consequence, it is infrequently used for *Candida* esophagitis.

○ **True/False: It is reasonable to empirically treat an HIV-infected patient with dysphagia but without oropharyngeal Candidiasis with fluconazole.**

True. Even in the absence of oral thrush, *Candida* esophagitis is the most common cause of dysphagia in HIV.

○ **How should a cancer patient with granulocytopenia and clear evidence of *Candida* esophagitis be treated?**

Intravenous amphotericin B can prevent and treat disseminated infection and it is also effective for systemic aspergillosis. Flucytosine may need to be added to amphotericin in life-threatening disease. Parenteral fluconazole is adequate for the treatment of Candidiasis but does not cover aspergillosis.

○ A 37-year-old woman, 4 months out from an allogeneic stem cell transplant, presents complaining of a 10-day history of severe odynophagia and 4 kg weight loss. Endoscopy demonstrates a single superficial ulceration near the esophagogastric junction. Biopsies are obtained. What is the most likely diagnosis?

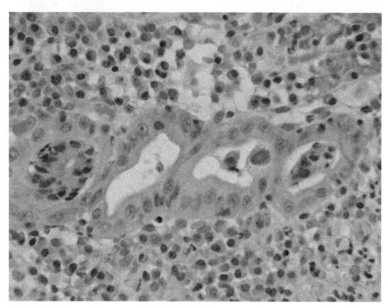

Figure 9-2 See also color plate.

CMV esophagitis. Demonstrated in the figure is a cytomegalic cell characterized by the presence of a large eosinophilic intranuclear inclusion with basophilic intracytoplasmic inclusions (hematoxylin and eosin staining).

○ **True/False: Non-*Candida* fungal infections (eg, *Aspergillus*, *Blastomyces*, *Cryptococcus*, and *Histoplasma*) of the esophagus occur only in severely immunocompromised individuals.**

True.

○ **True/False: Acyclovir is the preferred drug for treatment of *Herpes simplex* esophagitis in both immunocompetent and immunosuppressed patients.**

True. Acyclovir (400 mg po five times a day or 5 mg/kg body weight IV) should be given for 7–10 days for immunocompetent patients and for 2–3 weeks in immunosuppressed patients. The intravenous dosage is used when a patient is unable to tolerate oral medication or if disseminated *Herpes* infection is demonstrated or suspected.

○ **True/False: Biopsies of esophageal ulcers looking for *Herpes simplex* infection should be targeted toward the center of the ulcer, as the heaped-up margins are typically composed of normal epithelial cells.**

False. The opposite is true. *Herpes simplex* preferentially infects the epithelial cells, which are present at the ulcer margins.

○   **True/False: The endoscopic appearance and location of the ulceration seen in the figure would be consistent with CMV esophagitis.**

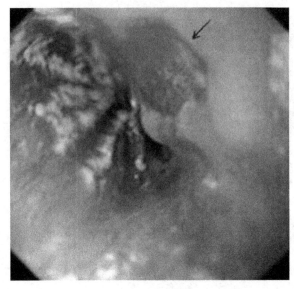

Figure 9-3 See also color plate.

True. CMV esophagitis usually causes one or more large but relatively superficial ulcers at the level of the distal esophagus and may have associated smaller surrounding ulcers. It less often appears as a diffuse esophagitis.

○   **True/False: In the absence of immunosuppression, an individual with nasolabial herpetic lesions and concurrent esophageal symptoms should have endoscopic biopsies and cultures done before a diagnosis of *Herpes* esophagitis is made.**

False. In this situation, a clinical diagnosis of *Herpes* esophagitis is likely enough to justify empiric treatment.

○   **Describe the typical endoscopic appearance and location of *Herpes* esophagitis.**

Herpes esophagitis usually presents as multiple erosions or shallow ulcers, usually in the proximal or mid-portion of the esophagus.

○   **True/False: A patient with known CMV infection who presents with new symptoms of dysphagia and odynophagia should be treated empirically for a diagnosis of CMV esophagitis without further diagnostic evaluation.**

False. Nausea, vomiting, epigastric pain, fever, and weight loss are usually the more prominent symptoms rather than classic symptoms of esophageal infection. Endoscopy should be done to rule out a separate explanation for esophageal symptoms.

○   **True/False: Biopsies and culture specimens of esophageal ulcers, looking for CMV infection, should be targeted toward the center of the ulcer, as the heaped-up edges are typically normal epithelial cells.**

True.

○ **True/False: ART, while of clear benefit in preventing opportunistic infections such as CMV, also substantially reduces mortality when initiated after the onset of CMV esophagitis.**

True. Mortality is reduced by 35%–40%.

○ **What are the main oral and intravenous medications used to treat CMV esophagitis?**

Oral valganciclovir or intravenous foscarnet is used for induction therapy for 3–6 weeks, usually starting with valganciclovir because of lower cost and toxicity, with the duration being based on clinical response and tolerance of the medication. Treatment failures are switched to the other of these agents or a combination of both. Once symptoms have responded, some practitioners will switch to oral valganciclovir combined with ART in HIV-infected patients. Recurrent CMV infection is treated with reinduction then maintenance with oral ganciclovir in conjunction with ART in HIV-infected patients. Cidofovir is only used if a patient has failed therapy with the combination of ganciclovir and foscarnet, or if these medications are not tolerated.

○ **True/False: Patients with reactivation of *Herpes zoster* infection on the chest wall who also have esophageal symptoms should be suspected of having zoster-associated esophagitis.**

True. Zoster-associated esophageal ulcers that endoscopically resemble those of *Herpes simplex* infection have been reported in this setting. These ulcers generally resolve with resolution of the skin eruptions.

○ **What is the most common pathophysiology of esophageal involvement in tuberculosis?**

Esophageal tuberculosis is most often the result of contiguous spread from an infected mediastinal lymph node. Infection reaches the esophagus by way of a fistula or due to lymphatic obstruction. This infection has become more common as a complication of AIDS.

● ● ● SUGGESTED READINGS ● ● ●

Pappas PG, Kauffman CA, Andes D, et al. Clinical practice guidelines for the management of candidiasis: 2009 update by the Infectious Diseases Society of America. *Clin Infect Dis.* 2009;48:503.

Chen LI, Chang JM, Kuo MC, Hwang SJ, Chen HC. Combined herpes viral and candidal esophagitis in a CAPD patient: case report and review of literature. *Am J Med Sci.* 2007 Mar;333(3):191-193.

Amaro R, Poniecka AW, Goldberg RI. Herpes esophagitis. *Gastrointest Endosc.* 2000 Jan;51(1):68.

CHAPTER 10
Esophageal Motility Disorders

Michael D. Crowell, PhD, FACG, AGAF and Brian E. Lacy, PhD, MD

○ **True/False: Dysphagia is the most common upper gastrointestinal symptom in the elderly.**

True. Dysphagia is present in 16% of the elderly population living in the community and swallowing dysfunction is present in as much as 50% of residents living in nursing homes.

○ **What is presbyesophagus?**

This is a benign condition seen in the elderly. There is usually a weakening of primary peristalsis and some contractions may not be transmitted (nonperistaltic). Patients are generally asymptomatic and this is most commonly identified on an upper gastrointestinal series or barium swallow performed for other reasons.

○ **A 46-year-old man develops solid food dysphagia 2 months following laparoscopic Nissen fundoplication. What is the most appropriate initial investigation?**

Barium esophagography with a solid food (barium-soaked bagel or marshmallow) or barium pill (13 mm) challenge is the best initial study. If this study does not show evidence of obstruction, a "slipped" Nissen or an overly tight Nissen, then endoscopy and manometry may be required.

○ **A 48-year-old woman with severe reflux symptoms is being considered for laparoscopic fundoplication. She is found to have facial telangiectasias and Raynaud's phenomenon. What further investigation(s) would be absolutely essential prior to surgery?**

Esophageal manometry. A diagnosis of scleroderma is a contraindication to a 360° fundoplication.

○ **What is the prevalence of esophageal dysmotility in systemic sclerosis (scleroderma)?**

As many as 70% of patients with scleroderma will have involvement of the esophagus.

○   **What two major manometric abnormalities seen in systemic sclerosis are shown in the figure?**

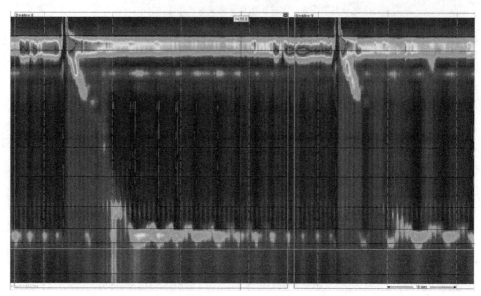

Figure 10-1 See also color plate.

Diminished lower esophageal sphincter (LES) tone (hypotensive LES) and decreased or absent contraction wave amplitude in the smooth muscle portion of the esophagus. Proximal esophageal peristalsis remains normal.

○   **Why do patients with scleroderma develop dysphagia?**

Dysphagia usually occurs as a result of poor bolus transit due to weak peristalsis; however, it can also be due to a stricture resulting from severe reflux that occurs in many of these patients secondary to very low LES resting pressure and poor esophageal acid clearance.

○   **What are two common radiological signs seen in scleroderma patients with esophageal involvement?**

Moderately dilated aperistaltic distal esophagus and free reflux. Peptic strictures may be seen in as much as 30% of patients.

○   **True/False: The distal esophagus is affected in dermatomyositis and polymyositis.**

False. The wall of the proximal one-third of the esophagus is composed of striated muscle, whereas the distal two-thirds consist of smooth muscle. The proximal one-third can be affected by any condition affecting striated muscle function, such as dermatomyositis and polymyositis.

○   **True/False: Diffuse esophageal spasm is the most common abnormality observed during esophageal manometry in patients with noncardiac chest pain.**

False. Esophageal motor disorders are an uncommon cause of noncardiac chest pain, and manometry is usually normal in these patients. Early studies reported that hypertensive peristalsis (nutcracker esophagus) was the most common manometric abnormality found in patients with noncardiac chest pain, but later studies have not demonstrated a clinical correlation between pain events and hypertensive peristalsis. The most common esophageal causes of noncardiac chest pain appear to be gastroesophageal reflux disease (GERD) and visceral hypersensitivity.

○ **What esophageal motility abnormality is commonly seen in gastroesophageal reflux disease?**

Ineffective esophageal motility (IEM) or hypocontracting esophagus is a common esophageal motility abnormality; however, most people with GERD will have a normal esophageal manometry.

○ **What are the manometric diagnostic criteria for IEM?**

Mean distal esophageal peristaltic wave amplitude less than 30 mmHg, or failed peristalsis in which the peristaltic wave does not traverse the entire length of the distal esophagus or simultaneous contractions with amplitudes less than 30 mmHg on at least 30% of wet swallows.

○ **True/False: A decreased frequency of transient lower esophageal sphincter relaxations (tLESR) is the primary pathophysiologic abnormality associated with GERD.**

False. An increase in tLESR frequency is the primary pathogenic mechanism in mild-to-moderate GERD. tLESR can only be detected during prolonged studies using a manometry catheter incorporating a sleeve sensor or during high-resolution esophageal manometry using an eSleeve.

○ **A 76-year-old woman with progressive solid and liquid dysphagia is found to have an absence of lower esophageal relaxation and esophageal peristalsis on manometry and a bird beak deformity of the gastroesophageal junction on barium swallow. Other than achalasia, what condition should be considered in the differential diagnosis?**

Pseudoachalasia. This condition has similar symptoms and manometric findings to achalasia; however, the underlying cause is typically a malignancy. Carcinoma-induced achalasia is responsible for 3% of all cases of achalasia and up to 9% in patients older than 60 years.

○ **What symptoms besides dysphagia and regurgitation occur commonly in patients with achalasia?**

Chest pain and weight loss are reported in as many as 50% of patients.

○ **What is the frequency of pulmonary complications in achalasia?**

As many as 10% of patients with achalasia will present with bronchopulmonary complications including aspiration pneumonia.

○ **What is the most common cancer associated with achalasia (pseudoachalasia)?**

Adenocarcinoma of the gastroesophageal junction accounts for more than 50% of cases of pseudoachalasia.

○ **What infectious disease can mimic achalasia?**

Chagas disease can produce a clinical picture identical to classical achalasia. Usually other tubular organs are also involved in Chagas disease. The presence of antibodies to *Trypanosoma cruzii* is diagnostic. Treatment is identical to the idiopathic form of achalasia.

○ **What is the most effective therapeutic option for achalasia?**

The best outcomes have been reported following Heller myotomy (80%–90% long-term success). Alternative approaches include pneumatic dilation (60%–90% long-term success) and botulinum toxin injection (60%–70% short-term success), both of which often require multiple treatments. The median duration of therapeutic response after botulinum toxin injection is approximately 10 months.

○ **A 50-year-old man has classical achalasia. He is considering either pneumatic dilation or laparoscopic Heller myotomy. He would rather not have surgery and would like to know the risks associated with pneumatic dilation. Describe the risks.**

Esophageal perforation is the main complication associated with pneumatic dilation. It occurs in 2%–5% of cases. There are no absolute risk factors associated with an increased occurrence of perforation.

○ **When is an ambulatory esophageal pH study indicated in a patient with noncardiac chest pain?**

Recent guidelines suggest that an ambulatory esophageal pH study is only indicated in patients who have not responded to a trial of a proton pump inhibitor (PPI). In patients with a low pretest probability of having acid reflux as the cause of their symptoms, pH monitoring should be performed off PPI therapy. In patients with a moderate to high probability of having acid reflux as the cause of their symptoms, those not responding to acid inhibition should undergo pH testing while on acid suppression in order to document the persistence of acid reflux and its association with symptoms.

○ **True/False: Recent studies have reported improved diagnostic yield with combined esophageal pH and impedance monitoring compared with conventional esophageal pH monitoring alone in patients studied while on acid suppression.**

True.

○ **Esophageal propulsion of swallowed food involves coordinated peristaltic activity within the longitudinal and circular muscle layers. What structure must relax in synchrony with the peristaltic wave to allow passage of the food bolus?**

Relaxation of the LES is coordinated with the peristaltic activity in the esophageal body through a vagally mediated reflex pathway.

○ **What are the two key manometric features of achalasia?**

1. Incomplete LES relaxation with swallowing.
2. Aperistalsis of the esophageal body.

○ **What other manometric findings may be present in patients with achalasia?**

- Low amplitude, mirror image simultaneous contractions.
- High amplitude esophageal contractions, which are usually not mirror image (vigorous achalasia).
- Increased tone of the LES (present in about 60% of cases).
- Resting intraesophageal pressure greater than intragastric pressure.

○ **A 73-year-old woman with Parkinson's disease develops liquid dysphagia with frequent coughing and choking. What is the most appropriate initial test?**

A videoesophagram is the best test for the initial investigation of suspected oropharyngeal dysphagia.

○ **Describe typical symptoms of oropharyngeal dysphagia.**

Coughing, choking, gagging, or nasal regurgitation with the ingestion of a liquid swallow.

○ **A 23-year-old man presents with odynophagia of 3-month duration. How would you investigate this?**

Odynophagia typically is associated with mucosal damage. An endoscopy would be the best initial investigation. GERD, esophageal candidiasis, and viral infections (eg, HSV and CMV) are the most common causes of odynophagia in this age group. Pill esophagitis may also present with symptoms of odynophagia, but rarely would it be this long in duration.

○ **A 40-year-old woman complains of a constant feeling of a lump in her throat. What is the likely diagnosis?**

The patient is describing globus sensation. It is differentiated from oropharyngeal dysphagia by being present continuously regardless of whether the patient is swallowing or not. The etiology of this condition is controversial. Gastroesophageal reflux, hypertensive upper esophageal sphincter, incomplete upper esophageal sphincter (UES) relaxation, and anxiety have all been suggested as possible causes. Treatment options include reassurance, education, antisecretory medications, and/or anxiolytics.

○ **Based on conventional esophageal manometry, what are typical manometric features of diffuse esophageal spasm?**

Simultaneous esophageal contractions occurring in more than 30% (controversial) of 5 mL water bolus swallows and repetitive or prolonged (>6 seconds) contractions, which are frequently of high (>180 mmHg) amplitude. The more abnormalities present, the more specific the diagnosis.

○ **A patient with severe GERD is being considered for laparoscopic fundoplication. What is the most important test to be performed to rule out gastrointestinal contraindications to the procedure?**

Esophageal manometry—to confirm good esophageal peristaltic activity and to rule out scleroderma. While controversial, very weak esophageal peristalsis may be a predictor of postoperative dysphagia.

○ **A 59-year-old man is referred for esophageal manometry because of chest pain and solid food dysphagia. He is found to have a high resting LES tone (45 mmHg) but 90% relaxation of the LES with deglutition and normal peristaltic activity in the body of the esophagus. What is the diagnosis?**

Hypertensive LES. The clinical significance of this finding is unclear.

○ **In patients with a hypertensive LES, what is often seen on barium swallow?**

A lower esophageal muscular ring at the level of the cephalad part of the LES. This is also referred to as a Schatzki's A ring.

○ **How are a hypertensive LES and its accompanying muscular ring treated?**

Esophageal dilatation with a large (17–20 mm) bougie is temporarily effective. Alternatively, botulinum toxin injection has been reported to be effective in some patients.

○ **A 50-year-old man is referred from cardiology for the evaluation of noncardiac chest pain. He only gets chest pain when swallowing crusty bread and baked potatoes. He has no associated dysphagia and has had a normal barium esophagram recently. A representative figure from his esophageal manometry is shown. All 10 water swallows are peristaltic but the mean amplitude of contraction in the distal esophagus is 287 mmHg. What is the diagnosis?**

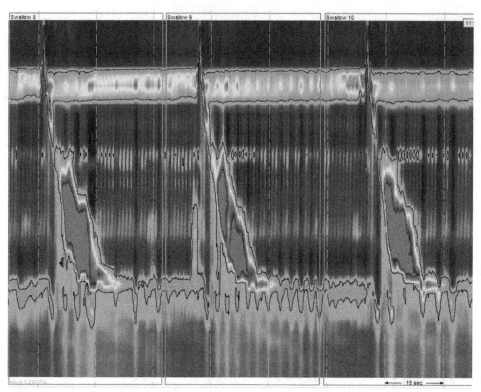

Figure 10-2 See also color plate.

Nutcracker esophagus. Nutcracker esophagus is a finding of unclear clinical relevance that is characterized by hypertensive (>180 mmHg) esophageal contractions with normal peristalsis and LES function. Peristaltic contractions of long duration (>6 seconds) are commonly found although they are not required for the diagnosis. This is a benign condition and of unlikely pathogenic importance in noncardiac chest pain.

○ **An elderly smoker develops progressive solid food dysphagia over a month and a 10-pound weight loss. What is your initial investigation?**

Endoscopy. Progressive solid dysphagia in an older patient raises concern for an obstructive neoplasm. Alternatively, a barium esophagram could be done but would not provide the opportunity for tissue biopsy and dilatation.

○ **A 35-year-old woman complains of severe heartburn that has not responded to multiple trials of twice-daily PPI therapy. Two separate endoscopies have been normal. What diagnostic test would be most useful at this point?**

Ambulatory esophageal pH testing (with or without impedance testing). In this situation, 48-hour wireless ambulatory pH monitoring or 24-hour pH monitoring off PPI therapy will determine whether she has significant acid reflux. If the pretest probability of having abnormal acid reflux is high, then ambulatory 48-hour esophageal pH monitoring or 24-hour monitoring with or without esophageal impedance while continuing to take the PPI would be the best test in order to determine whether her symptoms are associated with acid reflux and if the drug has successfully suppressed acid secretion. The addition of esophageal impedance to the 24-hour pH-metry may help to assess symptom association with weakly acidic or nonacidic reflux events while on PPI therapy.

○ **An 83-year-old man is referred because of regurgitation of undigested food, recurrent aspiration pneumonia, and chronic halitosis. He admits to frequent choking while eating, to a sense of difficulty initiating swallows and to food getting stuck in his throat. A barium swallow shows a large pharyngoesophageal diverticulum. What is the diagnosis?**

Zenker's diverticulum.

○ **How is Zenker's diverticulum formed?**

Zenker's diverticula are pulsion diverticula formed in the hypopharyngeal region (above the cricopharyngeus muscle) by high intraswallowing pressures resulting from a poorly compliant upper esophageal sphincter.

○ **What is the effect of a hiatus hernia on LES tone?**

None. LES tone is related to the myogenic and neurogenic properties of the sphincter, not its location relative to the diaphragmatic hiatus. However, competence of the antireflux barrier at the LES is, in part, maintained by contraction of the diaphragm.

○ **What location of a cerebrovascular accident most commonly results in swallowing difficulties?**

Brainstem. Dysphagia is much less common with cortical strokes. Fortunately, most dysphagia improves following a cerebrovascular accident.

○ **What is the mechanism of dysphagia in amyotrophic lateral sclerosis (ALS)?**

ALS is characterized by motor neuron degeneration. Dysphagia is common in the later phases of the disease. The tongue is first involved followed by the pharynx and the larynx. Aspiration is common. Patients usually eventually require placement of a gastrostomy tube to maintain nutrition.

○ **What is the main manometric abnormality seen in Parkinson's patients with dysphagia?**

Diminished pharyngeal propulsive forces are almost always present. Incomplete upper esophageal relaxation is seen in 21% of dysphagic Parkinson's patients.

○ **A 47-year-old man with ptosis develops progressive dysphagia and aspiration. What is the most likely diagnosis?**

Oculopharyngeal muscular dystrophy, a syndrome characterized by progressive dysphagia and palpebral ptosis. This type of muscular dystrophy is linked to chromosome 14 abnormalities and is more common, but not limited to, patients of French–Canadian lineage. Failure of pharyngeal motility leads to aspiration. Myasthenia gravis may also cause similar symptoms.

○ **What is the clinical utility of esophageal manometry?**

The clinical usefulness of a test is commonly referred to as its utility. This is determined by asking how frequently the test makes a new diagnosis, changes the diagnosis, or changes patient management. Esophageal manometry has been shown to be clinically useful for patients with dysphagia and chest pain. It does not have much value in the routine gastroesophageal reflux patient other than to help accurately place a wireless pH capsule or a pH probe.

O   **What are the Chicago criteria for esophageal motor disorders?**

The Chicago criteria are a list of standards and definitions used to define manometric findings using high-resolution esophageal manometry (HREM).

O   **What is a key difference between the performance of conventional esophageal manometry and HREM?**

A conventional (solid state or water perfused) esophageal manometry catheter typically has between four and eight recording transducers that are spaced 3–5 cm apart (depending on how it is built). The distal transducer is circumferential, meaning that it measures a 360° view. The other transducers are radial in nature, and measure a smaller view (less than 360°). Using a station pull-through technique, the combination of radial transducers and the circumferential transducer can provide an accurate assessment of LES length, LES resting pressure, LES relaxation with water swallows, and motility (waveform and amplitude) in the body of the esophagus. However, the catheter has to be positioned several times in order to extract all of this information. The HREM catheter has 36 circumferential transducers spaced 1 cm apart. Once passed transnasally, accurate measurements of the LES, UES, and esophageal body can be easily obtained without having to move the catheter.

O   **Based on HREM, three subtypes of achalasia have been proposed. Representative tracings are presented below. Name the three subtypes of achalasia and their primary characteristics?**

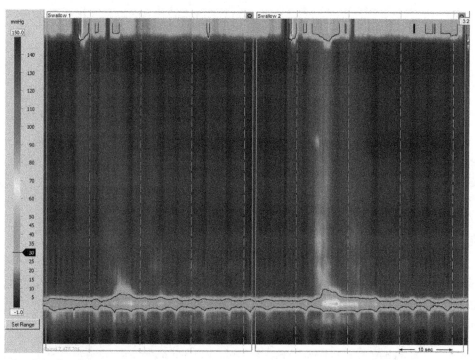

Figure 10-3 See also color plate.

Type I (classic) achalasia is defined by no distal esophageal pressurization >30 mmHg in 8 or more of the 10 test swallows.

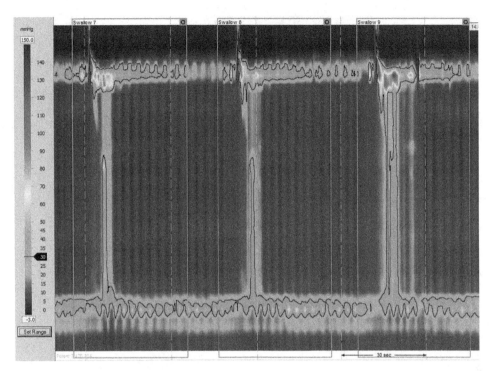

Figure 10-4 See also color plate.

Type II (esophageal pressurization) achalasia is defined by rapidly propagated compartmentalized pressurization that is localized to distal esophagus or includes the entire length of the esophagus with at least 2 of the 10 test swallows associated with panesophageal pressurization to >30 mmHg.

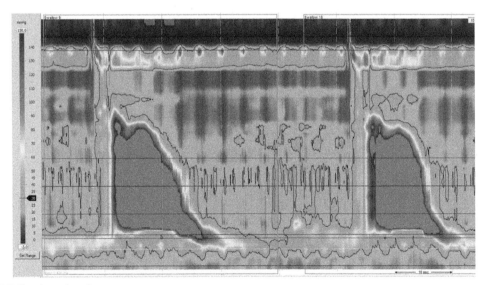

Figure 10-5 See also color plate.

Type III (spastic) achalasia is defined by rapidly propagated or simultaneous pressurization attributable to spastic contractions in at least 2 of the 10 test swallows.

● ● ● SUGGESTED READINGS ● ● ●

Pandolfino JE, Fox MR, Bredenoord AJ, Kahrilas PJ. High-resolution manometry in clinical practice: utilizing pressure topography to classify oesophageal motility abnormalities. *Neurogastroenterol Motil.* 2009;21(8):796-806.

Hirano I, Richter JE; Practice Parameters Committee of the American College of Gastroenterology. ACG practice guidelines: esophageal reflux testing. *Am J Gastroenterol.* 2007;102(3):668-685.

Pandolfino JE, Kwiatek MA, Nealis T, et al. Achalasia: a new clinically relevant classification by high-resolution manometry. *Gastroenterology.* 2008;135(5):1526-1533.

Kahrilas PJ, Sifrim D. High-resolution manometry and impedance-pH/manometry: valuable tools in clinical and investigational esophagology. *Gastroenterology.* 2008 Sep;135(3):756-769. Epub 2008 Jul 17. Review.

Kahrilas PJ, Shaheen NJ, Vaezi MF, et al. American Gastroenterological Association. AGA Medical Position Statement on the management of gastroesophageal reflux disease. *Gastroenterology.* 2008;135(4):1383-1391.

CHAPTER 11

Esophageal Miscellaneous Inflammatory Diseases

John K. DiBaise, MD

○ A 17-year-old woman with acne but otherwise healthy presents with persistent severe odynophagia. Endoscopy demonstrates the following finding in the mid esophagus. What is the most likely diagnosis.

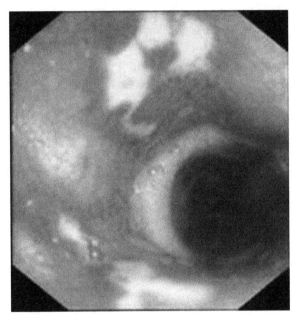

Figure 11-1 See also color plate.

Pill esophagitis. This patient recently began taking tetracycline for her acne.

○ **How common is pill-induced esophageal injury?**

The prevalence is very difficult to determine; however, the incidence is believed to be 3.9 per 100,000 populations per year based on one prospective Swedish study.

○ **Which patients are more likely to develop drug-induced esophageal injury?**

Most reports reveal predominance in elderly and female patients. The elderly are more prone due to a higher prevalence of esophageal motility disorders and obstructing lesions of the esophagus. In addition, the elderly ingest more drugs in general, produce less saliva, are more likely to forget proper dosing instruction, and spend more time in the recumbent position. Drug-induced injury is about twice as common in females due to greater use of potassium supplements and bisphosphonates.

○ **What are the major pathogenic factors contributing to drug-induced esophageal damage?**

The chemical content, formulation of the drug, and the manner in which the drug was taken by the patient are the major factors. Most patients with drug-induced esophageal injury have no detectable esophageal dysmotility or structural abnormality.

○ **What are the common locations in the esophagus for drug-induced esophageal injury?**

The level of the aortic-arch (more prevalent in older patients) and the distal esophagus.

○ **What are the most common clinical manifestations of drug-induced esophageal injury?**

Retrosternal chest pain is the most common manifestation (61%–72%) followed by odynophagia (50%–74%) and dysphagia (20%–40%). Symptoms can develop within hours to days after starting the medication. In almost all cases, the diagnosis can be determined on the basis of the history.

○ **What medications are commonly implicated in drug-induced esophageal injury?**

The most common is tetracycline or one of its derivatives. Other medications include nonsteroidal anti-inflammatory drugs, potassium chloride, iron sulfate, quinidine, corticosteroids, pancreatic enzymes, cloxacillin, dicloxacillin, oral contraceptives, and bisphosphonates.

○ **What is the best diagnostic modality in drug-induced esophageal injury?**

Although not necessary in every patient, endoscopy is the best diagnostic modality with considerable superiority in sensitivity over a barium contrast esophagogram.

○ **True/False: In chemotherapy-related esophagitis, esophageal involvement correlates with involvement of oropharyngeal mucosa (ie, presence of mucositis).**

True. It is very unusual to have esophageal damage in the absence of oral changes.

○ **True/False: The esophagus is the most common segment of the upper gut involved in acute graft versus host disease (GVHD).**

False. Acute GVHD of the upper gastrointestinal tract is most often characterized by anorexia, abdominal discomfort, nausea, and vomiting.

○ **A 35-year-old man with acute lymphocytic leukemia underwent bone marrow transplantation 120 days ago and now presents with dysphagia and retrosternal pain. Barium swallow reveals a mid-esophageal stricture. What is the most likely etiology?**

Chronic graft versus host disease (GVHD) is the most likely etiology and is manifested by webs, rings, and strictures of the upper and mid-esophagus. Esophageal dysmotility also appears to be common. Indeed, the clinical presentation resembles that of progressive systemic sclerosis. Dysphagia may also be precipitated by decreased oral saliva production. Immunosuppressive drugs are commonly employed in this situation and endoscopy with dilatation in selected cases may be helpful.

○ **True/False: The finding of esophageal parakeratosis should prompt a careful examination of the esophagus and head and neck for squamous cell cancer.**

True, although the clinical significance of the reported association between esophageal parakeratosis and esophageal and head and neck cancers remains unclear. Esophageal parakeratosis appears on endoscopy as whitish, membranous linear plaques that do not turn brown when sprayed with Lugol's solution. Biopsies reveal epithelial acanthosis, basal hyperplasia, and a dense compact layer of parakeratosis, often featuring cytoplasmic eosinophilia and pyknotic nuclei, covered by an outer layer of nonnucleated squamous cells.

○ **What condition is being demonstrated in the endoscopic image?**

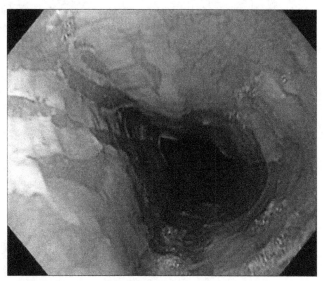

Figure 11-2 See also color plate.

Esophagitis dissecans superficialis. This is a rare condition characterized by sloughing of the esophageal mucosa, in severe cases appearing as tubular cast within or tethered to the esophagus. It has been seen in association with desquamating skin diseases such as pemphigus vulgaris.

○ **What is "black esophagus"?**

Acute esophageal necrosis is also referred to as black esophagus or necrotizing esophagitis. Patients typically present with upper gastrointestinal bleeding and usually have an underlying predisposing condition, most commonly, hypotension or gastric outlet obstruction. Its occurrence is in the absence of caustic or other injurious topical agents.

○ **True/False: The mortality rate in "black esophagus" approaches 90%.**

False. Most patients recover; however, mortality due to the underlying cause ranges from 25% to 30%.

○ A 37-year-old otherwise healthy man presents to the emergency department with a persistent esophageal food bolus impaction. Following endoscopic removal, the following endoscopic images are obtained and biopsies are taken. What is the diagnosis?

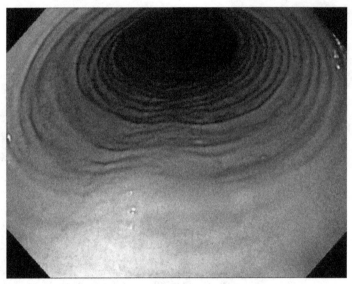

Figure 11-3 See also color plate.

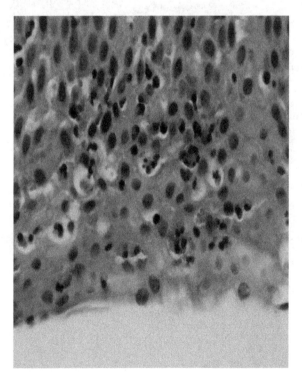

Figure 11-4 See also color plate.

Eosinophilic esophagitis. The diagnosis is based on symptoms, endoscopic appearance, and histological findings. Eosinophilic esophagitis should be considered in adults with a history of food impaction, chronic solid dysphagia, or with gastroesophageal reflux disease that fails to respond to medical therapy. In children, symptoms vary by age and include feeding disorders, vomiting, abdominal pain, dysphagia, and food impaction.

○ **True/False: Eosinophilic esophagitis (EoE) is more common in middle-aged women.**

False. It appears to be most common in young men. The pathogenesis of EoE is incompletely understood but includes both environmental and genetic factors. In particular, adaptive T-cell immunity driven by Th2 cells involving IL-13, IL-5, and IL-15 expression appears to play a major role.

○ **True/False: There is a strong association of EoE with allergic conditions such as food allergies, environmental allergies, asthma, and atopic dermatitis.**

True.

○ **Describe some endoscopic findings in EoE.**

Stacked circular rings ("feline" esophagus), linear furrowing that may extend the entire length of the esophagus, whitish papules representing eosinophil microabscesses, and a small caliber, poorly compliant esophagus. Importantly, the sensitivity and specificity of these findings is not good and often the endoscopic appearance is normal, reinforcing the need to biopsy when this condition is suspected.

○ **True/False: Biopsies of the distal esophagus are important in the diagnosis of EoE.**

False. Increased numbers of eosinophils in the distal esophagus may be due to gastroesophageal reflux. Biopsies for EoE should be taken from the mid- and proximal esophagus. A threshold of 15 eosinophils per high-power field is generally required for the diagnosis.

○ **True/False: Peripheral eosinophilia is present in about 10% of patients with EoE.**

False. Peripheral eosinophilia, usually mild, is seen in up to 40%–50%.

○ **Which one of the following has not been recommended for the treatment of EoE: swallowed fluticasone, inhaled fluticasone, swallowed viscous budesonide, elimination diet, proton pump inhibitor, and esophageal dilation?**

Inhaled fluticasone.

○ **True/False: Esophageal dilation in EoE is associated with a higher risk of mucosal tears and esophageal perforation.**

True. Indeed, endoscopy without dilation also appears to be at higher risk of tears and perforation.

○ **True/False: Esophageal lichen planus (ELP) is more common in middle-aged women.**

True. ELP is a rare manifestation of lichen planus, which is a common disease typically involving the scalp, nails, skin, and mucosa. Most patients with ELP will complain of dysphagia and will also have oral involvement. A recent review found that 87% of cases in the literature were women with a mean age of 62 years.

○ **True/False: Endoscopy with esophageal brushing/cytology is the diagnostic test of choice in suspected ELP.**

False. Mucosal biopsy at the time of endoscopy is needed. Endoscopy should be performed in all persons with mucocutaneous lichen planus who complain of esophageal symptoms and/or weight loss.

○ **True/False: Endoscopic findings in ELP are most commonly confined to the distal esophagus.**

False. The proximal and mid-esophagus are most commonly affected. The sparing of the distal esophageal may be a clue to the presence of ELP. Classical endoscopic findings include peeling tissue paper-like pseudomembranes. Friability of the mucosa is also common. Lacy white plaques, ulcerations, webs, and strictures have also been described.

○ **True/False: ELP is associated with an increased risk of esophageal adenocarcinoma.**

False. Malignant transformation of ELP to squamous cell cancer has been reported; however, its status as a premalignant condition remains unclear.

○ **What treatments are useful in the management of ELP?**

Systemic treatments are generally required and are usually effective. Systemic corticosteroids given over 4 to 6 weeks seem to be most effective. Cyclosporine, azathioprine, systemic retinoids, and biologic immunomodulators have also demonstrated benefit. Esophageal dilation(s) may also be needed, particularly once strictures have formed. Maintenance therapy with one of these agents in conjunction with an antisecretory agent has been recommended.

● ● ● SUGGESTED READINGS ● ● ●

Liacouras CA, Furuta GT, Hirano I, et al. Eosinophilic esophagitis: updated consensus recommendations for children and adults. *J Allergy Clin Immunol.* 2011;128(1):3-20.

Fox LP, Lightdale CJ, Grossman ME. Lichen planus of the esophagus: what dermatologists need to know. *J Am Acad Dermatol.* 2011;65:175-183.

Carpenter PA. Late effects of chronic graft-versus-host disease. *Best Pract Res Clin Haematol.* 2008;21(2):309-331.

Kikendall JW. Pill esophagitis. *J Clin Gastroenterol.* 1999;28(4):298-305.

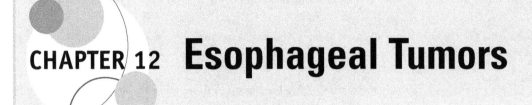

CHAPTER 12 Esophageal Tumors

Eric B. Goosenberg, MD

○ **True/False: Esophageal papillomas have been associated with squamous cell cancer and should be removed endoscopically when identified.**

True.

○ **True/False: Esophageal inlet patches are biologically similar to Barrett's esophagus and should be managed (eg, undergo routine endoscopic surveillance) similarly.**

False.

○ **What are risk factors for squamous cell carcinoma of the esophagus?**

Excessive alcohol use, smoking (of cigarettes more so than cigars or pipes) or chewing tobacco, ingestion of nitrosamines (from grilled meats, etc), pre-existing head and neck cancer, radiation exposure from prior cancer treatment, history of lye-induced esophageal strictures, long-standing achalasia, Plummer–Vinson syndrome, and tylosis. Tobacco and alcohol increase the risk in a dose-dependent manner and use of both is associated with a much higher incidence than with either substance alone. For unknown reasons, neither smoking nor alcohol is associated with esophageal cancer outside the United States. Family history only seems to be significant in regions of higher incidence of esophageal cancer.

○ **What are the most significant risk factors for adenocarcinoma of the esophagus?**

Barrett's esophagus is the strongest risk factor. Severe gastroesophageal reflux disease (independent of the presence of Barrett's), smoking, obesity (especially central obesity), older age, male sex, and low dietary intake of fruits and vegetables are other risk factors in the United States. Alcohol ingestion does not appear to be a risk factor, and wine ingestion may be protective.

○ **What demographic features are associated with squamous cell esophageal cancer in Americans?**

Males are more often affected than are females (ratio 3:1), African-Americans more often than Caucasians (ratio 4:1) and individuals of lower socioeconomic status have a greater incidence.

○ **True/False: The incidence and mortality related to esophageal cancer are highest in portions of China, Iran, and Africa.**

True. Environmental risk factors such as ingestion of foods and drinks (particularly tea) of higher temperatures are assumed but not proven to be responsible.

○ **True/False: People with tylosis have approximately a 50% likelihood of developing esophageal cancer during their lifetime.**

False. This rare condition presents with hyperkeratosis of the skin on the palms and soles and papillomas of the esophagus that progress to squamous cell cancer in virtually 100% of cases.

○ **How does achalasia influence the age of onset of esophageal cancer?**

It occurs 10 to 20 years earlier (mean age 52 years) than in patients without achalasia. The esophageal malignancy is squamous cell carcinoma in over 90% of achalasia patients and typically occurs about 20 years after the diagnosis of achalasia is made. The risk of squamous cell carcinoma in achalasia is about 10- to 30-fold greater than in the general population.

○ **When squamous cell esophageal cancer is diagnosed after the development of related symptoms, what can be predicted about its stage?**

Distant metastases will be present in 25%–30% of cases, lymph nodes will be affected in up to two-thirds of cases and it will be limited to the mucosa in only 2% of cases.

○ **What are the most common causes of hematemesis in patients with known esophageal cancer?**

Tumor ulceration and aorto-esophageal fistulization.

○ **True/False: The incidence of squamous cell carcinoma of the esophagus has fallen dramatically over the past several decades, such that squamous cell carcinoma and adenocarcinoma are now equally common in the United States.**

False. While it is true that these two cancers of the esophagus are now of roughly equal frequency in the United States, the incidence of squamous cell carcinoma has remained steady, but adenocarcinoma has increased markedly.

○ **What endoscopic tests can be done to distinguish benign from malignant esophageal masses?**

Endoscopic biopsies and brush cytology are the most commonly used techniques for confirmation of cancer. Endoscopic ultrasound (EUS) with or without fine needle aspiration is particularly useful. Endoscopically applied vital stains such as Lugol's solution may be helpful (with only normal tissue taking up stain) and concurrent magnification endoscopy may allow detection of features suggestive of metaplasia or dysplasia in Barrett's mucosa. Newer techniques such as optical coherence tomography (OCT) and spectroscopy have shown promise but are not widely available in clinical practice.

○ **True/False: When Barrett's esophagus without dysplasia is initially diagnosed and surveillance is planned, endoscopy should initially be repeated in 3 years.**

False. Endoscopy should be repeated in 1 year to confirm the absence of dysplasia. If this is confirmed, then the current recommendation is that endoscopy should be repeated at 3-year intervals.

○ **What tests should be done in the initial diagnosis and staging of esophageal cancer?**

Initial diagnosis should be made by endoscopy with biopsies (six are recommended). Cytologic brushings may be helpful in stenotic tumors where biopsies may be difficult to obtain. A barium swallow may be helpful in demonstrating high-grade luminal obstruction and in identifying esophagotracheal fistulae. A CT scan of the chest and upper abdomen should be done to look for distant metastatic disease or for contiguous involvement of adjacent structures. If distant disease is not detected, then positron emission tomography (PET) scanning is often utilized if available. PET scanning or combination "PET-CT" scans will identify distant metastatic disease in up to 20% of patients who otherwise might have unwarranted surgery based on the absence of metastases on CT scanning alone. If metastatic disease is not found with CT or PET scanning, then EUS is employed for local staging and, if necessary, for deeper biopsies of the primary tumor or of suspicious paraesophageal or celiac lymph nodes.

○ **True/False: If EUS demonstrates a very early tumor that is small (<2 cm), polypoid, elevated, and appears to be a T1a tumor (confined to the mucosa), then endoscopic mucosal resection (EMR) can be performed.**

True. EMR in this scenario may be curative in removing the tumor in its entirety, or may allow determination that the muscularis mucosae are involved, necessitating more aggressive treatment.

○ **What are the roles of EUS in esophageal cancer?**

Radial endosonography can determine the depth of esophageal wall invasion of cancer (T stage in the TNM system), the presence or absence of malignant paraesophageal lymph nodes (N stage) and to evaluate for celiac adenopathy (part of the M stage). Linear array instruments can be used to perform fine needle aspirates of submucosal lesions and of accessible lymph nodes. Endoscopic catheter probes are also available and may be used instead of or in addition to conventional EUS, particularly in the staging of stenotic tumors. The role of EUS to evaluate for evidence of malignancy in Barrett's esophagus is controversial. It does not seem to be an effective technique in evaluating the esophagus after radiation therapy because fibrosis can be difficult to distinguish from recurrent or residual cancer.

○ **What are the histologic equivalents of the five esophageal layers found by endoscopic ultrasonography?**

Layer 1 (white, hyperechoic)	superficial mucosa
Layer 2 (dark, hypoechoic)	deep mucosa
Layer 3 (white, hyperechoic)	submucosa
Layer 4 (dark, hypoechoic)	muscularis propria
Layer 5 (white, hyperechoic)	adventitia and paraesophageal fat

○ **What is the likely ultrasound T stage of the stenotic esophageal cancer shown in the figure?**

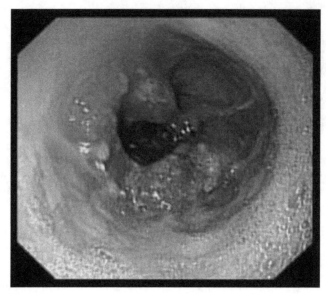

Figure 12-1 See also color plate.

Stenotic tumors are usually locally advanced—either T3 (invading the adventitia and paraesophageal fat) or T4 (invading adjacent organs).

○ **What is the EUS appearance (echogenicity, layer, or layers) of esophageal varices?**

Anechoic lesion of the submucosa (third ultrasonic layer).

○ **What is the EUS appearance (echogenicity, layer, or layers) of an esophageal lipoma?**

Hyperechoic lesion of the submucosa (third layer).

○ **What is the EUS appearance (echogenicity, layer, or layers) of an esophageal leiomyoma or leiomyosarcoma?**

Hypoechoic lesion of the muscularis propria (fourth layer).

○ **What is the EUS appearance (echogenicity, layer, or layers) of an esophageal gastrointestinal stromal tumor (GIST)?**

Fewer than 1% of GIST tumors occur in the esophagus (up to 60% occur in the stomach and 25%–30% are in the jejunum or ileum), but their EUS appearance is the same as that of a smooth muscle tumor, that is, an hypoechoic lesion of the muscularis propria (fourth layer).

○ **True/False: Smooth muscle tumors of the esophagus that cause dysphagia and bleeding are virtually always malignant (leiomyosarcomas).**

False. These symptoms, as well as chest pain, are indicators of a large tumor, but not necessarily of malignancy.

○ **How do squamous cell carcinomas and adenocarcinomas of the esophagus differ in terms of their natural history?**

Squamous cell carcinoma is more likely to be widespread at the time of diagnosis. Adenocarcinoma tends to progress by local extension. Accordingly, surgery has a more limited role in squamous cell carcinoma.

○ **Which form of endoscopic palliation would be most useful in the management of a tight stricture due to a leiomyosarcoma of the mid-esophagus?**

Stent placement is the only treatment mode that is useful in extrinsic stenoses due to submucosal or extrinsic tumors (such as lung cancer). Dilatation is usually ineffective, typically providing only transient relief of symptoms. Thermal devices have no role.

○ **Which form of endoscopic palliation would be most useful in the management of an esophageal carcinoma causing severe dysphagia before initiation of neoadjuvant chemotherapy and radiation?**

Dilatation with either Savary or hydrostatic balloon dilators often provides effective palliation before and during therapy. If there is a significant volume of exophytic tumor causing luminal stenosis, then a potentially removable self-expandable metal or plastic stent, or photodynamic therapy (PDT) are options. Fully covered metal stents can be removed, although they have a tendency to migrate. PDT has generally superceded endoscopic laser therapy because the former is easier to perform and is better tolerated.

○ **True/False: The palliative method shown in the figure represents the preferred management of tracheo-esophageal fistulae in esophageal cancer.**

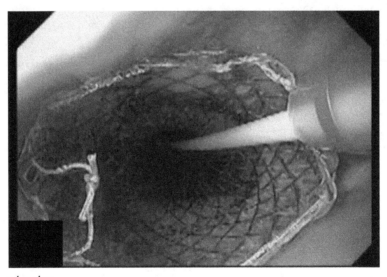

Figure 12-2 See also color plate.

True. Covered self-expanding metal stents are probably the best intervention in this setting. Low doses of radiation may also be effective, although larger doses may result in enlargement of a fistula.

○ **What are the most common complications of radiation therapy to the esophagus?**

Esophagitis (early) and esophageal strictures (late).

○ **What potentially curative endoscopic treatment options are available for early-stage esophageal cancer?**

EMR and PDT.

○ **How should nutritional support be provided to a patient with a resectable esophageal cancer during neoadjuvant therapy?**

In patients who cannot eat, a feeding jejunostomy tube is preferable to a gastrostomy tube because it will not affect the segment of the gut that needs to be mobilized (eg, gastric pull-up) after esophagectomy.

○ **True/False: Columnar epithelium with specialized intestinal metaplasia in the esophagus is associated with an increased risk of adenocarcinoma.**

True. This type of metaplastic mucosa is characterized histologically by the presence of goblet cells and defines "Barrett's esophagus."

○ **True/False: Short-segment Barrett's esophagus is not associated with an increased risk of adenocarcinoma.**

False. Short-segment Barrett's esophagus has been shown to be a risk factor for adenocarcinoma, although it appears to be of lesser relative risk compared to long-segment Barrett's (3 cm or longer).

○ **Describe an appropriate approach for a patient who has Barrett's esophagus and low-grade dysplasia (LGD)?**

Biopsies should be reviewed by a second expert pathologist and then, if the finding of LGD is confirmed, endoscopy with multiple biopsies should be repeated within 6 months. More recently, treatment with radiofrequency ablation (RFA) has shown good results with elimination of the dysplasia; however, the low rate of progression from low-grade dysplasia to cancer (less than 1% per patient-year) makes the subgroup that should be so treated difficult to determine.

○ **Describe an appropriate approach for a patient who has Barrett's esophagus and high-grade dysplasia (HGD).**

Confirmation of the diagnosis by a second expert pathologist is the first step. Because of the strong possibility that adenocarcinoma will already be present in patients whose biopsies show only HGD, patients who are surgical candidates should consider esophagectomy. Patients who refuse or cannot tolerate surgery should either be surveyed endoscopically every 3 months or undergo ablation with radio frequency ablation (RFA) or photodynamic therapy (PDT), preceded by EMR if there is a nodule with HGD or even intramucosal cancer.

○ **True/False: A potential limitation of ablative therapy in the management of Barrett's esophagus is that nonneoplastic mucosa may be restored over persistent submucosal neoplasia.**

True.

○ **What is the likelihood that endoscopic biopsies showing Barrett's esophagus and HGD but no cancer will contain cancer in an esophagectomy specimen?**

Up to 40%, historically. Recent data suggest the incidence to be much lower.

○ **What should be offered to a patient with nondysplastic Barrett's esophagus to reduce the likelihood of developing cancer?**

At present, only endoscopic surveillance, every 3 years, can be offered. Currently, there is no convincing evidence that any antireflux therapy will eliminate Barrett's esophagus or the risk of adenocarcinoma. The role of ablative therapy in this setting remains controversial given the low risk of progression, but it is generally not recommended.

● ● ● **SUGGESTED READINGS** ● ● ●

Wang KW, Wingkeesong M, Buttar NS. American Gastroenterological Association Technical Review on the Role of the Gastroenterologist in the Management of Esophageal Carcinoma. *Gastroenterology.* 2005;128:1471-1505.

Spechler SJ, Pharma P, Souze FR, Inadomi JM, Shaheen NJ. American Gastroenterological Association Technical Review on the Management of Barrett's Esophagus. *Gastroenterology.* 2011;140(3):e18-e52.

CHAPTER 13

Gastroesophageal Reflux Disease

Rajeev Vasudeva, MD, FACG

○ **True/False: Patients with gastroesophageal reflux disease (GERD) usually seek medical attention.**

False. While an extremely common problem, the majority of patients with GERD do not seek medical attention.

○ **How often is endoscopic evidence of erosive esophagitis and Barrett's esophagus seen in patients with symptoms suggestive of GERD?**

Up to one-half of patients with reflux symptoms and not receiving antisecretory medication will have erosive esophagitis, albeit usually mild, and about 11% will have Barrett's esophagus.

○ **What are the major physiologic mechanisms that protect against esophageal acid injury?**

Esophageal clearance mechanisms (peristalsis/saliva), esophageal mucosal/epithelial integrity, antireflux barrier (lower esophageal sphincter [LES]) competence, and gastric emptying are the four major physiologic mechanisms.

○ **What are the three mechanisms of LES incompetence and how often is each primarily responsible for GERD?**

Transient LES relaxation	65%
Increased intra-abdominal pressure	17%
Spontaneous free reflux	18%

○ **What factors are associated with severe esophagitis?**

Low LES pressure, esophageal motor abnormalities, and recumbent reflux are the most important determinants of severe endoscopic esophagitis. The presence of a hiatal hernia is also important.

○ **What esophageal histologic abnormalities are typical of GERD?**

The basal zone occupying more than 15% of the total thickness of the epithelium and the papillae extending more than two-thirds of the distance to the surface. Eosinophils and neutrophils are also commonly present. Unfortunately, the sensitivity and specificity of these findings, either individually or in combination, is only fair at best.

○   **What role does the hiatal hernia play in the pathogenesis of GERD?**

This has been a controversial issue for the past 4 decades. Initially thought to be the only mechanism by which reflux occurred, later it was considered to be unimportant. However, recently it has been shown that the right crus of the diaphragm contributes significantly to the antireflux barrier, thereby stressing the importance of a normally placed gastroesophageal junction. Some studies have shown that the hernia sac acts as a reservoir for gastric contents (acid trap) and is associated with complicated forms of GERD such as severe esophagitis and peptic strictures, suggesting that it is a major contributory factor.

○   **True/False: There is a clear correlation between abnormal esophageal acid exposure on ambulatory pH monitoring, clinical symptoms, and severity of esophagitis.**

False. It appears that all three are independent although related aspects of GERD. No clear relationship exists between symptom severity, amount of reflux, and presence of esophagitis.

○   **What is the cancer risk in Barrett's esophagus?**

Barrett's esophagus is the major risk factor for esophageal adenocarcinoma whose incidence has been rising dramatically over the past two decades. A recent meta-analysis suggests that patients develop esophageal adenocarcinoma at a rate of <0.5% per year (annual incidence rate). These patients have a 30 to 125 times increased risk of developing esophageal cancer compared to the general population.

○   **What are similarities and differences in demographics between patients with long-segment Barrett's esophagus (LSBE) and short-segment Barrett's esophagus (SSBE)?**

- In general, the prevalence of LSBE is 3 to 5 times less than that of SSBE.
- The mean age of diagnosis is similar (55 to 65 years) with a strong propensity for males in LSBE (>90%) and slightly less for SSBE (70%).
- Predominance of Caucasians is noted for both although more striking in LSBE.
- Both smoking and alcohol ingestion are more prevalent in LSBE than in SSBE.

○   **What are similarities and differences in pathophysiology and clinical presentation between patients with LSBE and SSBE?**

- Symptoms of heartburn are similar but duration of heartburn greater than 5 years appears to be a distinguishing feature of LSBE.
- The pathophysiology and degree of acid reflux is different. Patients with LSBE typically have a large hiatal hernia, very low LES pressure, and decreased distal esophageal amplitude as compared with SSBE patients. Additionally, patients with LSBE have a combination of upright and supine reflux and more proximal esophageal acid reflux, while SSBE have predominantly upright and distal esophageal reflux.

○   **What is the difference in dysplasia risk between patients with LSBE and SSBE?**

The dysplasia prevalence is 15%–24% in LSBE or 2 to 3 times higher than that in SSBE. The adenocarcinoma prevalence is 15% in LSBE or 7 to 15 times higher than that in the SSBE population.

○   **True/False: Intestinal metaplasia of the gastric cardia has the same malignant potential as SSBE.**

False.

○   **True/False: There is universal agreement among practice guidelines from the major GI societies in the developed nations that endoscopic screening for Barrett's esophagus is indicated for patients with chronic symptoms of GERD.**

False.

○   **True/False: Intestinal metaplasia is required for the diagnosis of Barrett's esophagus.**

True. This is the only of esophageal columnar epithelium that clearly predisposes to malignancy.

○   **What is the Prague classification system?**

This is a simple endoscopic method of recording the circumferential (C) and maximal extent (M) of metaplasia in centimeters that has been developed in hopes of promoting more uniformity in the reporting of Barrett's esophagus.

○   **True/False: Antireflux surgery has been repeatedly demonstrated to lead to a reversal of Barrett's esophagus and risk of esophageal adenocarcinoma.**

False. To date, no nonablative medical or surgical therapy has been convincingly shown to lead to reversal of Barrett's esophagus or the risk of esophageal adenocarcinoma.

○   **What are recommended guidelines for endoscopic surveillance in Barrett's esophagus?**

Although it is not clear that Barrett's esophagus adversely influences survival or that endoscopic surveillance can reliably detect early curable neoplasia, the following practice guidelines have been published:

- GERD should be treated aggressively prior to surveillance in order to minimize confusion due to inflammation.
- Random, four-quadrant biopsies taken with a large capacity forceps every 2 cm for standard histologic evaluation is recommended in those without dysplasia and every 1 cm in those with dysplasia. Specific biopsy sampling of mucosal irregularities should also be performed.
- For patients with no dysplasia at two endoscopies (at unspecified intervals), subsequent surveillance endoscopy is recommended at 3- to 5-year intervals.
- For patients with low grade dysplasia, the diagnosis should be confirmed by an expert pathologist and endoscopy should be repeated in 3–6 months and at yearly intervals thereafter if dysplasia has not progressed.
- For patients with high-grade dysplasia, the diagnosis should first be confirmed by an expert pathologist. Although esophageal resection is one option, given the morbidity and mortality of surgical approach is significant, an intensive endoscopic surveillance may also be considered depending on patient comorbidities and/or preference. A repeat endoscopy should be performed with special attention to any mucosal irregularity and multiple biopsies (or endoscopic mucosal resection) should be obtained with a large capacity forceps. Focal high-grade dysplasia (< 5 crypts) may be followed with 3-month intervals. Surgical intervention should be more strongly considered when multifocal high-grade dysplasia is confirmed. Ablative therapeutic modalities including radiofrequency ablation, photodynamic therapy, and endoscopic mucosal resection may also be considered; however, the completeness of their reversal and their durability remains uncertain.

○   **True/False: Chromoendoscopy is currently recommended for use during the routine surveillance of Barrett's esophagus.**

False.

○   **What is the natural history of high-grade dysplasia in Barrett's esophagus?**

The natural history is poorly defined and therefore management of this condition is disputed. On the one hand, some studies have shown that progression to cancer is frequent and rapid while other studies have shown no apparent progression to cancer and even regression. Therefore, management varies between esophageal resection, continued surveillance, and endoscopic ablative therapies.

○ **True/False: There is a relationship between GERD and a multitude of pulmonary and otorhinolaryngology symptoms.**

True. A number of uncontrolled studies and anecdotal reports link GERD with several symptoms including laryngitis, hoarseness, globus, laryngeal cancer, chronic cough, asthma, aspiration, bronchitis, sinusitis, and dental erosions; however, the association appears to be the strongest for chronic cough, hoarseness, and asthma.

○ **In patients with noncardiac (unexplained) chest pain, what percentage is due to GERD and how effective is treatment?**

Several studies show nearly 50% of patients may have underlying GERD. Uncontrolled studies reveal an improvement of 65%–100% in symptomatology utilizing proton pump inhibitors.

○ **What are the mechanisms by which GERD is thought to produce respiratory symptoms?**

Two mechanisms have been suggested: 1) microaspiration of refluxed gastric contents into the airway (reflux theory) and 2) reflux of gastric contents into the distal esophagus initiating a vagally-mediated reflex arc (reflex theory).

○ **In what way is the response to antireflux therapy in patients with extraesophageal symptoms different from classical GERD?**

Despite the lack of adequate controlled data, the therapeutic response appears to be less. Therefore, high-dose proton pump inhibitors and a longer duration (several months) of treatment are required. Additionally, remission may be more difficult to maintain. The optimal management strategy remains to be defined.

○ **What are the therapeutic recommendations in the management of confirmed or suspected reflux-related extraesophageal symptoms?**

A twice-daily proton pump inhibitor for at least 3 months should be attempted before considering a patient to have failed medical therapy or not to have GERD. Antireflux surgery may be considered as an alternative therapeutic modality in patients with documented GERD who have failed medical therapy. The efficacy of antireflux surgery in patients with extraesophageal GERD is unclear based on the published literature.

○ **In what situations should you consider diagnostic testing in patients with suspected GERD?**
  • Uncertain diagnosis.
  • Suspected atypical or extraesophageal symptoms (chest pain, ENT, pulmonary).
  • Symptoms associated with complications (dysphagia, odynophagia, unexplained weight loss, bleeding, anemia).
  • Inadequate response to therapy.
  • Recurrent symptoms.
  • Prior to antireflux surgery.

○ **What are the differences between the various diagnostic tests used in GERD?**

Diagnostic tests should be performed in individual patients to answer specific questions. While somewhat controversial, a barium swallow is the test of choice for evaluation of dysphagia given that its sensitivity is superior to endoscopy in identifying subtle mucosal rings and evaluating esophageal motility. Endoscopy with biopsy is the best study for evaluating mucosal injury as well as identifying Barrett's esophagus. Ambulatory pH monitoring is the best study to confirm GERD, quantify reflux, and allow symptom correlation. Combined impedance and acid testing can identify both acid and nonacid (volume) reflux, thereby identifying a subset of patients that do not respond to conventional acid suppression and may potentially benefit from alternative treatments. Esophageal manometry has a limited role but may be useful prior to antireflux surgery in order to identify severe esophageal peristaltic abnormalities.

○   **What are the indications for ambulatory esophageal pH monitoring?**
- Typical symptoms that do not respond to proton pump inhibitor therapy (on therapy).
- Atypical symptoms (noncardiac chest pain, ENT/pulmonary manifestations).
- Prior to antireflux surgery if confirmation of GERD is necessary (endoscopy-negative patients).
- Recurrent symptoms following antireflux surgery.

○   **True/False: A tubeless (ie, catheter-free) method of ambulatory esophageal pH monitoring is available for clinical use.**

True. A pH capsule that can be attached directly to the esophageal mucosa is available. This device may be more accurate than the catheter-based system due to its increased recording time (48 hours versus 24 hours) and comfort.

○   **True/False: Lifestyle modifications are extremely effective in the treatment of GERD.**

False. Lifestyle modifications are helpful in relieving symptoms in only about 20% of patients. No studies exist that demonstrate efficacy of lifestyle modifications in healing esophagitis, managing or preventing complications, or maintaining remission.

○   **True/False: An initial trial of empiric antisecretory therapy is appropriate in a patient with symptoms suggestive of uncomplicated GERD.**

True. It is also reasonable to assume a diagnosis of GERD in patients who respond to this therapy.

○   **Which class of drugs provides the best long-term remission rate in erosive esophagitis?**

Proton pump inhibitors. Of note, the maintenance dose requirement may increase with time.

○   **True/False: Large, population-based, epidemiological studies have demonstrated an association between proton pump inhibitor use and an increased risk of hip fracture and a decreased risk of infectious diarrhea including *Clostridium difficile* infection.**

False. While these studies have shown an increase in hip fracture risk, they have also shown an increased risk of infectious diarrhea including a doubling of the risk of *C. difficile*. Importantly, a causal relationship remains to be proven.

○   **How effective are promotility agents in GERD therapy?**

They are not ideal as monotherapy agents but can be used in selected patients as an adjunct to acid suppression. Their benefit comes mainly from enhancing gastric emptying rather than an effect on esophageal peristalsis or LES function.

○   **True/False: Agents targeting transient lower esophageal sphincter relaxation (tLESR) have been clearly shown to have clinical benefit in patients with GERD.**

False. Although baclofen, a gamma butyric acid (GABA-B) agonist, has been shown to have benefit in terms of reducing the frequency of tLESRs and acid reflux events, its symptomatic benefit in GERD patients has not been clearly demonstrated. Furthermore, it has significant side effects prohibiting its widespread use in clinical practice. Recent clinical trials using longer-acting, better tolerated agents targeting tLESRs are ongoing but, to date, have not shown convincing benefit.

○ **How effective are H_2 receptor antagonists as GERD therapy?**

They eliminate symptoms in up to 50% with twice-daily dosing. Healing of mild-to-moderate esophagitis requires at least twice-daily dosing and usually more frequent and higher dosing is often required. Remission of esophagitis healing occurs in only about 15%–25%. Although the addition of a nocturnal dose of these medications to twice-daily proton pump inhibitors received some popularity on the basis of pharmacodynamic studies, this practice has not been supported by studies using clinical endpoints.

○ **What is the recurrence rate of GERD on discontinuation of therapy?**

GERD is a chronic relapsing condition and, in one study, 80% of patients were symptomatic 6 months after discontinuation of antisecretory therapy.

○ **Where are peptic esophageal strictures usually located?**

The distal esophagus involving the squamocolumnar junction. Other etiologies should be considered if strictures are located elsewhere.

○ **True/False: Medical therapy is effective in preventing the need for subsequent stricture dilatation.**

True. While treatment with H_2 receptor antagonists and promotility agents does not decrease the need for subsequent dilatations, several studies have shown that proton pump inhibitors are effective in not only healing associated esophagitis but also decreasing the need for stricture dilatation.

○ **True/False: Medical intractability remains a major indication for antireflux surgery in the era of proton pump inhibitors.**

False. Although once the most frequent reason for antireflux surgery, it is currently not a major indication for surgery. True intractability is uncommon in the era of proton pump inhibitors and the physician should reconsider the diagnosis of GERD in those who do not respond to these drugs. Antireflux surgery today is best reserved for patients who respond well to medical therapy. However, there is a small group of high-volume, nonacid refluxers identified by impedance testing that may benefit from antireflux surgery.

○ **Describe potential postoperative gastrointestinal complications following antireflux surgery.**

Dysphagia, flatulence, inability to belch, gas-bloat, and diarrhea. These are usually mild and self-limited and rarely require surgical revision. Interestingly, many (if not the majority of) patients will require proton pump inhibitors on a daily basis for the management of postoperative dyspeptic complaints.

○ **True/False: Titrated dosing of proton pump inhibitor is equivalent to antireflux surgery in the long-term management of GERD.**

True.

○ **What are some of the reasons why proton pump inhibitors may fail to control gastric acidity?**

- Nonadherence to the medication regimen is likely the most common reason.
- There is significant intersubject variability in the bioavailability of proton pump inhibitors, which may be decreased even further when taken with food.
- The acid suppressive effect of proton pump inhibitors tends to be reduced in *Helicobacter pylori*–negative patients.
- Although uncommon, hypersecretors of acid may have a decreased effect.
- Rapid metabolizers, based on cytochrome P450 2C, show a decreased effect on acid control.

- True proton pump inhibitor resistance (rare).
- Incorrect diagnosis.
- Nonacid reflux.
- Factors including significant gastric stasis, LES dysfunction, or ineffective peristalsis may contribute to persisting symptoms.
- Many patients with GERD often have symptoms including bloating, distention, and nausea which may be unmasked by proton pump inhibitors even though the classic reflux symptoms have improved.

○ **What diagnostic study should be considered in patients with medically refractory GERD?**

Twenty-four hour simultaneous intraesophageal and intragastric pH-metry while on antisecretory medication. A similar study off medication may be considered if the diagnosis of GERD is in doubt.

○ **What are the best predictors of a good outcome after antireflux surgery?**

Age < 50 years and typical reflux symptoms that are resolved completely with medical therapy. The experience of the surgeon is also important for a good outcome.

○ **What are the indications for antireflux surgery?**

- Patient with severe GERD who are unwilling to accept life-long medical therapy.
- Patients with severe GERD who cannot tolerate proton pump inhibitors due to allergy or intolerable side effects.
- Patients who have GERD manifestations that require long-term high-dose proton pump inhibitor therapy.
- Patients who are young and require chronic proton pump inhibitor therapy for control of symptoms and complications of GERD.
- Patients with nonacid reflux and good symptom correlation unresponsive to aggressive medical treatment.

○ **True/False: Several endoscopic modalities to control GERD are clinically available and have shown comparable effectiveness as antireflux surgery.**

False. Several techniques have been developed but, for a variety of reasons, most are no longer available (eg, radiofrequency energy application, endoscopic sewing techniques, and injection of various substances into the LES region) and none are commonly used. Nevertheless, the development of endoscopic approaches to manage reflux continues.

● ● ● SUGGESTED READINGS ● ● ●

Altman KW, Prufer N, Vaezi MF. A review of clinical practice guidelines for reflux disease: toward creating a clinical protocol for the otolaryngologist. *Laryngoscope.* 2011;121(4):717-723.

Stefanidis D, Hope WW, Kohn GP, Reardon PR, Richardson WS, Fanelli RD. SAGES Guidelines Committee. Guidelines for surgical treatment of gastroesophageal reflux disease. *Surg Endosc.* 2010;24(11):2647-2669.

Kahrilas PJ, Shaheen NJ, Vaezi M. AGAI technical review: management of gastroesophageal reflux disease. *Gastroenterology.* 2008;135:1392-1413.

Spechler SJ, Sharma P, Souza RF, Inadomi JM, Shaheen NJ. AGA. American Gastroenterological Association technical review on the management of Barrett's esophagus. *Gastroenterology.* 2011;140(3):e18-e52.

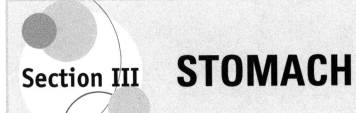

Section III   STOMACH

CHAPTER 14

Gastric Congenital and Structural Abnormalities

Ashok Shah, MD and Rene Rivera, MD

○ **What diagnosis should be considered in a newborn with postprandial nonbilious vomiting and an abdominal x-ray showing a distended stomach with an absence of air in the bowel?**

Gastric atresia. This condition most commonly affects the antrum and pylorus. Other symptoms include respiratory distress and drooling. The treatment is surgical.

○ **What condition during pregnancy is associated with gastric atresia?**

Polyhydramnios is common in gastric atresia, microgastria, and gastric teratoma.

○ **Gastric atresia can be associated with which of the following conditions?**

a. **Down's syndrome.**

b. **Junctional epidermolysis bullosa (JEB).**

c. **All of the above.**

d. **None of the above.**

c—Down's syndrome and JEB are both associated with gastric atresia. Other associated anomalies include absent gallbladder, vaginal atresia, tracheoesophageal fistula, atrial septal defect, and gut malrotation.

○ **True/False: The histology of the remnant stomach in microgastria is normal.**

True. This condition is extremely rare and is usually associated with congenital cardiac abnormalities. Most patients die within weeks to months of birth.

○ **True/False: Congenital hypertrophic pyloric stenosis may first become manifest as an adult.**

True. However, most cases of adult hypertrophic pyloric stenosis are acquired and occur most often in the setting of chronic peptic ulcer disease or cancer.

○ **True/False: The therapy of adult and infantile hypertrophic pyloric stenosis is the same.**

False. In neonates, the procedure of choice is a surgical pyloromyotomy. In adults, surgical resection of the pylorus is generally performed in order to rule out a small focus of cancer within the hypertrophied muscle.

○ **What classic physical finding may be found in infantile hypertrophic pyloric stenosis?**

"Palpable olive" or "palpable pyloric mass" plus visible peristalsis is found in 70%–90% of affected children.

○ **Which study has supplanted contrast radiography as the diagnostic study of choice for infantile hypertrophic pyloric stenosis?**

Abdominal ultrasonography of the pylorus.

○ **True/False: Gastric duplication occurs more commonly in women than in men.**

True. Duplication cysts are rare anomalies that arise during early embryonic development. Sixty-five percent of gastric duplications occur in women. When symptomatic, most (80%) become symptomatic in infancy or childhood.

○ **True/False: Duplication cysts most commonly involve the stomach.**

False. Duplication cysts most commonly involve the small bowel but may also involve the stomach, esophagus, and colon. There are two types of duplication cysts: one that lies adjacent to the bowel and does not communicate with the lumen and another that does communicate with the lumen.

○ **True/False: Gastric duplications are associated with gastric carcinoma.**

True. Malignant transformation has been documented in gastric duplications. Consequently, surgical excision has been recommended. Nevertheless, as most are asymptomatic and discovered incidentally, an expectant approach is often taken.

○ **Where are gastric diverticula most commonly located?**

Over 75% are located on the posterior wall within 2 cm of the gastroesophageal junction.

○ **Surgical treatment is recommended for distal gastric diverticula because of:**
a. High risk of bleeding.
b. High risk of perforation.
c. Associated risk of gastric obstruction.
d. Associated risk of malignancy.

d. Surgical treatment by amputation, invagination, or segmental resection has been recommended.

○ **True/False: Most gastric diverticula are acquired and symptomatic.**

False. Most are thought to be congenital, are asymptomatic, and are discovered incidentally.

○ **What congenital gastric tumor contains all three embryonic germ layers?**

Gastric teratoma. These tumors are rarely found in the stomach, occur almost exclusively in males, and are usually found extragastrically, near the greater curvature of the stomach.

○ **True/False: Gastric teratomas are usually associated with other congenital abnormalities.**

False. In most cases, gastric teratomas are an isolated finding. The prognosis of these tumors is good. Surgical excision is the treatment of choice.

⊛ ⊛ ⊛ SUGGESTED READINGS ⊛ ⊛ ⊛

Semrin MG, Russo MA. "Chapter 47-Anatomy, Histology, Embryology, and Developmental Anomalies of the Stomach and Duodenum." *Sleisenger and Fordtran's Gastrointestinal and Liver Disease: Pathophysiology/Diagnosis/Management.* 9th ed. Philadelphia, PA: Saunders; 2006:780-785.

Wyllie R. "Chapter 326 – Pyloric Stenosis and Congenital Anomalies of the Stomach. *Kliegman: Nelson Textbook of Pediatrics.* 18th ed. Philadelphia, PA: Saunders; 2007:1555-1558.

CHAPTER 15 Gastric Infectious Disorders

Kevin C. Ruff, MD

○ **What viral infections are associated with gastric ulcers?**

Cytomegalovirus and *Herpes simplex* type 1.

○ **A biopsy from a gastric ulcer reveals granulomas. What is the differential diagnosis?**

Infection (tuberculosis, histoplasmosis), Crohn's disease, sarcoidosis, and foreign body reaction.

○ **Menetrier's disease is associated with what viral infection?**

Menetrier's disease in childhood is usually associated with gastric cytomegalovirus infection.

○ **What other gastric infection is associated with the development of Menetrier's disease?**

Helicobacter pylori. (Note: *H. pylori* is covered further in the chapter on Peptic Ulcer Disease.)

○ **An acutely ill patient is found to have purulent gastric inflammation on endoscopy. What is the most likely diagnosis?**

Phlegmonous gastritis. Phlegmonous gastritis is a rare bacterial infection of the submucosa and muscularis propria of the stomach. Acute necrotizing gastritis (gangrene of the stomach) is a rare, often fatal disease that is now thought to be a variant of phlegmonous gastritis.

○ **What bacterial organism is most commonly associated with phlegmonous gastritis?**

Phlegmonous gastritis has been associated with alpha-hemolytic streptococcus in about 50% of the cases. *Escherichia coli*, *Enterobacter*, other Gram-negative bacilli, and *Staphylococcus aureus* have also been implicated.

○ **True/False: The mortality rate of phlegmonous gastritis approaches 25%.**

False. The mortality rate of phlegmonous gastritis is close to 70%, probably because it is so often misdiagnosed and treatment is initiated too late. The definitive treatment is resection or drainage of the stomach combined initially with broad-spectrum antibiotics.

○ **True/False: Emphysematous gastritis, a variant of phlegmonous gastritis, results from infection with gas-producing organisms.**

True. Predisposing factors are gastroduodenal surgery, ingestion of corrosive materials, gastroenteritis, or gastrointestinal infarction.

○ **What part of the gastrointestinal tract is most commonly involved in mucormycosis?**

The stomach. The typical lesion is a deep bleeding ulcer with black indurated edges.

○ **A 23-year-old woman develops severe abdominal pain after eating sushi. Upper endoscopy reveals a small worm protruding from the mucosa. What is the most likely diagnosis?**

Anisakiasis. This is acquired by eating sushi or other types of raw fish.

○ **True/False: Histoplasmosis of the gut mainly affects the stomach.**

False. The colon and the ileum are the most common sites. The stomach is rarely involved.

○ **Biopsies of the gastric antrum in a patient with diffusely congested and ulcerated mucosa show chronic active gastritis with inclusion bodies. What is the most likely diagnosis?**

Cytomegalovirus gastritis. The typical appearance of cytomegalovirus on histology shows intranuclear inclusion bodies often referred to as an "owl eye" appearance.

○ **Multiple small ulcerated plaques on endoscopic inspection of the stomach give a "cobblestone" appearance in which viral infections?**

H. simplex and *Varicella zoster*.

○ **A barium study of the upper GI tract shows evidence of a stricture in the mid gastric body with an "hourglass" shape on x-ray. Which bacteria is the most likely cause?**

Syphilis. Thickened gastric folds, mucosal nodularity, and irregular/serpiginous ulcers can also be present on endoscopic examination.

○ **True/False: Gastric infection with *Mycobacterium tuberculosis* is a rare entity that usually occurs in association with pulmonary tuberculosis.**

True.

○ ***Mycobacterium avium* complex (MAC), a common opportunistic bacterial infection among patients with AIDS, commonly affects the stomach.**

False.

○ **What risk factors contribute to the development of mucormycosis?**

Malnutrition, immunosuppression, antibiotic use, and acidosis (especially diabetic ketoacidosis).

○ **True/False: Gastric outlet obstruction can be a symptom of cryptosporidiosis.**

True. Strictures in the gastric antrum may cause substantial narrowing and limit gastric emptying.

○   **True/False: Ascariasis may cause gastric outlet obstruction.**

True. A high burden of *Ascaris lumbricoides* can lead to intermittent obstruction of the pylorus.

● ● ● SUGGESTED READINGS ● ● ●

Lee EL, Feldman M. Gastritis and Gastropathies. In: Feldman M, Friedman L, and Brandt L, eds. *Sleisenger and Fordtran's Gastrointestinal and Liver Diseases.* 9th ed. Philadelphia: Saunders-Elsevier; 2010:845-859.

Kim GY, Ward J, Henessey B, et al. Phlegmonous gastritis: case report and review. *Gastrointest Endosc.* 2005 Jan;61(1):168-174.

CHAPTER 16

Gastric Motility Disorders

Richard A. Wright, MD and John K. DiBaise, MD

○ **What pathways mediate the control of gastric emptying?**

Gastric motor activity is governed by extrinsic neural control from the parasympathetic nervous system, intrinsically by the enteric nervous system, and at the level of the smooth muscle by depolarization of the smooth muscle membrane.

○ **What are the major components of the enteric nervous system?**

The enteric nervous system consists of the myenteric (Auerbach's) plexus, which lies between the circular and longitudinal muscle layers, and the submucosal (Meissner's) plexus, which lies between the circular muscle layer and the mucosa.

○ **True/False: The stomach has two functional motor components.**

True. The proximal stomach represents the accommodating portion of the stomach. It is able to expand to allow large volumes of material to accumulate without causing a resultant increase in gastric pressure. It also receptively relaxes upon deglutition. In contrast, the distal stomach is responsible for trituration and emptying of gastric contents into the duodenum in a controlled manner.

○ **True/False: The gastric pacemaker is located near the incisura.**

False. The gastric pacemaker is located on the greater curvature of the stomach in the mid body. The pacemaker generates electrical potentials that sweep circumferentially and distally and correspond to peristaltic contractions during the appropriate stage of digestion.

○ **What is trituration?**

Trituration is the process of breaking down solid food to a size less than 1 mm by an antral grinding action. Large particles are repetitively propelled and retropulsed in the antrum, breaking them down to a size compatible with digestion and absorption.

○ **What are the interstitial cells of Cajal?**

These are specialized pacemaker cells present within the wall of the gut that transmit electrical signals throughout the gut smooth muscle.

○   **What receptors are present in the prepyloric region that help regulate emptying of materials into the duodenum?**

Size and osmole receptors. Size receptors will not allow particles greater than 1 mm to pass through the pylorus in the 2-hour postprandial period. Osmole receptors prevent the passage of hyperosmolar solutions into the duodenum. Hypertonic solutions must be diluted by gastric secretions to isotonicity before they are allowed to pass into the duodenum.

○   **What duodenal mechanisms cause feedback inhibition of gastric emptying?**

Acid stimulates the release of secretin from the duodenal mucosa which causes a decrease in gastric emptying. Lipids and amino acids cause release of cholecystokinin-pancreazymin from the duodenal mucosa, also resulting in the inhibition of gastric emptying, thus allowing for graded gastric emptying and preventing rapid transit of gastric contents into the duodenum.

○   **What is the effect of hyperglycemia on gastric emptying?**

Hyperglycemia delays gastric emptying in healthy individuals and patients with diabetes.

○   **What is the effect of vagotomy on the gastric fundus?**

Both receptive relaxation and accommodation are abolished. This may be partially responsible for the accelerated emptying that occurs after vagotomy (dumping syndrome). This is also the proposed mechanism for rapid gastric emptying that is sometimes seen in patients with diabetes mellitus.

○   **What abnormalities in gastric motor function have been described in patients with nonulcer (functional) dyspepsia?**

Altered accommodation, gastric dysrhythmias, antral hypomotility, and delayed gastric emptying have all been described.

○   **True/False: *Helicobacter pylori* plays a central role in the pathophysiology of nonulcer dyspepsia.**

False.

○   **True/False: Diabetic gastroparesis typically develops after diabetes has been present for at least 10 years.**

True.

○   **True/False: More individuals with type 1 diabetes with gastroparesis are seen in clinical practice compared with type 2 diabetes.**

False. Although gastroparesis appears to be more common in type 1 diabetics, given the higher prevalence of type 2 diabetes, more gastroparesis in type 2 diabetics is seen in clinical practice.

○   **What is the most common gastric motor defect observed in patients with diabetes mellitus?**

Autonomic neuropathy with "autovagotomy" results from long-standing diabetes mellitus. The clinical result is usually a delay in gastric emptying with the potential for bezoar formation; however, occasionally rapid emptying, especially of liquids, occurs and results in dumping syndrome.

○   **True/False: Idiopathic gastroparesis affects mostly men who are underweight at the time of diagnosis.**

False.

○ **True/False: Severe gastroparesis is typically associated with anorexia and vomiting.**

True.

○ **What connective tissue diseases are associated with gastroparesis?**

Scleroderma and systemic lupus erythematosus have been most commonly implicated.

○ **True/False: Patients with bulimia or anorexia nervosa and chronic vomiting frequently have gastric emptying abnormalities.**

True. In patients with anorexia nervosa or bulimia, impaired gastric emptying of solid foods has been reported, whereas liquid emptying is usually normal. Promotility drugs have been found to be helpful in alleviating gastroparetic symptoms in some of these patients.

○ **What tests are available to measure gastric emptying?**

Currently, the most common technique is scintigraphy using radionuclide-labeled meals. Both solid and liquid phases can be measured simultaneously by labeling the solids and liquids with different radionuclides; however, the solid phase seems to be most clinically useful. Transabdominal ultrasonography can be used to measure gastric emptying by determining serial measurements of antral size before and after a standard liquid meal. Magnetic resonance imaging is able to determine gastric emptying rates and the regional distribution of a meal within the stomach. Breath tests utilizing octanoic acid or spirulina, which do not contain radioactivity, are being developed to measure gastric emptying. Finally, an orally ingested capsule that continuously monitors time, pH, temperature, and pressure is available.

○ **What is the role of electrogastrography (EGG) in the evaluation of patients with dysmotilitylike symptoms?**

The exact role of EGG remains controversial. While certain dysrhythmias have been described in patients with these symptoms, there remains no consistent correlation between EGG findings, gastric emptying study results, and symptomatic response to promotility agents. EGG has been suggested to be complementary to the more conventional testing of gastric emptying.

○ **Name the abnormalities of the gastric rhythm.**

The normal discharge (normogastria) from the gastric pacemaker is 3 cycles per minute (cpm). Bradygastria is said to exist when the discharge rate is less than 2 cpm. Tachygastria is defined as a discharge rate of greater than 4 cpm.

○ **True/False: A succussion splash is the most common finding on physical examination in a patient with delayed gastric emptying.**

False. Most individuals with gastroparesis will have a normal examination; however, occasionally a succussion splash may be appreciated.

○ **What infectious diseases have been associated with delayed gastric emptying?**

Acute infection with Norwalk agent, a parvovirus, has been associated with a delay in gastric emptying. *Trypanosoma cruzi* causes delayed gastric emptying by damaging the myenteric plexus. Temporary delays in gastric emptying have also been noted in patients with varicella zoster, Epstein–Barr virus, cytomegalovirus, and *Clostridium botulinum* poisoning. While delayed gastric emptying has been described in patients with HIV infection, the mechanism is not clear. Patients with *H. pylori* infection have normal gastric emptying.

○ **True/False: Gastroparesis occurs commonly in patients with gastroesophageal reflux disease.**

True. Some studies have reported the presence of gastroparesis in up to one-half of these patients. The clinical significance of this delay in most patients remains disputed, however. Gastroparesis is not more prevalent in patients with Barrett's esophagus than in patients with erosive disease.

○ **What is the mechanism of action of metoclopramide?**

Metoclopramide is a centrally and peripherally acting dopamine (D_2 receptor) antagonist that enhances myenteric cholinergic transmission. It also has agonist activity at the 5-hydroxytryptamine (5-HT_4) receptor.

○ **What is the mechanism of action of domperidone?**

Domperidone is a selective dopamine antagonist similar to metoclopramide but with little penetration of the blood-brain barrier.

○ **What is the mechanism of action of erythromycin?**

Erythromycin is a motilin receptor agonist that causes stimulation of gastric smooth muscle directly and via cholinergic myenteric neural pathways. Erythromycin's use as a long-term promotility agent is limited by its antibacterial properties and tachyphylaxis caused by down-regulation of the motilin receptor.

○ **True/False: The risk of tardive dyskinesia with metoclopramide use relates to the dose but not the duration of therapy.**

False. The development of this potentially irreversible condition is directly related to the duration of metoclopramide use and the cumulative dose.

○ **What are other potential neurological side effects of metoclopramide?**

Pseudoparkinsonism, akathisia, and acute dystonic reactrions. These reactions typically respond to a reduction or cessation of metoclopramide use.

○ **True/False: The intramuscular injection of botulinum toxin into the pylorus has been shown in controlled studies to enhance gastric emptying and improve symptoms in patients with gastroparesis.**

False. Despite anecdotal reports and open trials suggesting otherwise, two recent randomized, controlled trials demonstrated no benefit of intrapyloric injections of botulinum toxin compared to placebo.

○ **True/False: Gastric electrical stimulation therapy derives its benefit from enhancing gastric emptying.**

False. Instead, its proposed mechanism of action has been suggested to be from a central neuromodulatory effect via vagal afferent stimulation.

○ **True/False: Gastric electrical stimulation is more likely to provide symptomatic benefit to those with idiopathic gastroparesis than those with diabetic gastroparesis.**

False. Factors suggested to predict a better outcome with this form of therapy include diabetes as the cause of gastroparesis, an absence of pain as a predominant symptom, and absence of chronic narcotic analgesic use.

○ **True/False: Gastrectomy should be offered to those with refractory gastroparesis.**

False. Gastrectomy should generally be reserved for those with refractory postsurgical causes of gastroparesis and, possibly, those with recurrent bezoar formation.

○ **True/False: Rapid gastric emptying (dumping) also commonly occurs in diabetics and produces symptoms virtually identical to those caused by delayed gastric emptying.**

True.

○ **What are the characteristic presentations of early and late dumping syndromes?**

Early dumping typically presents with gastrointestinal and vasomotor symptoms that occur shortly after eating. Late dumping typically presents with hypoglycemic symptoms. Both forms can be incapacitating.

○ **Describe the pathophysiology of early dumping syndrome.**

The enhanced rate of gastric emptying of solids and liquids allows higher volume hypertonic food boluses to be released into the small intestine. This induces a neurohumoral cascade responsible for the gastrointestinal and vasomotor symptoms seen.

○ **What is the primary factor in the pathogenesis of the symptoms of late dumping?**

Hypoglycemia resulting from the initial absorption of hyperosmolar carbohydrates producing hyperinsulinemia.

○ **True/False: The diagnosis of dumping syndrome is based on results of a gastric emptying test.**

False. Diagnosis is most commonly based on a suggestive symptom profile in the proper clinical context (eg, post gastric surgery).

○ **What is the initial treatment for dumping syndrome?**

Dietary maneuvers including low-sugar foods, smaller, more frequent meals, and consuming solids and liquids at separate times. The addition of soluble fiber to the diet to delay gastric emptying may also be of help. Medications that have demonstrated some efficacy in dumping include acarbose (late dumping) and short- and long-acting somatostatin analogues (early and late dumping).

● ● ● SUGGESTED READINGS ● ● ●

Parkman HP, Yates K, Hasler WL, et al. Clinical features of idiopathic gastroparesis vary with sex, body mass, symptom onset, delay in gastric emptying, and gastroparesis severity. *Gastroenterology.* 2011;140:101-115.

Camilleri M, Bharucha AE, Farrugia G. Epidemiology, mechanisms and management of diabetic gastroparesis. *Clin Gastroenterol Hepatol.* 2011;9:5-12.

Tack J, Arts J, Caenepeel P, De Wulf D, Bisschops R. Pathophysiology, diagnosis and management of postoperative dumping syndrome. *Nat Rev Gastroenterol Hepatol.* 2009;6:583-590.

CHAPTER 17 Gastric Tumors

Douglas O. Faigel, MD

○ **What is the most common type of malignant tumor of the stomach?**

Adenocarcinoma comprises 90% of all cases. Less common malignant neoplasms include lymphoma, stromal tumor, carcinoid, adenosquamous, and metastases.

○ **What are the two main histological types of gastric adenocarcinoma?**

Intestinal type and diffuse type.

○ **Germline mutations in which gene have been associated with diffuse type gastric adenocarcinoma?**

E-cadherin.

○ **True/False: *Helicobacter pylori* plays a role in the etiology of gastric cancer.**

True. *H. pylori* results in chronic gastritis which, presumably, may proceed to metaplasia, dysplasia, and cancer. It has been classified as a Class A carcinogen by the World Health Organization.

○ **What is a Krukenberg tumor?**

Gastric cancer metastatic to the ovary.

○ **What are the two most common sites of gastric cancer metastasis?**

The liver and lungs constitute about 40% of total cases.

○ **True/False: Most gastric cancer patients have signs of overt GI bleeding such as melena or hematemesis.**

False. Less than 20% have overt GI bleeding.

○ **True/False: Gastric ulcers require endoscopic follow-up to document healing.**

True. However, it has been suggested that extensive biopsies from the ulcer taken at the time of the initial endoscopy may obviate the need for follow-up endoscopy, if the biopsies were negative/not suspicious for malignancy.

○   **A 64-year-old man with gastric cancer presents with velvety, pigmented lesion in the axilla. What is the diagnosis?**

Acanthosis nigricans is considered a paraneoplastic manifestation.

○   **True/False: Endoscopic ultrasound (EUS) is the best modality to assess the extent of local disease in gastric cancer.**

True. This can be combined with a CT scan to allow for complete staging.

○   **What is the best prognostic factor in gastric cancer?**

The TNM (Tumor, Node, Metastasis) stage at the time of diagnosis.

○   **A patient with gastric adenocarcinoma undergoes EUS which demonstrates invasion into the left lobe of the liver. What is the T-stage?**

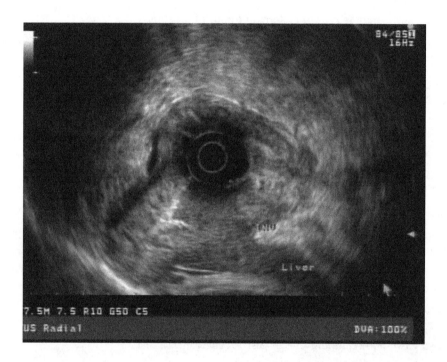

Figure 17-1

Invasion of an adjacent organ is T4.

○   **What treatment has the best curative potential for gastric adenocarcinoma?**

Surgical resection. Unfortunately, two-thirds of Western patients present with advanced disease and are not surgical candidates for cure.

○   **True/False: Perioperative chemoradiotherapy improves outcome in gastric adenocarcinoma?**

True. Three recent studies of perioperative chemoradiotherapy and at least four meta-analyses have shown improved disease-free and overall survival in the treated groups.

○ **What is the most common type of gastric malignancy after adenocarcinoma?**

Primary gastric lymphoma.

○ **What are the two most common types of gastric lymphoma?**

Diffuse large B cell lymphoma and low-grade B cell mucosa-associated lymphoid tissue (MALT) lymphoma.

○ **True/False: *H. pylori* is associated with gastric lymphoma.**

True. Ninety percent of low-grade MALT lymphomas are positive for *H. pylori*. Additionally, tumor remission has been documented after eradication of *H. pylori* in a number of cases.

○ **True/False: A 45-year-old man is found to have a B-cell lymphoma of the stomach. Based on the EUS image shown, he is likely to respond to anti-*H. pylori* therapy.**

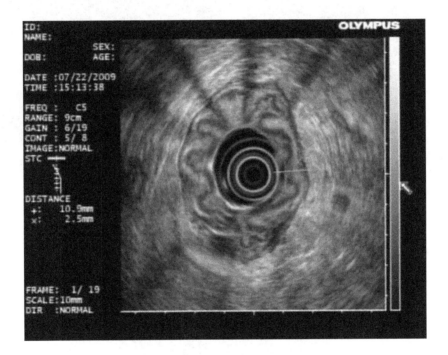

Figure 17-2

False. The EUS shows diffuse and deep invasion of the gastric wall. This is consistent with an aggressive diffuse large B-cell lymphoma. Antibiotic therapy would be inadequate.

○ **What part of the gastrointestinal tract is the most common site for a primary gastrointestinal lymphoma?**

The stomach is the site in 70% or more of the cases. The remaining cases are equally divided between the small and large intestine.

○   A 62-year-old woman with abdominal pain undergoes endoscopy and a submucosal tumor is found (see Figures 17-3 and 17-4). What is the most likely diagnosis based on the EUS image shown?

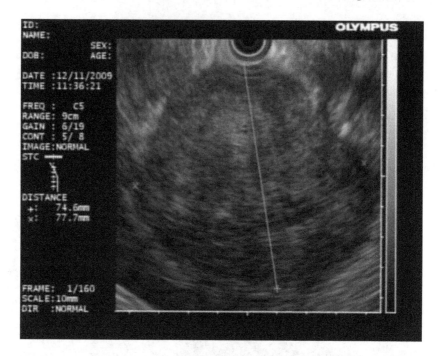

Figure 17-3

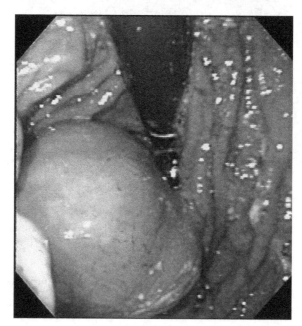

Figure 17-4 See also color plate.

Gastrointestinal stromal tumor (GIST).

○ **True/False: Discovered on GIST-1 (DOG1) is the most commonly used immunohistochemical marker for GIST.**

False. cKit is the most commonly used marker. DOG1 is reserved for suspicious tumors that are cKit negative.

○ **What proportion of GISTs are located in the stomach?**

Fifty percent. Most are in the proximal portion of the stomach.

○ **What is the Carney triad?**

Gastric stromal tumor, extra-adrenal paraganglioma, and pulmonary chondroma.

○ **Which features of a gastric stromal tumor indicate a higher likelihood of recurrence after resection?**

The mitotic index of 5 or more mitoses per 50 high-power fields, and size ≥5 cm.

○ **Which patients have a higher incidence of gastric carcinoid?**

Patients with hypergastrinemia as occurs in pernicious anemia, atrophic gastritis with achlorhydria and Zollinger–Ellison syndrome.

○ **True/False: Gastric carcinoids are grouped into two categories (type 1 and type 2).**

False. Gastric carcinoids are grouped into three categories: those associated with atrophic gastritis (type 1), gastrinoma or multiple endocrine neoplasia (type 2), and neither (type 3).

○ **True/False: Treatment of gastric carcinoid differs depending on the type.**

True. Types 1 and 2 smaller than 1 cm are generally amenable to endoscopic resection, while type 3 (sporadic) gastric carcinoids require more extensive gastric resection.

○ **True/False: The stomach is the most common site for GI neuroendocrine tumors (carcinoids)?**

False. Less than 5% of GI neuroendocrine tumors (carcinoids) are found in the stomach.

○ **True/False: Thickened folds of the stomach may be caused by metastatic breast cancer.**

True. Although breast cancer, like other types of cancer, may metastasize to the stomach causing a focal mass lesion, infiltration and thickening of the gastric folds as shown in the figure may also occur in breast cancer. This appearance is indistinguishable from other infiltrating tumors such as diffuse-type gastric adenocarcinoma and high-grade lymphoma.

○ **What is the most common location for a gastric lipoma?**

The antrum. These are benign submucosal tumors. EUS is very useful for differentiation from other tumors.

○ **What are the two most common types of gastric polyps?**

Hyperplastic polyps and fundic gland polyps. Together, they represent 70%–90% of all gastric polyps.

○   **A 73-year-old woman with a history of melanoma undergoes upper endoscopy and a brownish-black nodule is present in the stomach. What is the diagnosis?**

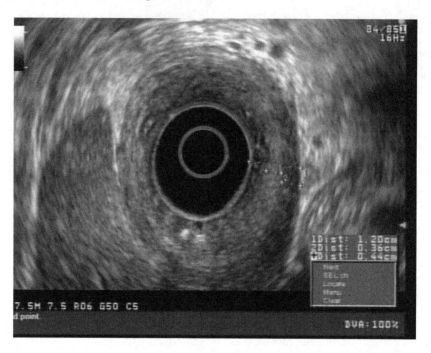

Figure 17-5

Metastatic melanoma involving the stomach.

○   **True/False: There is an association between fundic gland polyps and familial adenomatous polyposis (FAP).**

True. More than 60% of FAP patients have fundic gland polyps.

○   **True/False: Fundic gland polyps may be seen in patients on chronic proton pump inhibitor (PPI) therapy.**

True. Up to one-third of long-term users of PPIs have fundic gland polyps. The risk of histologic progression is negligible.

○   **What conditions are associated with hyperplastic polyps of the stomach?**

Atrophic gastritis and *H. pylori* infection.

○   **What is the most likely diagnosis of a 2-cm antral nodule with a central dimple?**

Pancreas rest (ectopic pancreatic tissue). This constitutes about 1% of gastric polyps.

○   **What is the only benign gastric polyp with significant malignant potential?**

Adenomatous polyp.

○   **True/False: The presence of invasive cancer in an adenoma correlates with size, villous histology, and degree of dysplasia.**

True.

○ **True/False: All gastric polyps should be biopsied and removed if possible.**

True. If multiple, a representative sample of polyps should be biopsied and the pathology identified. Those >1 cm should be removed whenever possible.

○ **True/False: Because adenomatous and hyperplastic polyps are associated with atrophic gastritis and *H. pylori* infection, the normal appearing antral and body mucosa should also be sampled.**

True.

● ● ● SUGGESTED READINGS ● ● ●

Hirota WK, Zuckerman MJ, Adler DG, et al. Standards of Practice Committee American Society for Gastrointestinal Endoscopy. ASGE guideline: the role of endoscopy in the surveillance of premalignant conditions of the upper GI tract. *Gastrointest Endosc.* 2006 Apr;63(4):570-580.

Ho MY, Blanke CD. Gastrointestinal Stromal Tumors: Disease and Treatment Update. *Gastroenterology.* 2011;40:1372-1376.

Khushalani NI. Cancer of the Esophagus and Stomach. *Mayo Clin Proc.* 2008;83(6):712-722.

CHAPTER 18 Peptic Ulcer Disease and Its Complications

Francisco C. Ramirez, MD

○ **What are the major factors that disrupt gastric mucosal resistance resulting in ulcer development?**

Nonsteroidal anti-inflammatory drugs (NSAIDs), *Helicobacter pylori*, diminished mucosal bicarbonate secretion, cigarette smoking, and gastric acid hypersecretion.

○ **What are the four most common causes of ulcer disease?**

H. pylori, NSAIDs, idiopathic, and hypersecretory states. About 50%–60% of *H. pylori*-negative ulcers are caused by aspirin or NSAID use, while about 10%–15% are idiopathic. It has been estimated that about 20% of peptic ulcers have false-negative *H. pylori* results.

○ **What is the main mechanism responsible for mucosal damage in patients taking NSAIDs?**

Inhibition of prostaglandin synthesis.

○ **What percent of NSAID users develop *asymptomatic* peptic ulcer disease (PUD) or gastropathy?**

20% in the first year.

○ **Who is more likely to develop an asymptomatic ulcer?**

The elderly and those taking NSAIDs.

○ **What percent of NSAID users develop symptomatic PUD or complicated PUD?**

3%.

○ **What are risk factors for developing NSAID-induced GI complications?**

History of PUD or complication of PUD (most important), age older than 60, high-dose NSAIDs, concomitant use of corticosteroids, concomitant use of anticoagulants, and concurrent *H. pylori* infection.

○ **True/False: Smoking is a risk factor for the development of NSAID-related ulcers.**

False. *H. pylori*-associated ulcers but not NSAID-induced ulcers are exacerbated by smoking.

○ **What is the annual incidence rate of PUD in *H. pylori*-infected individuals?**

1%.

○ **What is the lifetime prevalence of clinical PUD in the general population and in the *H. pylori*-infected population?**

10% and 20%, respectively.

○ **Which part of the stomach is predominantly involved in *H. pylori*-associated duodenal ulcer?**

Antrum (antral-predominant gastritis). In contrast, the body of the stomach is predominantly affected in *H. pylori*-associated gastric ulcer (corpus-predominant gastritis).

○ **True/False: The presence of *H. pylori* in the corpus of the stomach is associated with a lower gastric pH and a higher incidence of gastroesophageal reflux disease.**

False. Diffuse gastritis with *H. pylori* in this location is typically associated with an increase in gastric pH and may serve as a protective mechanism against reflux. In this situation, the eradication of *H. pylori* may result in a decrease in gastric pH and an increase in gastroesophageal reflux symptoms in susceptible individuals.

○ **True/False: The presence of pain and its relationship to meals does not accurately distinguish between gastric and duodenal ulcer patients.**

True. Nevertheless, as a reminder of the "classic" clinical presentations: Pain related to duodenal ulcers occurs about 2–5 hours after a meal and between 11 pm and 2 am (circadian acid stimulation is maximal), whereas pain related to a gastric ulcer occurs immediately after a meal.

○ **Which hypersecretory states may manifest with PUD?**

Hypergastrinemia-related: Zollinger–Ellison syndrome, antral cell hyperplasia, and retained antrum syndrome.

Nonhypergastrinemia-related: Systemic mastocytosis (increased histamine).

○ **Describe the nature of the relationship between *H. pylori* and NSAIDs in the pathogenesis of PUD (and bleeding ulcer).**

Synergistic.

○ **Describe the nature of the relationship between low-dose aspirin and cyclo-oxygenase (COX)-2 inhibitors in the pathogenesis of PUD.**

Synergistic. There is an increased risk of complications when taken concomitantly compared to when taking either drug alone.

○ **True/False: In a patient at high risk of PUD who needs to begin long-term NSAID therapy, the best strategy regarding *H. pylori* is to test and treat (if present) before initiation of the NSAID.**

True.

○ **True/False: In the patient with active PUD who has *H. pylori* infection and requires continuing long-term NSAID use, the best strategy for managing this patient is to treat the *H. pylori* and consider prophylactic antisecretory therapy.**

True.

○   **True/False: Endoscopically, an ulcer is differentiated from erosion by size alone.**

False. Depth is the primary feature differentiating the two. Histologically, an ulcer is defined by penetration of the muscularis mucosa.

○   **Describe instances when testing for *H. pylori* should be considered.**

Active PUD, documented history of PUD, gastric mucosa-associated lymphoid tissue (MALT) lymphoma, family history of gastric cancer, following resection of gastric adenocarcinoma, and uninvestigated dyspepsia in those <55 years of age and without "alarm" features. More controversial indications include naïve NSAID users, iron deficiency anemia, and idiopathic thrombocytopenic purpura (ITP).

○   **Describe the nonendoscopic tests used for the diagnosis of active *H. pylori* infection and their sensitivities and specificities.**

In-office antibody test (sensitivity: 88%–94%; specificity: 74%–88%)

ELISA on serum (sensitivity 86%–94%; specificity: 78%–95%)

Stool antigen (sensitivity 94%; specificity: 92%)

^{13}C or ^{14}C Urea breath test (sensitivity: 90%–96%; specificity: 88%–98%)

○   **Describe the endoscopic tests (requiring gastric biopsy) used for the diagnosis of active *H. pylori* infection and their sensitivities and specificities.**

Rapid urease test (sensitivity: 88%–95%; specificity: 95%–100%)

Histology (sensitivity: 93%–96%; specificity: 95%–100%)

Culture (sensitivity: 80%–98%; specificity: 100%)

○   **What precautions should be taken to avoid false-negative results when testing for *H. pylori*?**

Testing should be performed at least 4 weeks after stopping antibiotics, bismuth, and antisecretory medications.

○   **What is the duodenal ulcer recurrence rate after *H. pylori* eradication?**

Less than 10% (versus 65%–95% of those who remain infected).

○   **True/False: The re-infection rate after successful treatment of *H. pylori* in adults is about 5% per year.**

False. The re-infection rate is <2% per year.

○   **When is confirmation of eradication after *H. pylori* treatment recommended?**

Most guidelines now recommend that eradication be documented in all patients. Previously, this recommendation was limited to those with complicated PUD or those with persistent or recurrent symptoms following treatment.

○   **Which tests are useful to confirm eradication?**

Urea breath test, stool antigen, or gastric biopsy. In contrast, serologic antibody tests should not be used to confirm eradication as titers decrease slowly and may remain positive in approximately 40% of those successfully treated even after 18 months.

○ **What are the four main complications of PUD?**

Bleeding: 50–170/100,000 (as many as 30% of patients with PUD at some point in their lifetime)

Perforation: 1–10/100,000 (<5%)

Gastric outlet obstruction (rare)

Penetration (rare)

○ **In what locations of the stomach and duodenum are ulcers more likely to bleed?**

Ulcers located high on the lesser curve of the stomach or on the posterior inferior wall of the duodenal bulb are more likely to bleed.

○ **Name two high-risk ulcer stigmata at endoscopy that require endoscopic hemostasis and high-dose continuous infusion of a proton pump inhibitor (PPI).**

Actively bleeding vessel and nonbleeding visible vessel.

○ **True/False: Young age is a risk factor for ulcer bleeding-related death.**

False. Older age and failure to control bleeding endoscopically are risk factors for death within 48 hours of attempted endoscopic treatment.

○ **True/False: The incidence of duodenal ulcer has declined over the past 30 years.**

True. This decline is only partially explained by the introduction of potent antisecretory agents as it predated their availability. It may be partly explained by a decrease in smoking or possibly by an increase in antibiotic use.

○ **In patients with symptoms and endoscopically-documented PUD, what percent is present with upper gastrointestinal bleeding (UGIB)?**

Approximately 30% (often as the initial symptom).

○ **What is the major effect of administering high-dose PPI therapy prior to endoscopy in the patient presenting with UGIB?**

The effect seems to primarily be in the down-staging of endoscopic stigmata rather than modifying actual outcomes.

○ **The presence of an ulcer or ulcers in the distal duodenum or other atypical locations should raise suspicion for which conditions?**

Crohn's disease, ischemia, and Zollinger–Ellison syndrome.

○ **What characteristics should prompt extra awareness on the risk for gastric cancer in the patient with a gastric ulcer?**

Absence of *H. pylori* or NSAID use, large (>2 cm) size, and patient from an endemic area of gastric cancer (eg, Central America and East Asia).

○ **What is required to be present in the duodenum for *H. pylori* to cause duodenal ulcer?**

Gastric metaplasia. Hyperacidity from colonization of the gastric antrum causes gastric metaplasia of the duodenum which can in turn become colonized with the organism and lead to inflammation and ulceration.

○ **What is a unique and striking characteristic of the *H. pylori* organism?**

Production of urease (breath test and rapid urease testing on tissue are based on this characteristic).

○ **Name two *H. pylori* genotypes associated with increased morbidity in patients with PUD (ie, associated with increased virulence).**

vacA-positive (vacuolating cytotoxin) and cagA-positive (cytotoxin-associated gene A).

○ **Name the two main risk factors associated with clinically significant bleeding from stress-related mucosal disease (SRMD).**

Mechanical ventilation for >48 hours (OR: 15.6) and the presence of coagulopathy (OR: 4.3).

○ **True/False: Mortality in patients with SRMD and bleeding is high and usually relates to the underlying condition.**

True.

○ **Prophylaxis for SRMD-related bleeding is indicated in which circumstances?**

Severe trauma, burns involving >1/3 body surface area, major intracranial disease, severe illness requiring mechanical ventilation >48 hours, and the presence of coagulopathy.

○ **True/False: Prophylaxis for SRMD is associated with decreased risk of bleeding.**

True. The risk of bleeding, but not mortality, is reduced.

○ **What medications have been shown to have benefit in SRMD prophylaxis?**

Histamine receptor antagonists type 2, PPIs, and sucralfate.

○ **What are the two most important factors determining the speed of healing of a duodenal ulcer with antisecretory medications?**

Duration of time that the gastric pH is >3.0 and the number of weeks of treatment.

○ **True/False: Multiple endocrine neoplasia type 2 (MEN type 2) is associated with gastrinoma.**

False. About 20%–25% of patients with a gastrinoma have MEN type 1 (tumors of pancreas, parathyroid, and pituitary or "3 P's").

○ **True/False: A duodenal bulbar ulcer is the most common type of ulcer associated with gastrinoma.**

True.

○ **Describe three clinical situations where a gastrinoma should be considered in the differential diagnosis.**

1. Presence of multiple duodenal ulcers and esophagitis refractory to medical therapy.
2. Presence of duodenal ulcer(s) and diarrhea (malabsorption due to acid overload and inactivation of pancreatic enzymes).
3. Presence of duodenal ulcer(s) and hypercalcemia (hyperparathyroidism related to MEN type 1).

○ **True/False: A secretin stimulation test is the screening test of choice in the evaluation of a gastrinoma?**

False. Serum gastrin level is the screening test of choice. A level >1000 pg/ml strongly suggests gastrinoma.

○ **What test should be considered when the serum gastrin is markedly elevated but below 1000 and achlorhydria has been ruled out?**

Secretin stimulation test. A positive test is an increase of at least 200 pg/ml over baseline gastrin level. This test can be done in the presence of PPI use.

○ **True/False: Gastrinoma is the most common cause of hypergastrinemia.**

False. Achlorhydria, usually in the setting of atrophic gastritis, is the most common cause of achlorhydria.

○ **How can antral G-cell hyperplasia be differentiated from a gastrinoma?**

Like gastrinoma, it is associated with hypergastrinemia and the development of duodenal ulcers. However, it can be differentiated from a gastrinoma on the basis of a negative secretin test.

● ● ● SUGGESTED READINGS ● ● ●

Malfertheiner, P, Chan FKL, McColl KEL. Peptic Ulcer Disease. *Lancet.* 2009;374:1449-1461.

Yeomans, ND. The ulcer sleuths: the search for the causes of peptic ulcers. *J Gastroenterol Hepatol.* 2011;26(Suppl 1):35-41.

Arora G, Singh G, Triadafilopoulus G. Proton pump inhibitors for gastroduodenal damage related to nonsteroidal anti-inflammatory drugs or aspirin: twelve important questions for clinical practice. *Clin Gastroenterol Hepatol.* 2009;7:725-735.

Barkun A, Leontiadis G. Systematic review of the symptom burden, quality of life impairment and costs associated with peptic ulcer disease. *Am J Med.* 2010;123:358-366.

Gralnek IM, Barkun AN, Bardou M. Management of acute bleeding from a peptic ulcer. *N Engl J Med.* 2008;359:928-937.

Moller MH, Adamsen SV, Wojdemann M, Moller AM. Perforated peptic ulcer: how to improve outcome? *Scand J Gastroenterol.* 2009;44:15-22.

McColl KEL. Helicobacter pylori-negative non-steroidal anti-inflammatory drug negative-ulcer. *Gastroenterol Clin N Am.* 2009;38: 353-361.

Marik PE, Vasu T, Hirani A, Pachinburavan M. Stress ulcer prophylaxis in the new millennium: a systematic review and meta-analysis. *Crit Care Med.* 2010;38:2222-2228.

Barkun AN, Bardou M, Kulpers EJ, et al. International Consensus recommendations on the management of patients with nonvariceal upper gastrointestinal bleeding. *Ann Intern Med.* 2010;152:101-113.

CHAPTER 19

Surgical Aspects of Peptic Ulcer Disease

Joseph J. Cullen, MD and Jessica K. Smith, MD

○ **What are the indications for operative treatment of peptic ulcer disease?**

Perforation, obstruction, and bleeding. Traditionally, intractability was included but with the decrease in the incidence of peptic ulceration, the development of potent H2-receptor antagonists and proton pump inhibitors (PPIs), and increasing evidence regarding the role of *Helicobacter pylori* and nonsteroidal anti-inflammatory drug (NSAID)-induced ulceration, intractability has become rare.

○ **Chest radiographs demonstrate pneumoperitoneum in what percentage of patients with perforated duodenal ulcer?**

75%. In a minority of patients, omentum or liver seals the perforation and pneumoperitoneum is not seen.

○ **What is the principal cause of death from peptic ulcer disease?**

Hemorrhage, although the majority of patients who have acute hemorrhage from ulcers stop bleeding spontaneously.

○ **Which patients with a bleeding ulcer may be appropriate for radiologic embolization as an alternative to surgery?**

Poor surgical candidates or patients that have had multiple previous operations in the upper abdomen, making access to the duodenum exceedingly difficult.

○ **Bleeding must be at least at what rate in order to be visualized angiographically for embolization?**

1 ml/min.

○ **What are the indications for emergent surgical intervention for bleeding duodenal ulcer?**

Failure of initial endoscopic or radiologic therapy; bleeding refractory or inaccessibility to endoscopic control; high-risk findings for rebleeding at initial endoscopy such as large, pulsatile vessel; persistent hemodynamic instability or transfusion requirement exceeding 6 units of blood in a 24-hour period.

○   **Three-point suture ligation (see Figure 19-1) of the gastroduodenal artery (GDA) complex includes the proximal and distal gastroduodenal artery and what other branch?**

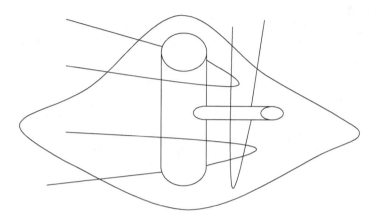

Figure 19-1

Transverse pancreatic branch.

○   **Why are fewer postgastrectomy complications seen following Billroth I reconstruction compared to other types of reconstruction?**

Preservation of the duodenal passage eliminates early dumping and malabsorption seen with the other types.

○   **What surgical treatment of dumping or enterogastric reflux after Billroth II reconstruction should be considered after failure of conservative (dietary and medical) management?**

Conversion to Roux-en-Y gastrojejunostomy.

○   **What is the mortality rate of partial gastrectomy for uncomplicated gastric ulcer?**

1%–2%.

○   **True/False: The risk of gastric cancer following partial gastric resection is greater than the general population.**

True. The overall magnitude of the relative risk has been estimated to be about 1.5 to 3.0 but depends on the type of surgery, duration of follow-up, and general location. The risk appears to be greatest after about 15 to 20 years postoperatively.

○   **What are the four major factors suggested to be involved in the pathogenesis of gastric stump cancer after partial gastrectomy for peptic ulcer disease?**

Enterogastric reflux, achlorhydria, bacterial overgrowth, and *H. pylori*.

○   **A patient, who is postoperative day 5 after antrectomy, vagotomy, and Billroth II gastrojejunostomy for an obstructing duodenal ulcer, develops an acute exacerbation of abdominal pain and fever. What is the most likely diagnosis?**

Patients who have leakage from a duodenal stump have an acute exacerbation of abdominal pain, typically on the fifth to seventh postoperative day. When the leak is sizeable, symptoms of an acute abdomen result.

○ **What is the mortality rate for duodenal stump blowout after an antrectomy and gastrojejunostomy for peptic ulcer disease?**

About 50%.

○ **True/False: Recurrent ulcers are more common after an operation for "intractable" duodenal ulcer than after an operation for gastric ulcer.**

True.

○ **What is the overall mortality rate for patients who undergo operation for perforated duodenal ulcer?**

3%–6%.

○ **What factors increase morbidity and mortality risk in patients with perforated duodenal ulcer?**

Serious comorbid illness, hemodynamic instability, perforations over 48 hours in duration at time of presentation, and age over 70.

○ **Figure 19-2 demonstrates a 46-year-old patient who presented with abdominal pain and pneumoperitoneum on upright chest x-ray. Rapid *H. pylori* testing was positive. The intraoperative findings are shown in the photograph. What operative intervention should be performed?**

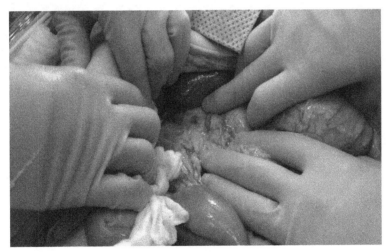

Figure 19-2 See also color plate.

Omental (Graham) patch closure of the perforated duodenal ulcer and treatment of *H. pylori* postoperatively.

○ **What is most commonly the first symptom of postoperative recurrent ulcer?**

Upper gastrointestinal bleeding is frequently the first symptom of postoperative recurrent ulcer, occurring in 40%–60% of patients.

○ **True/False: Perforation is a common presentation for recurrent ulcer in a postgastrectomy patient.**

False.

○ **Where are postoperative recurrent ulcers typically located?**

Recurrent ulcers nearly always occur within 1–2 cm of the gastrointestinal anastomosis.

○ **A postgastrectomy patient presents with recurrent ulceration. Serum gastrin levels are elevated. What are some of the possible causes?**

Gastrinoma, retained antrum, G-cell hyperplasia, or administration of PPIs.

○ **What are the characteristic endoscopic findings of stress ulceration?**

The lesions of stress ulceration are superficial, rather than deep, multiple rather than single, gastric rather than duodenal, fundic rather than antral, and usually bleed rather than perforate.

○ **A patient who underwent an antrectomy, vagotomy, and gastrojejunostomy for peptic ulcer disease complains of crampy abdominal pain, diaphoresis, dizziness, and palpitations 25 minutes after a meal. What is the diagnosis?**

The patient has dumping syndrome, which occurs in response to the ingestion of a hyperosmolar carbohydrate-rich meal.

○ **What percentage of chronic duodenal ulcers heal after highly selective vagotomy? What is the ulcer recurrence rate following this elective procedure?**

About 90% heal; 10%–20% recur.

○ **What common side effects of truncal vagotomy with antrectomy or pyloroplasty are rarely seen after highly selective vagotomy?**

Diarrhea, delayed gastric emptying, dumping syndrome, and bile reflux.

○ **What are the mechanisms that lead to the dumping syndrome?**

Loss of gastric reservoir function and rapid emptying of hyperosmolar carbohydrates into the small intestine.

○ **Which enteric hormones contribute to the vasomotor symptoms of early dumping?**

Serotonin, gastric inhibitory peptide, vasoactive intestinal peptide, and neurotensin.

○ **What is the incidence of the dumping syndrome after Billroth II gastrectomy?**

The incidence of the dumping syndrome may exceed 50% because the operation bypasses both pyloric control and duodenal inhibiting mechanisms.

○ **True/False: Long-acting somatostatin analogues are effective in improving the symptoms of dumping in patients unresponsive to other medical therapy.**

True. These agents improve the symptoms in 90% of patients with early dumping.

○ **Which type of vagotomy is responsible for the highest incidence of postvagotomy diarrhea—truncal, selective, or proximal?**

Truncal vagotomy has the highest incidence (20%), followed by selective vagotomy (5%) and proximal gastric vagotomy (4%).

○ **What percentage of postgastrectomy patient exhibit histologic gastritis?**

Over 60% exhibit histologic gastritis; however, the vast majority remain asymptomatic.

○ **The highest incidence of alkaline gastritis occurs after which operation for peptic ulcer disease?**

Billroth II gastrojejunostomy has the highest incidence, followed by loop gastrojejunostomy, Billroth I gastroduodenostomy, and then pyloroplasty.

○ **What is the surgical treatment in refractory cases of alkaline reflux gastritis?**

Although rarely necessary, conversion to Roux-en-Y gastrojejunal anastomosis.

○ **What medical disorders increase the risk of gastric atony?**

Preoperative gastric outlet obstruction, diabetes mellitus, hypothyroidism, and autonomic neurologic disorders.

○ **What percentage of patients who have the combination of vagotomy, antrectomy, and Roux-en-Y gastrojejunostomy develop epigastric fullness, abdominal pain, nausea, and vomiting—the so-called Roux stasis syndrome?**

Up to 50%.

○ **A patient who had an unknown gastric operation for peptic ulcer disease presents with epigastric fullness, nausea, and vomiting. Upper gastrointestinal barium radiographs demonstrate a mass in the gastric remnant. What is the most likely diagnosis?**

A bezoar is the most likely diagnosis; however, endoscopy is needed to distinguish the bezoar from a neoplasm.

○ **What percentage of patients have abnormal bone loss following gastric resection?**

About 25%.

○ **True/False: The large majority of patients who require treatment for perforation or bleeding due to duodenal ulcer do not have an antecedent history of ulcer pain.**

False. Only about 20% of patients who require treatment for bleeding or perforation do not have a history of ulcer pain.

○ **Which factor does NOT predict death in perforated duodenal ulcer: preoperative shock, perforation for longer than 24 hours, concomitant medical illness, or age?**

Age is not an independent predictor of death in perforated duodenal ulcer.

○ **True/False: A second hospitalization for ulcer hemorrhage is an indication for operation in the treatment of bleeding from duodenal ulcer.**

True, depending on the treatment and prevention recommendations performed previously.

○ **Which artery is primarily responsible for bleeding duodenal ulcers?**

Gastroduodenal artery. Operative management for bleeding from duodenal ulcer includes proximal and distal ligation of the gastroduodenal artery and ligation of the transverse pancreatic branch. (see Figure 19-1).

○   **True/False: Operative treatment of a gastric polyp is indicated for a sessile lesion of 3 cm in diameter.**

True. Operative treatment is indicated for sessile lesions over 2 cm in diameter, when tissue removed endoscopically arouses a question of malignancy, or when definitive treatment cannot be completed endoscopically.

○   **What are the two most common side effects after vagotomy for treatment of peptic ulcer disease?**

Diarrhea and delayed gastric emptying.

○   **What percentage of patients with early dumping do not respond to nonoperative measures and what treatment options exist for these patients?**

About 1%. Jejunal interposition or conversion to Roux-en-Y gastrojejunostomy.

○   **What is the typical presentation of the afferent loop syndrome? What is the treatment?**

Epigastric pain after eating relieved by bilious vomiting. Surgical correction is the only treatment.

○   **What is the recurrence rate of peptic ulcers in patients with retained antrum syndrome? How can this be diagnosed?**

Up to 80%; technetium scan.

○   **True/False: Most marginal ulcers after laparoscopic Roux-en-Y gastric bypass are associated with previously undiagnosed *H. pylori* infection.**

False.

○   **In Figure 19-3, the patient has undergone laparoscopic Roux-en-Y gastric bypass and has developed a marginal ulcer. What commonly associated finding is being demonstrated in Figure 19-4?**

Gastro-gastric fistula.

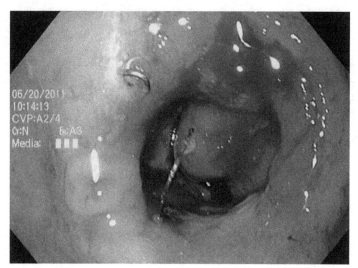

Figure 19-3 See also color plate.

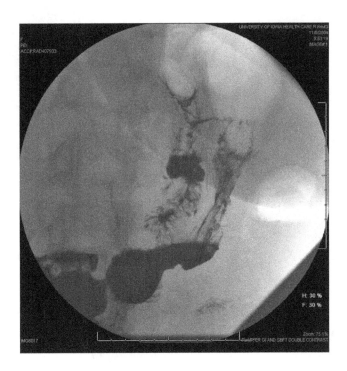

Figure 19-4

● ● ● SUGGESTED READINGS ● ● ●

Yeo CJ. *Shackelford's Surgery of the Alimentary Tract*. 6th ed. Philadelphia, PA: Saunders Elsevier, 2007; 791-939.

Gumbs AA, Duffy AJ, Bell RL. Incidence and management of marginal ulceration after laparoscopic Roux-Y gastric bypass. *Surg Obes Relat Dis*. 2006 Jul-Aug;2(4):460-463.

Gralnek IM, Barkun AN, Bardou M. Management of acute bleeding from a peptic ulcer. *N Engl J Med*. 2008 Aug 28;359(9): 928-937.

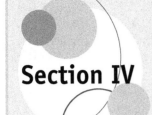

Section IV   SMALL INTESTINE

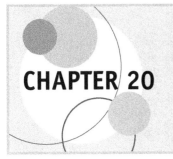

CHAPTER 20

Small Intestinal Congenital and Structural Abnormalities

Ashok Shah, MD and Rajiv Sharma, MD

○ **What is the difference between true and false diverticula?**

False diverticula do not include the muscularis propria in the sac wall.

○ **True/False: Juxtapapillary diverticula have a strong association with gallstones.**

True. Also known as extraluminal duodenal diverticula or periampullary diverticula, they occur within 2 cm of the ampulla of Vater.

○ **True/False: Intraluminal duodenal diverticula are lined by duodenal mucosa on the inside and outside of the structure.**

True. Also known as a windsock diverticulum, this is a single saccular structure that originates in the second portion of the duodenum. They may be connected to the entire circumference or only part of the duodenal wall.

○ **Jejunal diverticula are associated with what disorders?**

They are typically seen in disorders of small intestinal motility such as progressive systemic sclerosis and visceral myopathies and neuropathies.

○ **True/False: Recurrent asymptomatic, nonsurgical pneumoperitoneum may be seen in jejunal diverticulosis?**

True. The presence of free intraperitoneal gas usually warrants emergent surgery; however, some conditions such as jejunal diverticulosis and pneumatosis intestinalis may result in asymptomatic pneumoperitoneum and do not require surgical intervention.

○ **A Meckel's diverticulum is the remnant of what embryological structure?**

The omphalomesenteric or vitelline duct.

○ **True/False: A Meckel's diverticulum occurs on the mesenteric border of the gut.**

False. It occurs on the antimesenteric border.

○ **True/False: The most common location for Meckel's diverticulum is 10 cm from the ileocecal valve.**

False. Most commonly they are 100 cm from the ileocecal valve.

○ **Describe the "rule of two's" as relates to Meckel's diverticulum.**

The rule of two's best describes Meckel's diverticulum. It occurs in 2% of the population with a male-to-female ratio of 2:1, is found within two feet of the ileocecal valve, is two inches long, and approximately 2% develop a complication over the course of their lives.

○ **True/False: Heterotopic tissue is present in one-half of all Meckel's diverticula.**

True. The most common types are gastric mucosa, pancreatic tissue, or a combination of the two.

○ **True/False: Detection of Meckel's diverticula by technetium-99m pertechnetate radionucleotide scanning is dependent on the presence of gastric mucosa within the diverticula.**

True. Technetium-99m pertechnetate scan is considered the standard method for preoperative diagnosis of Meckel's diverticulum. It has a specificity of 95% and a sensitivity of 85%. Technetium-99m is taken up by the ectopic gastric mucosa and may be enhanced by blocking anion secretion from the mucosa with histamine type 2 receptor antagonists administered 24 to 48 hours before the scan.

○ **What is the most common complication of a Meckel's diverticulum in children? In adults?**

In children, usually in infants and those younger than 5, gastrointestinal bleeding occurs most commonly. In adults, intestinal obstruction is more common.

○ **What complications may result from a Meckel's diverticulum in the adult population?**

Complications include obstruction, bleeding, diverticulitis, perforation, and carcinoma.

○ **True/False: Intestinal duplications are hypothesized to develop from aberrant recanalization of the gut during morphogenesis and share the same blood supply with the native intestine.**
True.

○ **True/False: Duplications of the gastrointestinal tract are located on the mesenteric border of the gut.**
True.

○ **True/False: The most common segment of the gut involved in intestinal duplication is the colon.**
False. The ileum is the most common segment followed by the jejunum.

○ **True/False: Intestinal duplication may range from single cystic structures that do not communicate with the native bowel to tubular structures that share the lumen with the native bowel.**
True.

○ **True/False: Gastric mucosa may line intestinal duplications.**
True.

○ **True/False: Intestinal atresia with occlusion of the gut lumen is a common cause of intestinal obstruction in the neonate.**
True.

○ **Duodenal atresia and stenosis are frequently associated with what congenital abnormalities?**

Esophageal atresia, midgut malrotation, imperforate anus, annular pancreas, and Down's syndrome.

○ **Acute pancreatitis occurring in an adult patient with a history of congenital duodenal atresia is most likely related to what condition?**

Annular pancreas is a rare cause of acute pancreatitis in the setting of duodenal atresia.

○ **True/False: The distribution of gut atresia can range from the esophagus to the rectum.**

True.

○ **What is the incidence of small bowel atresia?**

1 in 3000 to 5000 live births.

○ **True/False: Small intestinal atresia is more common in a woman who has had multiple pregnancies compared with a woman with a single pregnancy.**

True.

○ **Describe the four types of intestinal atresia.**

Type I– diaphragm of mucosa and submucosa obstructs the lumen but the bowel wall and mesentery are intact.

Type II – two blind bowel ends connected by a fibrous cord.

Type IIIA – two blind bowel ends separated by a mesenteric gap.

Type IIIB – "apple peel" atresia—proximal small bowel atresia and absence of the distal superior mesenteric artery.

Type IV – "string of sausages"—multiple atretic regions throughout the small bowel.

○ **Duodenal atresia is thought to develop at what gestational age?**

Recanalization of the intestinal lumen from the solid cord stage occurs at 4 to 8 weeks of gestation.

○ **True/False: Polyhydramnios is frequently associated with gastrointestinal atresia of the distal gut.**

False. Proximal gut atresia is associated with polyhydramnios.

○ **A double-bubble sign on abdominal radiograph or ultrasound in a neonate is classic for what type of intestinal atresia?**

Duodenal atresia.

○ **True/False: Common presenting signs of a proximal (duodenal or proximal jejunum) atresia include jaundice and bilious vomiting.**

True. Distal atresias often present with abdominal distension.

○ **What are the two major complications of gut malrotation?**

Volvulus around the vascular pedicle and duodenal obstruction secondary to Ladd bands.

○ **True/False: Ladd bands are peritoneal bands that pass from the cecum across the duodenum to the right upper quadrant or to the duodenum and form after malrotation of the gut.**

True.

○ **The Ladd procedure is undertaken for management of what condition?**

Intestinal malrotation. The Ladd procedure involves division of the Ladd bands, if present, widening of the base of the mesentery by dividing any adhesions between the duodenum and cecum at the base of the mesentery, passing a tube through the duodenum to rule out any associated duodenal obstruction (in the newborn), appendectomy, and placing viable bowel in a position of nonrotation.

○ **Describe the gut anatomy following nonrotation.**

The small intestine (jejunum and ileum) lies on the right side of the abdomen and the colon is entirely on the left. The cecum lies in the left iliac fossa.

○ **What is reversed rotation of the gut?**

The gut rotates clockwise, instead of the normal 270-degree counterclockwise rotation, resulting in the colon entering the abdominal cavity first. The colon then takes a position posterior to the superior mesenteric artery and the duodenum. The small bowel mesentery passes in front of the transverse colon.

○ **True/False: Less than half of midgut malrotations present in infancy.**

False. Fifty percent to 80% present in infancy.

○ **True/False: Biliary atresia and congenital heart disease are associated with gut malrotation.**

True.

○ **True/False: Omphaloceles are sac-covered abdominal viscera herniating through the umbilical ring.**

True.

○ **True/False: Gastroschisis is a small defect in the abdominal wall usually to the right of the closed umbilical ring through which there is massive evisceration of the intestines with direct exposure to amniotic fluid.**

True. It requires immediate operation because a membrane does not cover the bowel.

○ **What is the gestational age when gastroschisis or omphaloceles develop?**

Between the fifth and tenth week of gestation.

○ **True/False: An elevated alpha-fetoprotein level in maternal serum is associated with ventral fetal abdominal wall defects such as omphalocele and gastroschisis.**

True.

○ **True/False: Long-term morbidity and mortality of gastroschisis are high because of the high risk of necrotizing enterocolitis, bowel perforation, or necrosis and the need for prolonged parenteral nutrition complicating the course.**

True.

○ **True/False: Omphaloceles are associated with extraintestinal birth defects, whereas gastroschisis is rarely associated with other defects.**

True.

○ **True/False: Volvulus of the small bowel in the absence of preexisting defects is more common in Africa, the Middle East, and India because of the ingestion of bulky foods after periods of fasting.**

True. Volvulus of the small bowel is rare in the United States without preexisting defects.

○ **True/False: Intussusception is one of the most common causes of bowel obstruction in children under the age of 2.**

True.

○ **What is the cause and frequency of a pathologic lead point in pediatric intussusception?**

Most are idiopathic. Approximately 8%–12% will have a structural abnormality such as a polyp, leiomyoma, or lymphoma. Benign lymphoid tissue has also been suggested as a potential lead point.

○ **True/False: The classic triad of pain, a palpable sausage-shaped abdominal mass, and currant-jelly stool occurs in most children who present with intussusception.**

False. This triad is seen in less than 15% of patients at the time of presentation.

○ **True/False: Intussusception may complicate the course of Henoch–Schonlein purpura.**

True. The vasculitic bowel may result in an intramural hematoma that acts as a lead point for intussusception.

○ **True/False: Small bowel intussusception is a major cause of intestinal obstruction in adults in the Western world.**

False. Approximately 5% of adult intestinal obstructions are caused by intussusception.

○ **What is the frequency of a pathologic lead point in adult intussusception?**

Approximately 90% of adult intussusceptions will have an identifiable cause such as a polyp, tumor, Meckel's diverticulum, and celiac disease with flaccid bowel.

○ **What is the most common bowel segment involved in cases of intussusception occurring in the pediatric population?**

Ileocolic intussusception is the most common.

○ **True/False: Reduction of an ileocolic intussusception in a stable pediatric patient should first be attempted by barium enema.**

True. Pneumatic or hydrostatic (eg, barium) enema is often successful in reducing an intussusception in a child.

○ **True/False: In adults with intussusception, the proper surgical management, in the absence of infarcted or gangrenous bowel, is manual reduction.**

False. Since many lead points in the adult population are malignant, manual reduction is not recommended. Instead, bowel resection of the affected segment is recommended.

○   **What clinical findings may be found in intestinal lymphangiectasia?**

Steatosis, malabsorption, lymphocytopenia, hypogammaglobulinemia, protein-losing enteropathy, chylous ascites, chlyous pleural effusion, and peripheral edema.

○   **What medical conditions may lead to secondary lymphangiectasia?**

Abdominal/retroperitoneal carcinoma/lymphoma, retroperitoneal fibrosis, pancreatitis, tuberculosis, Crohn's disease, celiac disease, systemic lupus erythematosus, and congestive heart failure.

○   **Congenital lymphangiectasia is also referred to as what?**

Milroy's disease.

○   **True/False: Wilkie syndrome is caused by compression of the third portion of duodenum by superior mesenteric artery.**

True. Superior mesenteric artery syndrome is also known as both Wilkie syndrome and Cast syndrome.

○   **Chronic postprandial abdominal pain and radiographic evidence of celiac artery compression should make one think of what diagnosis?**

Median arcuate ligament syndrome (MALS). Also known as celiac artery compression syndrome, MALS is caused by abnormally low insertion of the median fibrous arcuate ligament and muscular diaphragmatic fiber resulting in luminal narrowing of the celiac trunk.

○   **What is the traditional treatment of MALS?**

Surgical division of the median arcuate ligament and complete celiac ganglionectomy.

○   **How can a definite diagnosis of MALS be achieved?**

Lateral aortography of the visceral aorta and its branches during inspiration and expiration.

● ● ● SUGGESTED READINGS ● ● ●

Berrocal T, Lamas M, Gutieerrez J, Torres I, Prieto C, del Hoyo ML. Congenital anomalies of the small intestine, colon, and rectum. *Radiographics.* 1999 Sep–Oct;19(5):1219-1236.

Morikawa N, Kuroda T, Honna T, et al. A novel association of duodenal atresia, malrotation, segmental dilatation of the colon, and anorectal malformation. *Pediatr Surg Int.* 2009 Nov;25(11):1003-1005.

Vaos G, Misiakos EP. Congenital anomalies of the gastrointestinal tract diagnosed in adulthood–diagnosis and management. *J Gastrointest Surg.* 2010 May;14(5):916-925.

CHAPTER 21

Small Intestinal Infectious Disorders

Kevin C. Ruff, MD

○ **A 36-year-old man presents with chronic diarrhea, glossitis, and peripheral neuropathy. He returned several months ago from a 6-month mission to Haiti. What is the most likely diagnosis?**

Tropical sprue.

○ **What is the cause of tropical sprue?**

Current evidence suggests that tropical sprue results from an infectious disease of the small intestine caused by several offending agents, all of which are toxigenic strains of coliform bacteria, including *Klebsiella pneumoniae*, *Enterobacter cloacae*, and *Escherichia coli*. Travelers who acquire tropical sprue persist with bacterial contamination after return to a temperate climate until antibiotic treatment is given.

○ **What is the treatment of tropical sprue?**

Tetracycline or nonabsorbable sulfonamides given for several months. Additionally, daily oral folic acid and weekly parenteral B12 should be given when megaloblastic anemia is present.

○ **What symptoms may precede gastrointestinal complaints in Whipple's disease?**

Arthralgias and fever. Migratory arthralgias of the large joints may precede the onset of diarrhea by several years.

○ **What is the diagnostic procedure of choice for Whipple's disease?**

Upper endoscopy with multiple biopsies of duodenum or proximal jejunum. Biopsies show infiltration of the lamina propria with periodic acid-Schiff (PAS)-positive macrophages containing Gram-positive, acid-fast negative bacilli.

○ **In the absence of histologic evidence of Whipple's disease on small bowel biopsy, what further testing can be used to detect *Tropheryma whippelii*?**

Polymerase chain reaction of biopsied tissue.

○ **Why should rectal biopsy not be used to diagnose Whipple's disease?**

PAS-positive macrophages resembling those seen in Whipple's disease may be found in the rectal lamina propria of healthy individuals and in patients with benign conditions such as melanosis coli and colonic histiocytosis.

○ **What condition resembles Whipple's disease histologically?**

Intestinal infection with *Mycobacterium avium intracellulare*. The histologic lesions in these two conditions are similar; however, *T. whippelii* will not take up acid-fast stain.

○ **What is the most serious sequela in a patient with Whipple's disease?**

Neurologic sequelae, including irreversible dementia, may occur several months or years after successful treatment. This suggests that, unless an antibiotic that readily penetrates the blood-brain barrier is used, the central nervous system may provide a safe haven for residual Whipple's bacilli.

○ **What is the treatment of Whipple's disease?**

Double-strength trimethoprim-sulfamethoxazole twice daily for a year. This antibiotic readily crosses the blood-brain barrier and should effectively eradicate central nervous system involvement. For patients intolerant of this drug, a third-generation cephalosporin can be used.

○ **What is the treatment of a central nervous system relapse in Whipple's disease?**

Repeat initial therapy with double-strength trimethoprim-sulfamethoxazole. If unsuccessful, chloramphenicol, which also results in high central nervous system concentrations, is given at a dose of 250 mg four times a day.

○ **What is the appearance of *Cryptosporidium* on mucosal biopsy specimens?**

On light microscopy, the trophozoites appear as multiple, round, tiny basophilic bodies lying on the brush border of enterocytes.

○ **After successful treatment of intestinal cryptosporidiosis in immunocompromised patients, what causes recurrence?**

Seeding from the biliary tract, where *Cryptosporidia* can also reside.

○ **How is *Isospora belli* detected in the stool?**

Oocysts in the stool fluoresce bright yellow with auramine-rhodamine stain and appear pink with red-purple sporocysts on a modified acid-fast stain.

○ **What segment of the intestinal tract is most commonly involved in histoplasmosis?**

Terminal ileum.

○ **True/False: Histoplasmosis can occur in an immunocompetent host.**

True. Histoplasmosis is a very common infection in the midwestern and south-central United States, where 80% of inhabitants are infected. However, gastrointestinal disease is seen only in immunocompromised individuals.

○ **When should infection with microsporidiosis be considered?**

When no other pathogens are identified in an immunocompromised patient with severe diarrhea, malabsorption, and weight loss.

○ **What is the most specific diagnostic tool for detecting *Microsporidia* in intestinal biopsy specimens?**

Electron microscopy. Under light microscopy, the organism is difficult to identify.

○ **Why should patients with underlying liver disease be warned about eating raw seafood, especially raw oysters?**

Vibrio vulnificus infection can be acquired through direct consumption of seafood, usually raw oysters. Subsequent septicemia has a 50% mortality rate. This infection can be lethal in patients with underlying liver disease.

○ **What severe intestinal complications may occur in typhoid fever?**

Perforation (3% of cases) and hemorrhage (20% in pre-antibiotic era). These events are not related to the severity of the disease and tend to occur in the same patient, with bleeding serving as a harbinger of a possible perforation.

○ **True/False: The distal ileum and cecum are the most common sites of intestinal involvement with tuberculosis.**

True.

○ **What small intestinal parasite, once ingested, has part of its life cycle in the lungs?**

Ascaris lumbricoides. Duodenal larvae migrate through the epithelium into portal venous blood and eventually reach the lungs causing a pneumonitis. Larvae then migrate up the bronchioles to the pharynx, are swallowed, and develop into adults in the small intestine.

○ **What tapeworm may cause vitamin B12 deficiency?**

Diphyllobothrium latum. The worm ingests vitamin B12 and competes with the host for available vitamin B12.

○ **What parasitic infestation may result in variceal bleeding?**

Schistosomiasis. Granulomatous fibrosis occurs around entrapped ova in prehepatic portal venules with relative sparing of hepatic parenchyma. This results in presinusoidal portal hypertension.

○ **True/False: Rotavirus, Norovirus, and Enterovirus are causes of enteritis that occur primarily in children.**

False. Rotavirus and Enterovirus are most common in young children. Norovirus affects all ages and is responsible for outbreaks in camps, cruise ships, hospitals, and nursing homes.

○ **What Gram-negative curved rod with a single flagella can cause 15–20 liters of stool per day?**

Vibrio cholera.

○ **True/False: Bloody diarrhea is a common symptom caused by *Vibrio cholera* due to the invasive nature of this organism.**

False. "Rice water" stools are typical, not blood. *V. cholera* causes diarrhea by attaching to the intestinal epithelium and releasing a toxin which increases cAMP, leading to a secretory diarrhea.

○ **True/False: *Yersinia* enterocolitis typically occurs in children over the age of 5 years and may be confused with acute appendicitis.**

True. Radiographic imaging studies may be useful to distinguish between the two.

○ **True/False: There is no substantial evidence that antibiotics alter the course of *Yersinia* gastrointestinal infection, even in immunocompromised patients.**

True, although antibiotic treatment is mandatory in the latter.

○ **Daycare centers and well water are risk factors for which protozoal infection?**

Giardia lamblia (also known as *G. intestinalis* and *G. duodenalis*). Infective cysts are ingested and the flagellated trophozoites become active after excystation due to gastric acid exposure.

○ **Which treatment for *Giardia* may be most appropriate for pregnant women?**

Paromomycin is not absorbed and so poses less risk to the developing fetus than metronidazole or nitazoxanide.

○ **What is the most likely route of transmission for *Cyclospora cayetanensis*?**

Contaminated water or produce, especially during wet summer months. There is no person-to-person spread.

○ **Charcot-Layden crystals are found in stool analysis for which protozoal infection?**

Isosporidia. Individuals may also have peripheral eosinophilia.

○ **A serpiginous, pruritic rash known as cutaneous larva migrans occurs in which nematode infection?**

Hookworm. Exposure to soil contaminated with human waste allows entry through the skin, causing this characteristic rash.

○ **True/False: *Trichenella* is identified primarily on stool testing.**

False. Eggs are laid after invasion of the intestinal villae and larvae mature in striated muscle. Diagnosis is made by serology or muscle biopsy.

○ **Which cestode is the largest human parasite?**

Diphyllobothrium latum (fish tapeworm). It can grow up to 40 feet long.

○ **Cysticercosis is caused by which parasitic organism and how is it treated?**

Taenia solium. Albendazole is the treatment of choice with steroids as needed for inflammation that develops during treatment.

○ **What is the most common tapeworm in humans?**

Hymenolepis nana (dwarf tapeworm). It is the smallest but most common tapeworm in humans due to the ease of person-to-person transmission, self-inoculation, and internal autoinfection.

○ **What intracellular parasitic infection is a common cause of diarrheal outbreaks in chlorinated pools?**

Cryptosporidiosis. *Cryptosporidium* is chlorine resistant in the spore form with excystation occurring in the small intestine due to bile salt exposure.

○ **What is the treatment of choice for cryptosporidiosis?**

Nitazoxanide is the only known drug with consistent efficacy in treating *Cryptosporidium*.

○ **What host mechanisms prevent against the development of small intestinal bacterial overgrowth (SIBO)?**

Intestinal motility, gastric acid production, intestinal epithelial mucus layer, bile and pancreatic secretions, as well as the intestinal immune system.

○   **True/False: An intact ileocecal valve is the most important anatomical factor predisposing to the development of SIBO.**

False. Blind loops and strictures are more important anatomical factors. In fact, the role of the ileocecal valve in preventing SIBO in nonshort bowel syndrome patients remains unclear.

○   **What are the most common presenting signs and symptoms of SIBO?**

The most frequent presenting symptoms are abdominal pain, diarrhea, weight loss, bloating, excess flatulence, malabsorption, and anemia (usually macrocytic).

○   **True/False: Elevated vitamin B12 and decreased folate levels are classic findings in SIBO.**

False. The opposite is true; albeit, uncommon.

○   **True/False: Given the limitations in diagnostic testing for SIBO, empiric antibiotic therapy is the recommended "diagnostic" tool of choice in suspected SIBO.**

False. Although this approach appears to be commonly followed in clinical practice, it is not recommended due to the difficulty in determining the response and the cost and side effects of antibiotic treatment. (Note: Additional questions regarding SIBO, diagnostic testing for SIBO in particular, are in the Chapter 22 "Small Intestinal Motility Disorders.")

○   **Describe the major treatment modalities used in SIBO.**

Treatment of the underlying disease and antibiotics represent the major treatment modalities. Although modification of the diet to include high-fat, low-carbohydrate, and low-fiber elements has been recommended, there is no evidence from controlled trials to support this approach.

○   **True/False: Antibiotic therapy in SIBO should focus on anaerobic organisms.**

False. Effective antibiotic treatment should cover both aerobic and anaerobic enteric bacteria given the usual broad-spectrum of the microbes involved. Similarly, bacterial culture and sensitivity testing is often not helpful since various bacterial species with different antibiotic sensitivities coexist.

○   **What organisms are commonly implicated in traveler's diarrhea?**

E. coli (ETEC), *Shigella*, *Campylobacter*, and *Salmonella* are the most common bacterial causes. Viruses and parasites also may be responsible and include such organisms as rotavirus, *Giardia*, *Cryptosporidia*, and *Cyclospora*.

○   **True/False: Parasitic causes of traveler's diarrhea are common in traveler's to Mexico.**

False. Parasitic traveler's diarrhea is rare.

○   **True/False: Traveler's diarrhea follows a benign, self-limited course in the vast majority of cases.**

True. However, dehydration can occur and may be serious.

○   **True/False: A college student on spring break to Cancun has an equal risk of contracting traveler's diarrhea as a business executive attending an industry conference in Mexico City.**

False. Traveler's diarrhea is more common in younger adults than older adults and more common in traveling students or tourists than business professionals or people visiting relatives.

○ **Since traveler's diarrhea is generally self-limited, treatment is often symptomatic and initiated without documenting an etiologic agent. When should treatment be considered and what are the main treatment modalities?**

If symptoms are severe and associated with toxicity or if they persist beyond 48 to 72 hours, intervention may be necessary. Fluid replacement is the mainstay of treatment. Antibiotics and antidiarrheal agents may also be needed.

○ **True/False: Stool culture should always be done prior to antibiotic treatment in cases of suspected traveler's diarrhea.**

False.

○ **True/False: Antibiotic therapy reduces the duration of illness by about 1 day.**

True. Antibiotics are warranted to treat diarrhea in those who develop moderate to severe diarrhea as characterized by more than four unformed stools daily, fever, blood, pus, or mucus in the stool. Common antibiotic agents used include fluoroquinolones, azithromycin, and rifaximin. Quinolones are usually given for 1 or 2 days after the onset of diarrhea, while the others are typically given for 3 days.

○ **True/False: Bismuth subsalicylate can be an effective prophylaxis for traveler's diarrhea.**

True. Greater than 50% of cases of traveler's diarrhea can be prevented by daily use of bismuth subsalicylate. Antibiotics may be more effective but are expensive and have a greater risk of side effects. Bismuth can also be used to treat an episode of traveler's diarrhea; however, large doses are generally required with the potential for salicylate toxicity.

○ **True/False: Prophylactic antibiotics are recommended for all travelers to developing countries.**

False. Although prophylactic antibiotics prevent the majority of diarrheal disease in travelers, they are generally not recommended unless the complications of diarrhea or an underlying medical condition make the consequence of dehydration so severe that the benefits of using antibiotic prophylaxis outweigh the risks.

● ● ● **SUGGESTED READINGS** ● ● ●

Hill DR, Beeching NJ. Travelers' diarrhea. *Curr Opin Infect Dis.* 2010 Oct;23(5):481-487.

Quigley EM, Abu-Shanab A. Small intestinal bacterial overgrowth. *Infect Dis Clin North Am.* 2010 Dec;24(4):943-959.

Nath SK. Tropical sprue. *Curr Gastroenterol Rep.* 2005 Oct;7(5):343-349.

Afshar P, Redfield DC, Higginbottom PA. Whipple's disease: a rare disease revisited. *Curr Gastroenterol Rep.* 2010 Aug;12(4):263-269.

Gianella R. Infectious Enteritis and Proctocolitis and Bacterial Food Poisoning. In: Feldman M, Friedman, L, Brandt L, eds. *Sleisenger and Fordtran's Gastrointestinal and Liver Diseases.* 9th ed. Philadelphia, PA: Saunders-Elsevier; 2010:1843-1886.

CHAPTER 22   Small Intestinal Motility Disorders

Rejy Joseph, MD and
Robin D. Rothstein, MD

○ **What is the migrating motor complex (MMC)?**

The migrating motor complex is a cyclical pattern of gastrointestinal motility occurring during the fasting period that consists of three phases that repeat every 90 to 120 minutes. Phase I is a period of absent motor activity (motor quiescence) lasting 40 to 70 minutes. Phase II lasts 20 to 30 minutes and is characterized by irregular motor activity. Phase III consists of a 5- to 10-minute period of intense lumen-occluding contractions that begin in the body of the stomach and sequentially propagate aborally through the small intestine.

○ **What physical finding is usually present in a scleroderma patient with gastrointestinal dysmotility?**

Raynaud's phenomenon.

○ **What complications may occur in a scleroderma patient with small bowel involvement?**

Malabsorption, pseudo-obstruction, pneumatosis cystoides intestinalis, bacterial overgrowth, and malnutrition.

○ **True/False: The abnormalities in small bowel motility that may occur in scleroderma occur secondary to a myopathic process.**

False. Both myopathic and neuropathic abnormalities are responsible. The neurologic changes typically occur first followed by myopathic alterations.

○ **Subcutaneous octreotide has been used to manage small bowel motor complications of scleroderma. What is a common long-term complication of this therapy?**

The development of biliary sludge and gallstones.

○ **What effect does low dose octreotide have on small bowel motility as detected by intestinal manometry?**

Stimulates phase III of the migrating motor complex. However, higher doses of octreotide actually inhibit gastrointestinal motility.

○ **What developmental abnormality of the gastrointestinal tract may occur in children with familial pseudo-obstruction syndromes?**

Intestinal malrotation or nonrotation.

○ **In general, surgery is not performed in patients with chronic idiopathic intestinal pseudo-obstruction; however, surgery may be considered in certain circumstances. What surgical procedures are occasionally performed in these patients?**

Placement of venting gastrostomy and/or jejunostomy tubes, ileostomy or colostomy, and intestinal transplantation.

○ **What complication of gut dysmotility is associated with an increased risk of spontaneous bacterial peritonitis in patients with end-stage liver disease?**

Small bowel dysmotility is associated with bacterial overgrowth that may lead to bacterial translocation resulting in systemic infection.

○ **A 36-year-old man with short bowel syndrome as a result of vascular injury during an exploratory laparotomy presents with persistent foul-smelling diarrhea despite various dietary maneuvers and antidiarrheal agents. What small intestinal condition is likely to be responsible for the diarrhea?**

Small intestinal bacterial overgrowth.

○ **The use of proton pump inhibitors may further increase what complication in patients with chronic intestinal pseudo-obstruction?**

Small intestinal bacterial overgrowth. While the hypochlorhydria caused by potent antisecretory agents does not generally result in clinically significant bacterial overgrowth (with clinically significant types of bacteria) in otherwise healthy individuals, it may in patients with chronic intestinal pseudo-obstruction.

○ **List some causes of mechanical obstruction that may occur in patients with chronic intestinal pseudo-obstruction.**

Adhesions from prior surgery or bezoars related to hypomotility.

○ **What endocrine conditions may cause small intestinal dysmotility?**

Diabetes mellitus, hypothyroidism, hyper- and hypoparathyroidism, and adrenal insufficiency.

○ **When should antibiotics be considered for use in cases of chronic intestinal pseudo-obstruction?**

Antibiotics may be considered if there is bacterial overgrowth and can be used on a rotational schedule to delay/prevent the development of antibiotic resistance.

○ **What are nonendocrine causes of pseudo-obstruction?**

Amyloidosis, paraneoplastic syndrome, connective tissue diseases (scleroderma), degenerative neuropathies, viral diseases, radiotherapy, and medications.

○ **What medications are associated with the development of chronic intestinal pseudo-obstruction?**

Narcotics, tricyclic antidepressants, phenothiazines, ganglionic blockers, calcium-channel blockers, and anti-Parkinson's medications are a few of the more common medications associated with this condition.

○ **What clinical tests are available to diagnose intestinal dysmotility?**

First and foremost, it is essential to rule out mechanical obstruction. Nuclear scintigraphy may be used to evaluate transit through the stomach, small intestine, and colon. Stationary or ambulatory small bowel manometry may be performed using a water-perfused or solid-state catheter.

○ **What features on small bowel manometry suggest myopathic or neuropathic causes of chronic intestinal pseudo-obstruction?**

In myopathy, there are low amplitude contractions and in neuropathic conditions, there is organizational disarray of the phase III complex (intrinsic neuropathy) or fed pattern (extrinsic neuropathy).

○ **Why is it important to differentiate mechanical obstruction from pseudo-obstruction and how is this best accomplished?**

Treatment of the two conditions is significantly different. Barium contrast studies, including small bowel follow-through or enteroclysis, may indicate a transition point. The latter is the more sensitive of the two. CT enterography is also useful and has generally superseded barium contrast studies in the diagnosis of bowel obstruction. Small bowel manometry may also be helpful as patterns suggestive of mechanical obstruction have been described and include simultaneous or rapidly propagating clustered contractions and/or high amplitude, prolonged, or giant contractions.

○ **What tumors and associated autoantibodies occur with paraneoplastic visceral neuropathy?**

The most common tumor causing paraneoplastic visceral neuropathy is small cell cancer of the lung, which may also be associated with a generalized sensory neuropathy. Histologically, there may be degeneration of neurons and a lymphoplasmacytic infiltration in the bowel, but no evidence of tumor. Associated antibodies that can be detected in the serum are anti-Hu, aka ANNA-1 (type 1 antineuronal nuclear antibody).

○ **What tests are useful for the diagnosis of bacterial overgrowth and what are their potential shortcomings?**

Culture of small intestinal aspirate is the gold standard in the diagnosis of bacterial overgrowth; however, both false positives (contamination) and false negatives (difficulties in culturing anerobes) may occur. Alternatively, a ^{14}C-xylose breath test, which measures expired CO_2 production, can be used. However, it requires the use of radiolabeled material and is not widely available. Hydrogen breath testing using either glucose or lactulose as a substrate is also widely available and does not involve radiation; however, its sensitivity and specificity have been questioned.

○ **What are the shortcomings of hydrogen breath tests?**

Interpretation may be difficult in some cases when there are altered transit times. In these cases, the hydrogen peak occurring from SIBO may be difficult to discriminate from the normal peak from colonic bacteria. False negative results occur in patients with low bacterial counts or those who do not have hydrogen-generating bacteria (8%–20%).

○ **What findings are suggestive of small bowel bacterial overgrowth on the breath hydrogen test?**

An increase in breath hydrogen (usually > 20 ppm) expired during the first 2 hours of ingestion of substrate or an elevation of the fasting breath hydrogen (also usually > 20 ppm). The classical double-peak described in the lactulose hydrogen breath test is infrequently seen and does not appear to reliably distinguish small bowel bacterial overgrowth.

○ **What measures could improve the reliability of breath testing for bacterial overgrowth?**

Certain foods (bread, pasta, fiber) should be avoided prior to testing as they cause prolonged hydrogen secretion. Cigarette smoking or vigorous physical exercise may also affect hydrogen secretion and needs to be avoided for 2 hours prior to testing. Oral bacteria may lead to an early hydrogen peak; thus, pretest mouthwashing with an antiseptic should be considered.

○ **What disturbances in small bowel motility may be seen in amyloidosis?**

Dysmotility seems to correlate with the degree of amyloid deposition in the gut. Small bowel loops may be dilated and transit can be delayed. Small bowel motility studies may reveal findings consistent with either a myopathic or a neuropathic disturbance.

○ **What small bowel motility abnormalities have been described in irritable bowel syndrome?**

Most studies do not indicate any specific abnormality; however, some patients have discrete clustered contractions in the duodenum and jejunum that are associated with symptoms.

○ **What is the utility of a full-thickness intestinal biopsy in a patient with suspected pseudo-obstruction?**

To completely evaluate the neuromuscular apparatus of the gut, a full-thickness intestinal biopsy with special stains for muscle, nerves, and connective tissue can be obtained. The clinical utility of this information, however, remains unclear and opportunities to obtain this tissue are infrequently encountered.

○ **What factors play a role in the pathophysiology of ileus?**

The lack of intestinal activity is most likely related to increased sympathetic inhibitory activity (imbalance of autonomic nervous system) and a resultant loss of normal coordination of activity. Nitric oxide, vasoactive intestinal polypeptide, and possibly substance P act as inhibitory neurotransmitters in the gut and may also play a role. Finally, decreases in motilin and increases in the inhibitory factor's calcitonin gene-related peptide and corticotropin-releasing factor have also been implicated in the pathophysiology of ileus.

● ● ● **SUGGESTED READINGS** ● ● ●

Stanghellini V, Cogliandro RF, de Giorgio R, Barbara G, Salvioli B, Corinaldesi R. Chronic intestinal pseudo-obstruction: manifestations, natural history and management. *Neurogastroenterol Motil.* 2007;19(6):440-452.

Millar AJ, Gupte G, Sharif K. Intestinal transplantation for motility disorders. *Semin Pediatr Surg.* 2009;18(4):258-262.

Bures J, Cyrany J, Kohoutova D, et al. Small intestinal bacterial overgrowth syndrome. *World J Gastroenterol.* 2010;16(24):2978-2990.

CHAPTER 23

Small Intestinal Tumors

Suryakanth R. Gurudu, MD, FACG, FASGE

○ **What percentage of primary gastrointestinal tumors originate in the small bowel?**

Less than 5%.

○ **What clinical conditions are associated with an increased risk of small bowel tumors?**

- Crohn's disease of the small intestine (adenocarcinoma)
- Familial adenomatous polyposis (adenoma and adenocarcinoma, particularly periampullary)
- Celiac sprue (lymphoma and adenocarcinoma)
- AIDS (non-Hodgkin's lymphoma and Kaposi's sarcoma)
- Neurofibromatosis (leiomyoma and adenocarcinoma)
- Ileal conduit or ileocystoplasty (adenocarcinoma)
- Ileostomy after colectomy (adenocarcinoma at ileocutaneous junction)
- Immunoproliferative small intestine disease (non-Hodgkin's lymphoma)
- Nodular lymphoid hyperplasia (non-Hodgkin's lymphoma)

○ **What is the most common benign small bowel tumor?**

Adenoma. Followed in descending order by leiomyoma, Brunner's gland hamartoma, and lipoma. As in the colon, adenomas of the small bowel are considered premalignant.

○ **What is the most common malignant small bowel tumor?**

Adenocarcinoma. Followed in descending order by carcinoid, lymphoma, and leiomyosarcoma.

○ **What is the most common presentation of malignant periampullary tumors?**

Jaundice is seen in up to 80% of cases.

○ **What is the most common clinical presentation of benign small bowel tumors?**

While most remain asymptomatic, mechanical small bowel obstruction, usually related to luminal constriction or intussusception, is the most common clinical presentation.

○ **What nongastrointestinal malignancy has the highest rate of metastasis to the small bowel?**

Melanoma.

○ **Which benign small bowel tumor has the highest propensity for malignant change?**

Villous adenoma. They are often sessile, located in the second portion of the duodenum and 40%–45% have undergone malignant degeneration at the time of diagnosis.

○ **What is the most common cause of intussusception in adults?**

Benign small bowel tumors. Lipomas are the leading cause.

○ **Where are lipomas of the small intestine most often located?**

Ileum.

○ **What is the initial therapy of choice for small bowel adenomas?**

Endoscopic mucosal resection (EMR) is safe and effective; however, the presence of a villous adenoma or the presence of malignant changes on biopsy warrants surgical resection. The size and sessile nature of most villous adenomas make complete resection by endoscopic methods almost impossible. High rates of cancerous transformation also make surgery a preferred option.

○ **What is the most appropriate treatment of small bowel adenomas that cannot be resected endoscopically?**

Laparotomy with segmental resection.

○ **What symptoms are most commonly produced by duodenal villous adenomas?**

Most symptomatic duodenal villous adenomas are 3 cm or more in diameter. The usual clinical presentations include partial gastric outlet obstruction, pancreatitis, bleeding, and obstructive jaundice.

○ **What is the leading cause of cancer death in patients who have undergone proctocolectomy for familial adenomatous polyposis?**

Adenocarcinoma of the proximal small bowel.

○ **True/False: Endoscopic surveillance of the upper gastrointestinal tract is indicated in individuals with familial adenomatous polyposis.**

True.

○ **What is the diagnostic test of choice in the evaluation of patients with a suspected small bowel tumor?**

CT or MR enterography; particularly in patients with obstructive symptoms. Capsule endoscopy and balloon-assisted enteroscopy may play a complementary role in the evaluation.

○ **Which benign small bowel tumor has the highest predilection for severe gastrointestinal bleeding?**

Gastrointestinal stromal tumor (GIST). As these tumors grow, they can undergo necrosis and bleeding which is sometimes severe.

○ **What radiographic or endoscopic feature is commonly seen in GIST?**

Central ulceration of the lesion may be seen as umbilication on barium radiograph or endoscopy.

○ **What is the cell of origin of a GIST?**

The interstitial cell of Cajal, an intestinal pacemaker cell.

○ **What is the most common location for a GIST?**

Stomach followed by small bowel.

○ **What endoscopic ultrasound (EUS) findings are suggestive of a benign natural history of a GIST?**

Regular margins, tumor size less than 3 cm, and a homogeneous echogenicity pattern. Presence of cystic spaces and irregular margins predict malignant potential.

○ **What is the therapeutic agent of choice for unresectable or metastatic GIST?**

Imatinib.

○ **True/False: Peutz–Jeghers syndrome affects the small bowel.**

True. Patients with this syndrome develop hamartomatous polyps throughout the gut. These polyps are especially common in the jejunum. Malignant degeneration can occur but is rare.

○ **Which small bowel malignancy has the slowest rate of growth and metastasis?**

Carcinoid. The average time from onset of symptoms to death from metastases is 9 years.

○ **What organs are most frequently involved by metastases from small bowel carcinoid tumors?**

Liver, bone (especially bones of the orbit and the eye itself), female breast, and ovary.

○ **How do small bowel carcinoid tumors lead to intestinal ischemia?**

Spread of disease into mesenteric and celiac lymph nodes produces encasement of the mesenteric artery causing ischemia and eventually small bowel infarction. This is a surprisingly frequent cause of death with small bowel carcinoids.

○ **Malignant carcinoids are most commonly found in which portion of the small bowel?**

Forty-four percent of all gastrointestinal carcinoids arise in the small bowel. The ileum is the most frequent location for gastrointestinal carcinoids.

○ **What is the most important factor that influences whether a carcinoid tumor is metastatic?**

Size of the primary lesion. Metastasis is found in only 6% of tumors less than 1 cm in diameter. Conversely, tumors over 2 cm have metastases in over 80% of cases.

○ **What is the surgery of choice for an appendiceal carcinoid tumor more than 2 cm in size?**

Right hemicolectomy is appropriate for tumor size more than 2 cm, extension into muscularis propria, or evidence of lymph node metastasis. Appendectomy alone is adequate for tumor size <2 cm in size. Appendiceal carcinoids are often found incidentally at the time of appendectomy and have the best prognosis of all types of carcinoids.

○   **True/False: Small bowel carcinoids commonly present with gastrointestinal bleeding.**

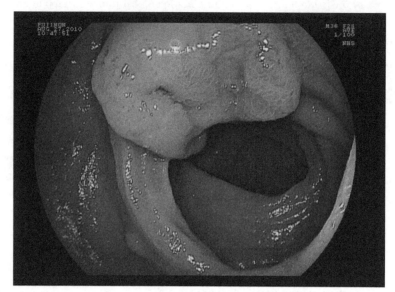

Figure 23-1 See also color plate.

False. Gastrointestinal bleeding from ulcerated tumors as shown in the figure is uncommon. Intermittent obstructive symptoms are more common. Presentation with the carcinoid syndrome is rare.

○   **What are the most common symptoms of carcinoid syndrome?**

Flushing, diarrhea, and abdominal pain. Asthma, pellagra, and cardiac valvular lesions are uncommon.

○   **When do patients with small bowel carcinoid tumors develop the carcinoid syndrome?**

Typically only when hepatic metastasis is present. Even with hepatic lesions, 30%–50% of patients with carcinoid tumors do not develop the carcinoid syndrome.

○   **What laboratory test can be used to diagnose carcinoid syndrome?**

Urinary 5-hydroxyindoleacetic acid (HIAA) level. Levels greater than 20 mg in 24 hours are diagnostic.

○   **When do 5-HIAA levels elevate in carcinoid tumors?**

5-HIAA is cleared by the liver after the first-pass from the primary tumor. Thus, it is not elevated until hepatic metastases are extensive.

○   **What serotonin-containing foods should be avoided when collecting urine for 24-hour 5-HIAA?**

Walnuts, bananas, pecans, butternuts, pineapples, and tomatoes.

○   **What nuclear medicine scans can be used to diagnose carcinoid tumor?**

[123]I-labeled Tyr3-octreotide (TOCT, a somatostatin analog) or ^{123}I-labeled metaiodobenzylguanidine. These scans take advantage of the large number of somatostatin receptors expressed by most carcinoid tumors.

○ **True/False: Small bowel carcinoid tumors are almost always solitary.**

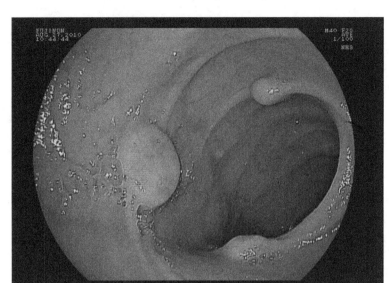

Figure 23-2 See also color plate.

False. Multicentric carcinoid tumors, as shown in the Figure 23-2, are seen in up to 33%.

○ **What medical therapy is available for treating the symptoms of carcinoid syndrome?**

Octreotide, a synthetic somatostatin analog, injected subcutaneously in doses of 50–250 µg BID-TID. Symptoms improve in more than 90% of patients; however, disease progression is not altered. If effective, a long-acting depot form may be substituted.

○ **What can be done to prevent carcinoid crisis caused by invasive procedures?**

The use of octreotide before invasive procedures is an important step to prevent carcinoid crisis in patients with known carcinoid syndrome. A bolus dose of 250–500 µg should be given subcutaneously 1 to 2 hours before the surgery and followed by an infusion of 50–200 µg/hour during the surgery.

○ **Weight loss is usually most severe in what type of malignant small bowel tumor?**

Lymphoma.

○ **What small bowel lymphoma is seen exclusively in underdeveloped countries?**

Immunoproliferative small intestinal disease (IPSID), also known as alpha-chain disease and Mediterranean lymphoma. Microbial colonization of the small bowel is of major etiologic significance in IPSID.

○ **What small bowel tumor should be suspected in a patient with long-standing celiac disease who develops a relapse of symptoms despite strict adherence to a gluten-free diet?**

Intestinal lymphoma, which occurs in 7%–12% of patients with long-standing celiac disease. The cells of this secondary lymphoma are of T-cell origin.

○ **What cell type is present in the majority of primary gastrointestinal lymphomas?**

B-cell.

○ **List the criteria for the diagnosis of a primary gastrointestinal lymphoma.**

- Absence of palpable peripheral lymphadenopathy on initial presentation
- Absence of mediastinal lymphadenopathy on chest radiography
- A normal peripheral blood smear
- At laparotomy, involvement of only the gut and regional lymphadenopathy
- Absence of liver and spleen involvement except by direct spread from a contiguous focus

● ● ● SUGGESTED READINGS ● ● ●

Oberg K. Gastrointestinal Carcinoid Tumors (Gastrointestinal Neuroendocrine Tumors) and the Carcinoid Syndrome. In: Feldman LS, Friedman LS, Brandt LJ, eds. *Sleisenger and Fordtran's Gastrointestinal and Liver disease.* Philadelphia, PA: Elsevier; 2010:475-490.

Paski SC, Semrad CE. Small Bowel Tumors. *Gastrointest Endosc Clin N Am.* 2009;19(3):461-479.

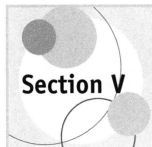

Section V   LARGE INTESTINE

CHAPTER 24

Large Intestinal Congenital and Structural Abnormalities

Ashok Shah, MD and Rajiv Sharma, MD

○ **The colon and the rectum account for what percentage of all gastrointestinal duplications.**

Five percent and 10%, respectively.

○ **True/False: Asymptomatic rectal duplication should undergo surgical resection because of an increased risk of neoplasia.**

True.

○ **A child presents with chronic constipation, abdominal distension, volvulus, and perforation. What is the most likely diagnosis?**

Hirschsprung's disease.

○ **What percentage of Hirschsprung's disease involves the rectosigmoid colon?**

75%–80%.

○ **True/False: Anorectal manometry typically reveals a normal sphincter profile and an abnormal rectoanal inhibitory reflex in Hirschsprung's disease.**

True.

○ **What cell type is absent in the submucosa and myenteric plexus of patients with Hirschsprung's disease?**

Ganglion cells that migrate from the neural crest region.

○ **What pull-through operations have been used to surgically treat Hirschsprung's disease?**

Swenson technique, Duhamel procedure, and Soave procedure.

○ **True/False: Hirschsprung's disease may occur in combination with colonic atresia.**

True.

○ **True/False: Colonic atresia has been linked to congenital varicella syndrome.**

True.

○   **True/False: Malrotation of the colon occurs if the midgut fails to complete the 180-degree counterclockwise rotation as it returns from herniation during the 10th to 12th week gestational period.**

False. It is a 270-degree counterclockwise rotation.

○   **What associated anomalies have been reported in 30%–60% of patients with malrotation?**

Small bowel atresia, intussusception, Hirschsprung's disease, and abdominal wall defects.

○   **An infant presents at 1 month of age with a proximal small bowel obstruction, volvulus, or colonic ischemia. What is the most likely diagnosis?**

Malrotation.

○   **True/False: Operative treatment of malrotation also includes an appendectomy because future diagnosis of appendicitis would be difficult.**

True.

○   **True/False: The midgut volvulus formed by malrotation is reduced by untwisting it in a clockwise rotation.**

False. Reduction is performed in a counterclockwise rotation.

○   **True/False: Gut nonrotation is not as dangerous as gut malrotation.**

True. Because the base of the mesentery is wider than in malrotation, the risk of volvulus is less.

○   **True/False: Imperforate anus occurs in 1:1,000,000 live births.**

False. It occurs in about 1:20,000 live births.

○   **True/False: Congenital abnormalities such as genitourinary, cardiac, and gastrointestinal anomalies are rarely associated with imperforate anus.**

False. These anomalies occur in up to 50% of cases of imperforate anus.

○   **What are three common chromosomal abnormalities associated with imperforate anus?**

Down's syndrome, trisomy 8 mosaicism, and fragile X syndrome.

○   **True/False: Infants with imperforate anus cannot pass meconium at birth.**

True. Some may have fistulae by which meconium can pass.

○   **True/False: Imperforate anus is classified as either a high or a low lesion according to the relation of the rectum to the levator ani muscle.**

True.

○   **True/False: For the complete evaluation of the patient with imperforate anus, an intravenous pyelogram and voiding cystourethrogram are recommended.**

True. Genitourinary defects are occasionally seen in association with imperforate anus.

○ **Surgical treatment of high imperforate anus is successful in what percentage of the time?**

70%–80%.

○ **What are the prerequisites for colonic volvulus formation?**

A dilated, redundant colon, and a narrow-based mesocolon.

○ **True/False: Common symptoms of colonic volvulus are abdominal pain, obstipation, and abdominal distension.**

True.

○ **What percentage of colonic obstructions in the United States are caused by a volvulus?**

Less than 10%.

○ **True/False: A colonic volvulus occurs when a stool-filled segment of bowel twists about its mesentery.**

False. A volvulus occurs when an air-filled segment forms a twist.

○ **True/False: The sigmoid colon is involved in 90% of all colonic volvuli seen in the United States.**

False. A more accurate range is from 40% to 70%.

○ **In which type of colonic volvulus is a "coffee bean sign" seen on abdominal x-ray?**

Cecal volvulus. It is seen in about 80% cases of cecal volvuli. In contrast, a "bird's beak sign" is an x-ray finding suggesting the presence of a sigmoid volvulus.

○ **What segments of the population are at risk for a colonic volvulus?**

The elderly, institutionalized, and neuropsychiatric patients.

○ **What action should be taken to reduce a colonic volvulus in a patient with peritoneal signs?**

Emergency exploratory laparotomy. In a stable patient without peritonitis, sigmoidoscopy or a barium enema may reduce the volvulus.

○ **What is the recurrence rate of a colonic volvulus after nonoperative reduction?**

Greater than 40%.

○ **True/False: Cecal volvulus generally occurs in younger patients.**

True.

○ **What percentage of all colonic volvuli involve the cecum?**

About 40%–50% depending on the age and geographic location.

○ **True/False: A cecal volvulus occurs because of an anomalous fixation of the right colon leading to a freely mobile cecum.**

True.

○ **What are some precipitating factors for a cecal volvulus?**

Pregnancy, adhesions, and an obstructing lesion of the left colon.

○ **What percentage of a cecal volvulus involves a full axial twisting of the associated mesentery and its blood vessels?**

90%.

○ **True/False: Cecal bascule and cecal volvulus refer to the same condition.**

False. A cecal bascule may form when redundant mesentery or hypofixation, in combination with massive distention, allows the cecum to fold onto itself. With the cecum flipped upward on itself, a deep crease across the bowel forms, and occlusion of the gut lumen with bowel obstruction may develop.

○ **True/False: The signs and symptoms of cecal bascule and cecal volvulus are similar.**

True. Although abdominal pain and massive distention are common to both entities, the presence of previous abdominal surgery, especially appendectomy, is more often associated with the cecal bascule.

○ **True/False: Plain films of the abdomen are similar in cecal bascule and cecal volvulus.**

False. Massive distention of the small bowel and cecum are commonly noted on the plain abdominal radiograph; however, neither the typical "coffee-bean sign" associated with cecal volvulus nor the "bird's beak" of sigmoid volvulus are present because there is no axial torsion of the bowel.

○ **True/False: Colitis cystica profunda is characterized by the presence of submucosal mucus-filled cysts.**

True.

○ **True/False: The rectum is rarely involved in colitis cystica profunda.**

False. Most lesions are found within 12 cm of the anal verge.

○ **True/False: It is rare for patients with colitis cystica profunda to have rectal prolapse.**

False. Rectal prolapse occurs about 50% of the time.

○ **A plain radiograph of the abdomen shows linear, curvilinear, or cystic lucencies in the bowel wall. What is the diagnosis?**

Pneumatosis intestinalis.

○ **True/False: The amount of hydrogen in the cysts of pneumatosis intestinalis can approach 50% of the gas present.**

True.

○ **True/False: Pneumatosis cystoides intestinalis is characterized by multiple, thin-walled, noncommunicating, gas-filled cysts with epithelial lining in the wall of the small or large intestines, or both.**

False. The gas-filled cysts have no epithelial lining.

○ **True/False: Pneumatosis cystoides intestinalis is associated with chronic obstructive pulmonary disease, intestinal obstruction, collagen vascular disease (scleroderma), and iatrogenic conditions such as postendoscopy or surgery.**

True.

○ **True/False: Pneumatosis intestinalis is one cause of prolonged recurrent asymptomatic pneumoperitoneum.**

True.

○ **What are successful treatments of pneumatosis intestinalis?**

High-flow oxygen breathing, hyperbaric oxygen, antibiotics, and surgical resection.

○ **True/False: Surgical treatment has been shown to be curative in most cases of pneumatosis intestinalis.**

False. Surgery is not always successful and more extensive pneumatosis may occur; therefore, surgery is indicated only in fulminant cases such as those with a likelihood of bowel necrosis, sepsis, and death.

○ **Histologic examination of a colonic lesion shows von Hansemann's cells and Michaelis–Gutmann's bodies. What is the diagnosis?**

Malakoplakia. A defect in macrophage phagocytic activity has been proposed as a mechanism for the pathogenesis of malakoplakia. Colonic malakoplakia is generally treated with antibiotics such as rifampicin, fluoroquinolones, and trimethoprim-sulfamethaxazole, which penetrate the cell membrane and concentrate within macrophages in combination with a cholinergic agonist like bethanechol to correct the lysosomal defect.

○ **True/False: Malakoplakia is a rare chronic, granulomatous, inflammatory disorder that can affect the genitourinary and gastrointestinal tract.**

True. It can also affect the skin, lung, bone, and brain.

○ **What are the most common sites of the large bowel affected by malakoplakia?**

Rectum, descending, and sigmoid colon. It can also affect appendix and stomach.

○ **What other diseases or conditions are associated with colonic malakoplakia?**

Colonic adenoma, carcinoma, chronic granulomatous disease, ulcerative colitis, and celiac disease.

○ **What are the peak ages of incidence of malakoplakia?**

The age of incidence is bimodal with an early peak at 13 years of age and a late peak around the age of 57.

○ **Name three predisposing conditions associated with malakoplakia.**

Chronic infection with *Escherichia coli*, sarcoidosis, and tuberculosis.

● ● ● SUGGESTED READINGS ● ● ●

Berrocal T, Lamas M, Gutieerrez J, Torres I, Prieto C, del Hoyo ML. Congenital anomalies of the small intestine, colon, and rectum. *Radiographics*. 1999 Sep-Oct;19(5):1219-1236.

Morikawa N, Kuroda T, Honna T, Kitano Y, Tanaka H, Takayasu H, et al. A novel association of duodenal atresia, malrotation, segmental dilatation of the colon, and anorectal malformation. *Pediatr Surg Int*. 2009 Nov;25(11):1003-1005.

Vaos G, Misiakos EP. Congenital anomalies of the gastrointestinal tract diagnosed in adulthood—diagnosis and management. *J Gastrointest Surg*. 2010 May;14(5):916-925.

Large Intestinal Infectious Disorders

Holenarasipur R. Vikram, MD, FACP, FIDSA

○ **What are the strains of diarrhea-causing *Escherichia coli*?**

Enterotoxigenic *E. coli* (ETEC), enteropathogenic *E. coli* (EPEC), enteroinvasive *E. coli* (EIEC), enterohemorrhagic *E. coli* (EHEC, also known as Shiga toxin-producing *E. coli* or STEC), and enteroaggregative *E. coli* (EAEC).

○ **What regions of the gastrointestinal tract do the strains of *E. coli* involve?**

Enterotoxigenic	- small intestine
Enteropathogenic	- small intestine
Enteroinvasive	- large intestine
Enterohemorrhagic	- large intestine
Enteroaggregative	- unknown

○ **What clinical syndromes are associated with ETEC?**

Dehydrating watery diarrhea in young children (< 2 years old) in the developing world, diarrhea in older individuals not previously exposed to this organism, and traveler's diarrhea. ETEC can readily survive in food and water supplies.

○ **How does EPEC cause disease?**

It leads to adherence and effacement of enterocytes.

○ **True/False: Stools from patients with ETEC are bloody.**

False. They are watery without blood or fecal leukocytes.

○ **What is the site of infection with EIEC?**

The colonic mucosa. Ulceration may occur as a result of this infection. Clinical manifestations resemble those of shigellosis.

○ **Which *E. coli* strain is associated with the hemolytic-uremic syndrome (HUS)?**

EHEC belonging to the serotype O157:H7. Several non-O157 strains of EHEC, particularly seen outside the United States, can also cause HUS.

○ **What are the clinical components of the classic triad of HUS?**

The classic triad of HUS includes: 1) acute renal failure, 2) thrombocytopenia, and 3) microangiopathic hemolytic anemia.

○ **What is the characteristic colonic histopathology in patients with EHEC infection?**

Hemorrhage and edema in the lamina propria of the colon. Focal necrosis, neutrophilic infiltration, and pseudomembranes may also be seen.

○ **What is the major virulence factor of EHEC?**

Shiga toxin. Following attachment to the intestinal epithelial cells, secretion of bacterial proteins into these cells and elaboration of Shiga toxins takes place. Shiga toxins enter the systemic circulation and are bound to polymorphonuclear leukocytes, which are responsible for endothelial cell injury in various organs, bloody diarrhea, and in some cases, manifestations of HUS.

○ **How is *E. coli* O157:H7 transmitted?**

The GI tract of cattle is the most important reservoir for *E. coli* O157:H7. Undercooked ground beef has traditionally been the major source of transmission. Other sources of food-borne transmission have included raw milk, green onions, shredded lettuce, and apple juice. Person-to-person transmission, as well as exposure to animals in county fairs, petting zoos, and farms, has led to O157:H7 outbreaks due to inadequate hand hygiene practices. The exact source of the May 2011 outbreak of O104:H4 in Germany remains uncertain.

○ **True/False: There is a seasonal pattern associated with EHEC infection.**

True. In the United States, majority of cases occur between the months of June and September.

○ **What is the infectious dose of *E. coli* O157:H7 for humans?**

Ten to 100 organisms are sufficient to cause infection. This is similar to *Shigella*, and is very low in comparison to other diarrhea-causing bacterial pathogens.

○ **What are the most common clinical manifestations of *E. coli* O157:H7 infection?**

The incubation period following exposure to EHEC is usually 3–4 days. Bloody diarrhea, leukocytosis, absence of fever, and abdominal tenderness are the most common clinical manifestations. Up to half of symptomatic patients might require hospitalization with a mortality rate of 1%–2%, especially the elderly and those who develop HUS.

○ **What percentage of patients infected with *E. coli* O157:H7 develop HUS?**

Approximately 6%–9% of all cases of EHEC infections (15% in those under the age of 10) are complicated by HUS. In 2008, two-thirds of all cases of postdiarrheal HUS occurred in children less than 5 years of age. In a recent outbreak of EHEC O104:H4 in Germany (May 2011), more than 80% of infected patients were >18 years of age, and HUS was observed in 30% of these infections.

○ **True/False: All individuals with *E. coli* O157:H7 should be treated with antibiotics.**

False. Observational studies have reported an increased risk of HUS if antibiotics are administered during the phase of bloody diarrhea, probably due to increased expression and release of Shiga toxin. Furthermore, antibiotic therapy does not alter the duration of illness. Likewise, antimotility drugs also seem to enhance the risk of HUS in patients with EHEC infection. Therefore, both antibiotics and antimotility agents should be avoided.

○ **What is the clinical outcome in patients with postdiarrheal HUS?**

Among those who develop postdiarrheal HUS, up to 50% of patients might require dialysis during the acute phase and 5%–10% may have residual renal or neurologic sequelae. Overall mortality is 3%–5%.

○ **How is *E. coli* O157:H7 detected in the laboratory?**

The Center for Disease Control and Prevention recommends all stool samples submitted for culture be screened for *E. coli* O157:H7. However, > 90% of positive stool cultures for *E. coli* O157:H7 come from visibly bloody stool or those with a recent history of bloody diarrhea. Sorbitol-MacConkey (SMAC) agar is the medium used for this purpose. *E. coli* O157:H7 produces colorless colonies on SMAC agar. The colonies can then be tested with antisera to the O157 antigen. Newer diagnostic techniques can directly detect Shiga toxins in stool.

○ **What are the four species of *Shigella*?**

Shigellae are nonmotile, facultatively anaerobic, nonlactose fermenting Gram-negative rods. The four species (and serogroups) are as follows:

1. *S. dysenteriae* (serogroup A)
2. *S. flexneri* (serogroup B)
3. *S. boydii* (serogroup C)
4. *S. sonnei* (serogroup D)

○ **Which species of *Shigella* is the most common isolate in the United States?**

S. sonnei accounts for about 75% of cases of Shigellosis in the United States, followed by *S. flexneri*.

○ **How does *Shigella* produce dysentery?**

Ingestion of as few as 10–100 viable organisms in contaminated food and water can cause disease. They multiply several-fold in the small intestine (relatively resistant to gastric acid) and reach the colon, where they invade the colonic mucosa causing cell death, an intense inflammatory reaction, ulcerations, and abscesses. *Shigella* strains also elaborate three distinct enterotoxins. Shiga toxin is produced by *S. dysenteriae* type 1. The relative contribution of these toxins to disease is unknown, as nontoxigenic strains of *Shigella* are also pathogenic.

○ **True/False: Blood cultures are usually positive with *Shigella* infection.**

False. The organism rarely invades beyond the mucosa. Although uncommon, bacteremia can occasionally be seen in children < 5 years of age who present with severe disease.

○ **What is the typical clinical course of *Shigella* infection?**

The average incubation period is 3 days. Initial manifestations include fever and abdominal cramping followed by watery diarrhea. Subsequently, bloody mucoid diarrhea and tenesmus are noted. Disease severity also varies by serogroup: *S. dysenteriae* type 1 and *S. flexneri* commonly cause dysenteric symptoms, while *S. sonnei* often leads to a mild illness with watery diarrhea. The course of the disease is typically self-limited in healthy adults.

○ **What are the laboratory findings in patients with *Shigella* infection?**

The peripheral white blood cell count can be elevated. Microscopic evaluation of feces shows many polymorphonuclear leukocytes. Since *Shigella* does not ferment lactose, colonies appear colorless on lactose-containing media. Additional selective media can be utilized to work up suspicious lactose-negative colonies. Serologic studies are not helpful in establishing the diagnosis; however, they may serve as epidemiologic tools for defining the extent of an epidemic. *Shigellae* are nonmotile, indole-positive, urease- and oxidase-negative, and ferment glucose.

○ **What are some of the described intestinal and systemic complications of *Shigella* infection?**

Toxic megacolon, rectal prolapse, intestinal obstruction, and colonic perforation are uncommon intestinal complications in patients with severe disease. Profound dehydration, hyponatremia, protein-losing enteropathy, leukemoid reaction, bacteremia, seizures, and reactive arthritis are known systemic complications. HUS can be associated with shiga toxin-producing strains of *S. dysenteriae* type 1.

○ **True/False: Patients with *Shigella* infections should receive antibiotic treatment.**

True. Antibiotics have been shown to decrease the duration of fever and diarrhea by about 2 days. Even though *Shigella* infection is self-limiting in healthy individuals, treating anyone with a positive stool culture for *Shigella* is recommended to reduce the duration of shedding in the stool and to limit person-to-person spread.

○ **What antibiotics are used to treat *Shigella* infections?**

Ciprofloxacin (500 mg twice daily for 5 days) or another fluoroquinolone is the drug of choice for shigellosis acquired in the United States, while awaiting antimicrobial susceptibilities. Trimethoprim-sulfamethoxazole and azithromycin are alternatives (if susceptible). For strains of *Shigella* acquired in the Asian subcontinent, a third generation cephalosporin is preferable due to widespread resistance to ciprofloxacin. Trimethoprim-sulfamethoxazole and azithromycin are alternatives.

○ **Untreated, how long can patients with *Shigella* gastroenteritis excrete the microorganism?**

For up to 6 weeks.

○ **What host factor lowers the infectious dose required in *Salmonella* infections?**

Lack of gastric acid.

○ **What are the major clinical syndromes caused by *Salmonellae*?**

Gastroenteritis, enteric fever, chronic asymptomatic carrier state, endovascular infection (especially aortitis or vascular graft infections), and focal metastatic infections.

○ **What are the main modes of acquisition of nontyphoidal *Salmonella* infection?**

Eggs and poultry. *Salmonellae* can undergo transovarial transmission from chickens into intact shell eggs. Contaminated peanut butter, milk, ice cream, fresh produce, and meat have also been associated with outbreaks. Pet reptiles, snakes, frogs, iguanas, turtles, and rodents can also transmit *Salmonella*, especially to young children. Therefore, children under the age of 5 and immunocompromised hosts should avoid contact with reptiles.

○ **What host factors predispose patients to infections with *Salmonella*?**

AIDS, organ transplantation, chronic corticosteroid use, cancer chemotherapy, extremes of age, reduced gastric acidity, altered intestinal function due to prior antibiotic therapy or inflammatory bowel disease, impaired phagocytic function (eg, schistosomiasis, histoplasmosis, malaria, chronic granulomatous disease), and iron overload states (such as hemoglobinopathies) result in increased susceptibility to *Salmonella* infection.

○ **Describe the clinical features of *Salmonella* gastroenteritis?**

Symptoms (nausea, vomiting, and diarrhea) begin within 48 hours of ingestion of contaminated food or water. The diarrhea varies in volume; blood or mucus is usually absent. Fever and abdominal cramping are reported in about 90% of cases. Fever resolves in 2–3 days and the diarrhea is usually self-limiting.

○ **Who are at risk for cardiovascular complications following nontyphoidal *Salmonella* bacteremia?**

Older age (> 60 years), preexisting atherosclerotic disease or aortic aneurysm, and prosthetic cardiac valves predispose patients to develop mycotic (infected) aneurysms, aortitis, and endocarditis with resulting metastatic infection in the presence of *Salmonella* bacteremia. Older patients with *Salmonella* bacteremia and chest/abdominal/back pain should undergo urgent evaluation to exclude infective aortitis or aneurysm.

○ **What does laboratory investigation of a patient with *Salmonella* infection typically reveal?**

Fecal leukocytes are seen on microscopic evaluation of stools. *Salmonella* sp. are nonlactose fermenters; therefore, the colonies appear colorless on lactose-containing media. Less than 5% of immunocompetent individuals will have positive blood cultures with nontyphoidal *Salmonella* infections. *S. typhimurium* and *S. enteritidis* are the most frequently isolated serotypes in stool cultures in the United States. Most nontyphoidal salmonellae produce hydrogen sulfide.

○ **How long can patients excrete *Salmonella* in their stool after resolution of an episode of gastroenteritis?**

Asymptomatic fecal excretion of nontyphoidal *Salmonella* strains may occur for about 4–5 weeks. The influence of antimicrobial therapy on the risk of prolonged excretion is unclear. Stool shedding can be intermittent. The importance of hand washing cannot be overemphasized in healthcare workers and food handlers.

○ **What are the recommendations for antimicrobial treatment of *Salmonella* gastroenteritis?**

Otherwise healthy individuals with mild symptoms do not require antimicrobial therapy, as the illness is self-limited. Immunocompetent patients with severe diarrhea, persistent fever, and those requiring hospitalization should receive antibiotics. Immunocompromised patients, those at extremes of age, and patients with *Salmonella* bacteremia require antimicrobial therapy. Fluoroquinolones, trimethoprim-sulfamethoxazole and beta-lactam antibiotics are usually effective. Therapy can be modified based on antimicrobial susceptibility results.

○ **What are the common reservoirs of *Campylobacter jejuni*?**

Campylobacter is a zoonosis. It is most commonly acquired from poultry but also may be transmitted through raw milk, other dairy products, or undercooked meat. The two most important species are *C. jejuni* and *C. coli*.

○ **True/False: Campylobacter is one of the leading causes of acute diarrheal disease worldwide.**

True.

○ **What are the sites of tissue injury in *Campylobacter* infections?**

Jejunum, ileum, colon, and rectum. Histologic appearance is indistinguishable from shigellosis and salmonellosis.

○ **What does laboratory investigation of a patient with *C. jejuni* infection typically reveal?**

Gram stain of a stool specimen can reveal faint-curved, Gram-negative (gull-wing) bacteria. The sensitivity of stool Gram stain is 50%–75%. Stool culture must be undertaken with selective media under microaerophilic conditions. Blood cultures are positive in less than 1%.

○ **What are some of the unique manifestations of *C. jejuni* infection?**

Most patients have a self-limited diarrhea that lasts for a mean of 7 days. Some patients can manifest with bloody diarrhea and acute colitis that can be mistaken for inflammatory bowel disease. Acute ileocecitis from *Campylobacter* can mimic acute appendicitis. Other acute complications that can result from *Campylobacter* infections include massive hemorrhage, HUS, cholecystitis, pancreatitis, hepatitis, peritonitis in patients on continuous ambulatory peritoneal dialysis, and infected pseudoaneurysm. Patients with HIV/AIDS can develop long-term carriage leading to recurrent episodes of enteritis and sometimes bacteremia.

○ **What are the two major late sequelae following *C. jejuni* infection?**

Reactive arthritis and Guillain–Barrè syndrome (GBS). Reactive arthritis can also occur following other bacterial diarrheal infections, and is more common in patients with the HLA-B27 phenotype. Up to 40% of GBS cases are attributable to recent *Campylobacter* infection (overt or asymptomatic). The onset of GBS is usually 1–2 weeks after *Campylobacter* infection.

○ **Which antimicrobial agents are utilized to treat *Campylobacter* infections?**

Since *Campylobacter* gastroenteritis is a mild self-limited infection, most patients do not need antimicrobial therapy. However, antibiotics may be necessary in those with severe or extraintestinal disease, in the elderly, during pregnancy, and in the immunocompromised host. *C. jejuni* is inherently resistant to beta-lactams and trimethoprim. The incidence of fluoroquinolone resistance among *Campylobacter* is increasing throughout the world. Macrolides or tetracyclines are the preferred agents. If the person cannot tolerate oral medications, either an aminoglycoside or a carbapenem should be administered. The final choice of antibiotic therapy should be based on susceptibility testing.

○ **Describe the histopathologic findings in patients with intestinal *Entamoeba histolytica* infection (amebiasis).**

Majority of infections (up to 90%) are asymptomatic. It exists in two forms: a cyst stage (infective form) and a trophozoite stage (causes invasive disease). Colonic lesions range from nonspecific thickening of the mucosa to the classic flask-shaped ulcer. Twenty to 50% of patients have classic ulcers extending through the mucosa and muscularis layer into the submucosa. Colonoscopy is not routinely recommended in patients with active amebic colitis due to the risk of perforation.

○ **What tests are available to diagnose intestinal amebiasis?**

Stool examination to demonstrate cysts or trophozoites, fecal and serum antigen detection assays, and serology. Antigen detection is more sensitive than stool examination. It can help with diagnosis during early infection and in endemic areas where serology is of limited utility.

○ **Describe the extraintestinal manifestations of amebiasis.**

Amebic liver abscess is the most common extraintestinal manifestation, with infection reaching the liver via the portal venous system. Pleuropulmonary amebiasis can occur as a complication of amebic liver abscess. Intraperitoneal rupture of liver abscesses can also occur. Rarely, pericardial, genitourinary, and cerebral amebiasis have been described.

○ **How is infection with *E. histolytica* treated?**

The goal of therapy is to eliminate trophozoites causing invasive colitis and to eradicate intestinal cyst carriage. A 10-day course of metronidazole followed by a 7–10 day course of an intraluminal agent such as diloxanide furoate or paromomycin is recommended. Extraintestinal amebiasis may require a longer course of metronidazole therapy.

○ **What is the most common infectious cause of healthcare-associated diarrhea?**

Clostridium difficile is the most common cause of infectious diarrhea in healthcare settings. It accounts for 20%–30% of all cases of antibiotic-associated diarrhea.

○ **What are the risk factors for *C. difficile* infection (CDI)?**

Advanced age (> 64 years), duration of hospitalization, exposure to antimicrobial agents, cancer chemotherapy, gastrointestinal surgery, tube feeding, and gastric acid suppression are known risk factors for CDI.

○ **True/False: Alcohol-based hand sanitizers and hand washing with soap and water are equally effective in the prevention of nosocomial transmission of *C. difficile*.**

False. The spores of *C. difficile* are highly resistant to killing by alcohol. Therefore, alcohol-based hand sanitizers are ineffective. Hand washing with soap and running water mechanically removes *C. difficile* spores from the hands of healthcare workers and is the recommended option for hand hygiene in this setting.

○ **What are the various tests available for the diagnosis of CDI?**

C. difficile toxins A and B testing by enzyme immunoassay (EIA), polymerase chain reaction (PCR), cell cytotoxicity assay, toxigenic culture, and *C. difficile* common antigen (glutamate dehydrogenase) are available for the diagnosis of CDI.

○ **How is an initial episode of CDI treated?**

The offending antimicrobial agent should be discontinued as soon as possible. For an initial episode of CDI (mild-to-moderate), metronidazole 500 mg orally three times per day for 10–14 days is recommended. For an initial episode of severe CDI, vancomycin 125 mg orally 4 times per day for 10–14 days is the treatment of choice. With an initial episode of severe, complicated CDI (hypotension or shock, ileus, megacolon), vancomycin 500 mg 4 times per day by mouth (or nasogastric tube), PLUS metronidazole 500 mg every 8 hours intravenously is recommended. If there is complete ileus, rectal instillation of vancomycin should be considered. Colectomy can be life-saving for selected patients. The newly approved agent fidaxomicin was demonstrated to be noninferior to vancomycin for the treatment of CDI and was associated with a significantly lower rate of CDI recurrence. Antimotility agents and opiate antagonists should be avoided in patients with CDI as they may precipitate toxic megacolon.

○ **What options are available for the management of patients with recurrent CDI?**

The first step would be to minimize and avoid antimicrobial therapy in patients with a history of recurrent CDI. First recurrence of CDI can be treated with the same regimen as the initial episode. In patients with multiple recurrences, a tapered or pulsed regimen of vancomycin can be tried. Other modalities with reported success in patients with recurrent CDI include: a) oral vancomycin followed by rifaximin, b) nitazoxanide, c) intravenous immunoglobulin, and d) fecal transplantation from a "healthy" donor. The addition of human monoclonal antibodies against *C. difficile* toxins A and B to those receiving either oral vancomycin or metronidazole significantly reduced recurrent CDI. The newly approved agent fidaxomicin was demonstrated to be noninferior to vancomycin for the treatment of CDI and was associated with a significantly lower rate of CDI recurrence.

○ **Who are at risk for developing typhlitis?**

Typhlitis is a life-threatening enterocolitis that develops most often in patients with hematologic malignancies following chemotherapy. Patients are usually profoundly neutropenic and present with fever and abdominal pain. It is also referred to as "neutropenic enterocolitis." The cecum is almost always affected with involvement of the adjacent colon and ileum.

○ **Describe conditions that predispose patients to develop cytomegalovirus (CMV) colitis.**

AIDS, solid organ transplant recipients (especially those who are CMV mismatch [D+/R-]), following allogeneic stem cell transplantation, patients receiving chronic high-dose steroid therapy, and those with inflammatory bowel disease requiring high-dose immunosuppression can manifest CMV colitis. Colonoscopy with biopsy and immunohistochemical staining can provide a definitive diagnosis.

○ **What is *Strongyloides* hyperinfection syndrome?**

Strongyloides stercoralis can complete its entire life cycle within the human host. Such autoinfection can persist for decades and can be asymptomatic in immunocompetent hosts. However, in the setting of immunosuppression, the parasite burden is tremendously increased and can lead to hyperinfection syndrome. Filariform larvae penetrate the intestinal wall and enter the bloodstream with widespread dissemination. In the process, they can also cause bacteremia with enteric pathogens resulting in septic shock. Timely diagnosis can be life-saving. Stool examination, serology, or endoscopy can be utilized for diagnosis. Ivermectin and albendazole are the treatments of choice.

○ **What is the treatment of choice for *Balantidium coli* infection?**

B. coli is a protozoan that can cause acute colitis (trophozoite form) or lead to asymptomatic cyst excretion in humans. Tetracycline and metronidazole are the drugs of choice for *B. coli*.

○ **What are the gastrointestinal manifestations of Chagas disease?**

Chagas disease is caused by the protozoan *Trypanosoma cruzi* and is endemic in many South American countries. Gastrointestinal involvement is seen in the chronic phase of Chagas disease and manifests as megaesophagus and megacolon. This is due to a loss of neurons in the gastrointestinal tract. Most patients with gastrointestinal involvement also have concurrent chronic Chagas heart disease.

● ● ● **SUGGESTED READINGS** ● ● ●

Guerrant RL, Van Gilder T, Steiner TS, et al. Practice guidelines for the management of infectious diarrhea. *Clin Infect Dis.* 2001;32: 331-350.

Goldsweig CD, Pacheco PA. Infectious colitis excluding *E. coli* O157:H7 and *C. difficile. Gastroenterol Clin North Am.* 2001;30: 709-733.

Cohen SH, Gerding DN, Johnson S, et al. Clinical practice guidelines for *Clostridium difficile* infection in adults: 2010 update by the Society for Healthcare Epidemiology of America (SHEA) and the Infectious Diseases Society of America (IDSA). *Infect Control Hosp Epidemiol.* 2010;31:431-455.

Large Intestinal Motility Disorders

Edy E. Soffer, MD and
Claudia P. Sanmiguel, MD

○ **What segments of the colon are usually involved in volvulus?**

Sigmoid volvulus accounts for up to 70% of all cases of colonic volvulus followed by the cecum.

○ **How helpful are abdominal x-rays in making the diagnosis of colonic volvulus?**

Classic radiological features of sigmoid or cecal volvulus are observed in approximately 50% of patients. Water-soluble enemas and computed tomography scans are indicated when the diagnosis is unclear.

○ **How effective is endoscopic decompression in the management of colonic volvulus?**

Flexible sigmoidoscopy and rectal decompression tube placement for sigmoid volvulus is effective in 60%–80% of cases. In the case of cecal volvulus, nonoperative decompression is usually not successful.

○ **What is the recurrence rate of colonic volvulus after endoscopic decompression?**

Sigmoid volvulus recurs in approximately 50%. Therefore, surgical correction is often subsequently performed on an elective basis. Primary surgical correction of cecal volvulus is the treatment of choice.

○ **True/False: Hirschprung's disease may occur in adults.**

True. Hirschprung's disease may be diagnosed in young adults. Diagnosis should be suspected in patients who have history of constipation dating back to early childhood.

○ **True/False: Anorectal manometry can exclude Hirschprung's disease.**

True. The presence of a rectoanal inhibitory reflex (RAIR)—reflex relaxation of the anal sphincter with distention of the rectum—excludes Hirschprung's disease. In contrast, the absence of the RAIR does not necessarily prove the diagnosis of Hirschsprung's disease.

○ **True/False: A full thickness colon biopsy is always needed to confirm the diagnosis of Hirschsprung's disease.**

False. Rectal mucosal biopsy using either a large forceps or suction biopsy technique is the first step. If taken from the appropriate segment of the rectum and ganglion cells are present in the submucosa, Hirschprung's disease is excluded. The absence of ganglion cells using these techniques, on the other hand, requires a full thickness biopsy to establish a diagnosis.

○ **What are the predisposing factors for acute colonic pseudo-obstruction?**

This condition is typically seen in the elderly following trauma or recovery from surgery, particularly, orthopedic, obstetric, or abdominal surgery. It can also occur in the setting of any severe medical illness.

○ **What is the most effective drug therapy for acute colonic pseudo-obstruction?**

Neostigmine, 2 mg given intravenously by slow push, achieves rapid decompression in most patients.

○ **What are potential complications of intravenous neostigmine use in acute colonic pseudo-obstruction?**

The most common adverse effect is mild to moderate crampy abdominal pain. Excessive salivation and vomiting may also occur. Symptomatic bradycardia requiring atropine is possible and cardiac monitoring should be in place. Bronchospasm and hypotension have also been reported.

○ **When should colonoscopic decompression be attempted in the management of acute colonic pseudo-obstruction?**

In a patient without evidence of compromised bowel (eg, peritonitis, pneumoperitoneum), if initial measures such as nasogastric decompression, discontinuation of narcotics/anticholinergic medications, correction of electrolytes and hypoxemia, and pharmacological therapy are unsuccessful, colonoscopic decompression should be attempted. Standard recommendations suggest colonoscopy when the diameter of the cecum is greater than 11 or 12 cm. A colonic decompression tube may be left in place, although its utility remains debatable.

○ **True/False: A gender difference exists in the irritable bowel syndrome (IBS).**

True. IBS is twice as common in females.

○ **What pharmacologic therapy has recently been shown to induce a sustained effect in IBS?**

Antibiotics. A recent study has shown that a short course of treatment with an antibiotic (rifaximin) resulted in sustained improvement (over 12 weeks) in patients with diarrhea-predominant IBS. This differs from other therapies for IBS which tend to lose their effectiveness shortly after their discontinuation.

○ **True/False: IBS is associated with other gastrointestinal symptoms and nongastrointestinal conditions.**

True. Upper gastrointestinal symptoms such as heartburn, nausea, and vomiting are reported in up to 50% of patients with IBS. Urinary symptoms, dyspareunia, headaches, and fibromylagia are also more common in patients with IBS compared to patients with organic gastrointestinal diseases.

○ **True/False: IBS is associated with an identifiable gut motor abnormality.**

False. While a number of motor changes have been described in patients with IBS, no pathognomonic gastrointestinal motor abnormality has been defined thus far.

○ **Which laxatives are associated with melanosis coli?**

Anthranoid laxatives such as senna, cascara, and aloe. However, up to 30% of patients found to have melanosis coli during colonoscopy do not have history of laxative use—many of these are using herbal supplements that contain anthranoid derivatives.

○ **Where in the gut is melanosis seen?**

Melanosis can be seen throughout the colon; however, the proximal colon is usually more affected.

○ **True/False: Melanosis coli is a risk factor for colon cancer.**

False. Although melanosis coli has been associated with increased cellular apoptosis, no studies have shown an association between colon cancer and melanosis coli.

○ **What is the most common reason for fecal incontinence in children and institutionalized elderly?**

Fecal retention resulting in overflow soiling.

○ **What is the most common etiology of constipation?**

Idiopathic.

○ **What subtypes are included in idiopathic constipation?**

IBS, dyssynergic defecation, and slow transit constipation.

○ **What is dyssynergic defecation?**

In this condition, also referred to as anismus, pelvic floor dysfunction, or obstructed defecation, there is a paradoxical contraction rather than relaxation of the external anal sphincter and puborectalis in response to defecation.

○ **How is dyssynergic defecation diagnosed?**

Several tests are available. The more of these tests that are abnormal, the stronger the diagnosis. Digital exam of the anal canal may show contraction of the sphincter apparatus rather than relaxation when the patient is asked to bear down. Anorectal manometry and electromyography may show contraction rather than relaxation of the muscles during attempted defecation. Balloon expulsion test may demonstrate difficulty expelling the balloon from the rectum (ie, prolonged time or inability to expel the balloon). Finally, evacuation proctography (defecography) may demonstrate anorectal angle narrowing rather than widening during attempted defecation.

○ **What is the most appropriate treatment for this condition?**

Recent controlled trials have shown that pelvic floor retraining (biofeedback) is superior to laxatives and achieves up to 80% improvement (at least over the short term).

○ **What medications can cause or aggravate constipation?**

Opiate derivatives, anticholinergics, calcium- or aluminum-containing antacids, calcium channel antagonists, and clonidine are a few.

○ **True/False: Surgery is indicated if both a rectocele and difficult evacuation are present.**

False. Rectoceles are common, even in nonconstipated women. A history of applying digital pressure on the posterior wall of the vagina to help evacuation and a defecogram showing a large rectocele with residual barium at the end of defecation suggest that surgical repair may be helpful.

○ **True/False: Surgery is often helpful in the management of dyssynergic defecation.**

False. Operations such as division of the internal anal sphincter and puborectalis are usually not successful and may result in fecal incontinence.

○ **True/False: Botulinum toxin injection into the puborectalis is of proven benefit in the management of dyssynergic defecation.**

False. Although ultrasound-guided injection of botulinum toxin into the puborectalis has been reported to improve defecatory complaints in a small, open-label study, experience is limited and repeated injections may be needed.

○ **How is colonic transit measured in clinical practice?**

Transit study by radio-opaque markers is the most common method used. Radionuclide scintigraphic colon transit testing is also available but mainly in referral centers. A wireless motility capsule has also recently been approved for clinical use for this purpose but is not widely available at present.

○ **When should the use of a colon transit study be considered?**

In patients with severe intractable constipation. A normal colonic transit in such patients is associated with a higher prevalence of psychological distress when compared to patients with slow transit.

○ **True/False: Exercise is helpful in the treatment of constipation.**

False. While constipation is associated with inactivity, there are no convincing data to suggest that, in active subjects, bowel habits are affected by exercise.

○ **What is the recommended daily dose of fiber per day?**

Between 20 and 30 grams.

○ **True/False: Fiber is effective in patients with severe constipation.**

False. Fiber comes from different sources and its effect on colonic transit is variable. All patients with constipation should have an appropriate amount of fiber in their diet; however, while patients with mild constipation may improve with additional fiber, those with significant slow transit constipation can experience bloating and distension.

○ **What are the potential complications of mineral oil?**

Lipoid pneumonia, if aspirated. It can also cause anal seepage and there is a potential risk of malabsorption of fat soluble vitamins when used long term.

○ **How do stimulant laxatives work?**

Both anthranoid laxatives, such as senna and aloe, and the diphenylmethanes, such as phenolphthalein and bisacodyl, act by increasing colonic motility and by inducing secretion. Phenolphthalein compounds have been withdrawn from the market.

○ **How do osmotic laxatives work?**

Osmotic laxatives contain poorly absorbable ions, such as magnesium, and increase water content in the colon.

○ **True/False: Hypermagnesemia is a potential side effect of osmotic laxative use.**

True. This is mainly of concern only in those with renal insufficiency.

○ **True/False: Polyethylene glycol solution is useful in the management of chronic constipation.**

True. Polyethylene glycol is a nonabsorbable electrolyte solution. While normally given for bowel cleansing prior to colonoscopy, when taken in smaller amounts (250–750 ml per day), it can be extremely helpful in the treatment of chronic constipation in both children and adults.

○ **True/False: Lubiprostone, approved for the treatment of both chronic constipation and constipation-predominant IBS, selectively activates type 2 chloride channels in the apical membrane of intestinal epithelial cells, thereby stimulating chloride secretion along with passive secretion of sodium and water, and inducing peristalsis and laxation.**

True, although the exact mechanism of action of this drug remains unclear.

○ **What is the most common operation for patients with severe constipation and slow colonic transit?**

Subtotal colectomy with ileorectal anastomosis. Segmental colon resections in patients with severe slow transit constipation should be avoided.

○ **True/False: Prior to consideration of surgery for refractory slow transit constipation, an evaluation to exclude a more diffuse gut dysmotility syndrome (intestinal pseudo-obstruction) should be performed.**

True. The presence of diffuse gut dysmotilty predicts a less than optimal response to surgical removal of the colon. Gastric emptying test and intestinal manometry should be considered prior to surgery.

○ **How does narcotic use induce constipation?**

Constipation is frequently seen in patients using narcotics. There are several mechanisms involved in the development of constipation including increased anal sphincter tone, decreased peristalsis, increased water and electrolyte absorption, and impaired defecation response.

○ **True/False: Polyethylene glycol is more effective than lactulose for the treatment of narcotic associated constipation.**

False. A randomized, double-blind, crossover study showed no significant difference in effectiveness between these two medications.

○ **True/False: Methylnaltrexone, used for treating severe narcotic-induced constipation in the palliative care setting, is safe and effective and does not interfere with pain control.**

True. Several studies have shown that up to half of the patients who received methylnaltrexone experienced laxation within 4 hours of the initial dose. There were no significant side effects and there were no signs of opioid withdrawal or changes in pain scores during treatment.

○   **What is narcotic bowel syndrome?**

Narcotic bowel syndrome (NBS) is an opioid-induced bowel dysfunction that is characterized by chronic or frequently recurring abdominal pain that worsens with continued or escalating dosages of narcotics. This syndrome is frequently under-recognized. Narcotic bowel syndrome can occur in patients with no prior gastrointestinal disorder, patients with functional GI disorders, or patients with other chronic gastrointestinal diseases who receive narcotics for pain control.

○   **True/False: Amyloidosis affects the colon more frequently than other gastrointestinal segments.**

False. The small bowel is most frequently affected by amyloidosis. Macroglosia is almost pathognomonic but is seen only in 10%–23% of the patients with systemic immunoglobulin light chain (AL) amyloidosis.

● ● ● **SUGGESTED READINGS** ● ● ●

Rao SS. Constipation: evaluation and treatment of colonic and anorectal motility disorders. *Gastrointest Endosc Clin N Am.* 2009 Jan;19(1):117-139.

Bharucha AE. Treatment of severe and intractable constipation. *Curr Treat Options Gastroenterol.* 2004 Aug;7(4):291-298.

Lembo A, Camilleri M. Chronic constipation. *N Engl J Med.* 2003 Oct 2;349(14):1360-1368.

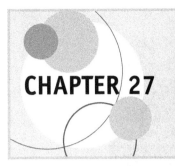

CHAPTER 27

Large Intestinal Miscellaneous Inflammatory Diseases

Reena Khanna, MD, FRCPC and John K. Marshall, MD, MSc, FRCPC, AGAF

○ **True/False: Lymphocytic and collagenous colitis are distinct clinical entities.**

This question continues to be debated. Although they differ slightly in the histologic criteria for diagnosis, growing evidence suggests that lymphocytic and collagenous colitis are two manifestations of the same disorder, with similar presentation, response to treatment and prognosis. Approximately half of the cases fulfill histologic criteria for both lymphocytic and collagenous colitis, representing a mixed disease variant.

○ **How does microscopic colitis typically present?**

Patients with microscopic colitis are typically middle-aged or elderly females (female to male ratio 4:1 for lymphocytic colitis and 1:1 for collagenous colitis) with large-volume, nonbloody, watery diarrhea. A prior history of nonsteroidal anti-inflammatory drug ingestion is common and was suggested to be a risk factor in a published case-control study. Clinical severity correlates with the degree of inflammation seen in histological samples.

○ **Which medications are associated with the development of microscopic colitis?**

The most consistent association has been with nonsteroidal anti-inflammatory drugs. Other medications linked to microscopic colitis include acarbose, aspirin, carbamazepine, flutamide, gold salts, proton pump inhibitors, paroxetine, sertraline, ranitidine, simvastatin, and ticlopidine.

○ **True/False: Rectal biopsy is highly sensitive for detecting collagenous colitis.**

False. Only 27% of cases of collagenous colitis are detected on rectal biopsy. To exclude the diagnosis, full colonoscopy is usually required. Histologic changes are seen in the cecum in 82% of patients and the transverse colon in 83%.

○ **True/False: Microscopic colitis can cause histologic changes in the small bowel.**

True. Increased intraepithelial lymphocytes have been seen in terminal ileal biopsies from patients with microscopic colitis. More than five intraepithelial lymphocytes per 100 epithelial cells in the terminal ileum has been suggested to have high predictive value for the diagnosis of microscopic colitis when compared with healthy controls or patients with inflammatory bowel disease (IBD).

○   **What are the classic histological features of lymphocytic and collagenous colitis?**

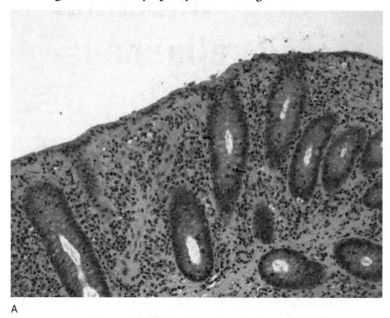

A

Figure 27-1A See also color plate. (Figure used with permission of Dr J. Radhi, McMaster University, Hamilton, ON, Canada.)

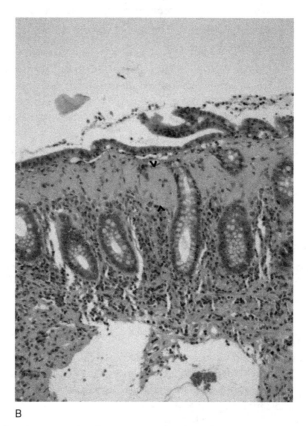

B

Figure 27-1B See also color plate. (Figure used with permission of Dr J. Radhi, McMaster University, Hamilton, ON, Canada.)

Lymphocytic colitis is defined as the presence of more than 15–20 intraepithelial lymphocytes per 100 epithelial cells (normal 3–5 intraepithelial lymphocytes per 100 epithelial cells), as shown in Figure 27-1A. Collagenous colitis is characterized by a thickening of the subepithelial collagen band to greater than 10 μm (normal 1–7 μm), which can be seen in Figure 27-1B. Although thickening of the collagen band is a hallmark feature of collagenous colitis, it is not pathognomic. Thickening of this band can also be seen with ischemia, trauma, or neoplasia. (See also color plate.)

○ **What are some proposed theories for the pathogenesis of collagenous colitis?**

Proposed mechanisms include abnormalities in collagen metabolism, effects of bacterial toxins, altered expression of transforming growth factor 1, and drug effects.

○ **What are six conditions associated with microscopic colitis?**

Celiac disease, irritable bowel syndrome, thyroid disease, diabetes mellitus, rheumatoid arthritis, and asthma/allergy.

○ **True/False: Approximately 5% of patients with celiac disease have features of lymphocytic colitis on colonic biopsies.**

False. Features consistent with lymphocytic colitis are seen in 20%–30% of patients with celiac disease undergoing colonoscopy with biopsy. The relative risk of microscopic colitis among patients with celiac disease is approximately 70.

○ **True/False: Lymphocytic colitis usually responds to a gluten-free diet.**

False.

○ **What laboratory abnormalities are associated with microscopic colitis?**

Laboratory abnormalities that have been associated with microscopic colitis include anemia, elevated inflammatory markers, and presence of autoantibodies (rheumatoid factor, antimitochondrial antibody, and antineutrophilic cytoplasmic antibodies [ANCA]).

○ **Characterize the natural history of lymphocytic/collagenous colitis.**

Lymphocytic and collagenous colitis usually enter remission spontaneously in the short term but may ultimately follow a chronic relapsing course. Between one-quarter and two-thirds of patients will require long-term medication for chronic intermittent diarrhea.

○ **What treatments may be prescribed for lymphocytic/collagenous colitis?**

Patients should be advised to avoid secretagogues such as caffeine and lactose. Medical treatment options include budesonide, bismuth subsalicylate, 5-aminosalicylate derivatives, cholestyramine, and systemic corticosteroids. Antidiarrheal agents such as diphenoxylate and loperamide are often ineffective. Refractory cases have required surgical diversion of the fecal stream.

○ **Which of the above treatment options is/are supported by evidence from controlled clinical trials?**

For *induction of remission*, a meta-analysis of randomized controlled trials found clinical response to occur in 100% of patients taking bismuth compared to 0% on placebo ($p = 0.03$). In three trials of budesonide, clinical response was seen in 81% of patients in the treatment arm compared to 17% in the placebo group ($p < 0.00001$), with an odds ratio of 12.32 (95% CI 5.53 to 27.46) and a number need to treat of 2. Clinical response to budesonide was associated with a significant histologic response. Small trials have failed to show the superiority of prednisolone, probiotics, or mesalamine with or without cholestyramine over placebo in the treatment of microscopic colitis ($p = 0.15$, $p = 0.38$, and $p = 0.14$, respectively).

For *maintenance of remission*, budesonide given at a dose of 6 mg daily for 6 months maintained clinical response in 83% of patients compared to 28% receiving placebo ($p = 0.0002$), with an odds ratio of 7.17 (95% CI 3.00 to 17.12) and a number needed to treat of 2. Similarly, histologic response occurred in 48% in the treatment arm and 15% among those receiving placebo ($p = 0.0002$).

○ **True/False: Collagenous/lymphocytic colitis is associated with an increased risk of IBD.**

False.

○ **True/False: Collagenous/lymphocytic colitis increases the risk of developing colorectal carcinoma.**

False.

○ **True/False: Diversion colitis occurs more commonly after colectomy for IBD than for cancer.**

True. Diversion colitis develops more frequently among patients who undergo surgery for IBD (89%) than for cancer (23%).

○ **How does the endoscopic appearance of diversion colitis differ from that of ulcerative proctitis?**

Diversion colitis cannot be differentiated endoscopically from ulcerative proctitis. Endoscopy typically reveals an erythematous and friable rectal mucosa with superficial ulceration.

○ **What causes diversion colitis?**

Diversion colitis occurs when a segment of bowel is excluded from the fecal stream. Current evidence implicates deficiency of luminal short-chain fatty acids (SCFAs) such as acetate, propionate, and butyrate. Butyrate normally provides 70% of the oxidative energy for colonocytes. SCFAs also regulate colonic motility, fluid and electrolyte balance, and blood flow. The absence of SCFAs is believed to alter colonic bacterial flora in the excluded segment resulting in fewer anaerobic and more nitrate-producing bacteria.

○ **How does diversion colitis present?**

Up to 40% of patients develop symptoms from diversion colitis, including tenesmus, rectal discharge (blood and mucous), abdominal pain, and diarrhea. Rarely, sepsis or rectal abscesses have been described.

○ **How is diversion colitis treated?**

The best treatment for diversion colitis is to restore the fecal stream. SCFA enemas induce remission in many patients but are not commercially available. A suggested formulation contains 60 mmol/L acetate, 30 mmol/L propionate, and 40 mmol/L butyrate. Hydrocortisone enemas are ineffective and there is little evidence to support the use of aminosalicylate preparations.

○ **What histologic feature, as shown in Figure 27-2, is the hallmark of diversion colitis?**

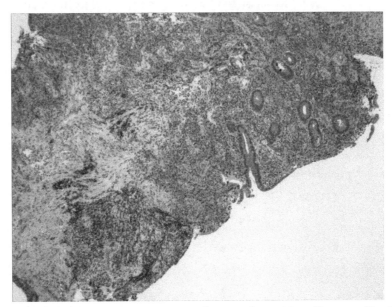

Figure 27-2 See also color plate. (Figure used with permission of Dr J. Radhi, McMaster University, Hamilton, ON, Canada.)

Lymphoid follicular hyperplasia with germinal centers is found in almost all cases. Cryptitis and neutrophil infiltration develop in at least 60% after 3 months.

○ **How does acute radiation proctosigmoiditis present?**

Acute injury presents with diarrhea and tenesmus during radiation treatment or within 6 weeks of exposure. The endoscopic appearance of the rectum is normal.

○ **What are the clinical manifestations of chronic radiation proctitis?**

The typical symptoms of chronic injury are rectal bleeding, diarrhea, and tenesmus. Rectal strictures may develop as can fistulae to the vagina, bladder, or uterus.

○ **True/False: Rectal biopsies may lead to fistula formation in chronic radiation proctitis.**

True, theoretically. Although evidence for a clear link between fistula formation and biopsy is lacking, a theoretical risk exists. A fistula is thought to develop from a site of necrosis. It is recommended to avoid taking biopsies from the rectal wall with greatest radiation exposure. For example, biopsies should be avoided from the anterior rectal wall in patients receiving radiation therapy for prostate cancer.

○ **Describe the typical endoscopic appearance of chronic radiation proctitis.**

Endoscopy typically reveals mucosal pallor, with friability and telangiectasia.

○ **How long after radiation exposure does chronic radiation proctitis develop?**

On average, symptoms develop after 1 year, fistulae after 18 months, and strictures after 3 years.

○ **True/False: Patients with IBD are more likely to develop radiation proctitis following radiation therapy.**

True.

○ **What other risk factors exist for the development of colonic radiation injury?**

Risk factors for radiation injury are thought to include previous lower abdominal surgery, diabetes, and concomitant vascular disease.

○ **What medical therapies may be helpful in preventing acute radiation colitis?**

Routine prophylactic therapy is not advised; however, potential therapies include amifostine, sulfasalazine, balsalazide, and selenium.

○ **What is the natural history of radiation colitis?**

One-third of patients with mild radiation proctitis will enter a spontaneous remission within 6 months, without requiring therapy.

○ **What treatments are effective in controlling hemorrhage from radiation proctitis?**

Oral 5-aminosalicylic acid (5-ASA) and corticosteroid enemas do not appear to control bleeding or tenesmus. Local instillation of 4% formalin, sucralfate, or 5-ASA may be effective. Nd:YAG, argon laser ablation or electrocoagulation of the rectal mucosa are useful endoscopic approaches. Hyperbaric oxygen therapy may also be beneficial by attenuating tissue hypoxia from obliterative endarteritis. Proctectomy may be considered for refractory cases but the colo-anal anastomosis is prone to leakage.

○ **At what age is the incidence of milk protein allergy highest?**

The peak incidence is at 6 weeks. Symptoms may include vomiting, colic, diarrhea, and rectal bleeding from colonic ulcers. Since the allergy is usually IgE-mediated, eczema, urticaria, and angioneurotic edema may also be seen.

○ **How is the diagnosis of milk protein allergy made?**

Resolution of symptoms with milk withdrawal and recurrence within 48 hours of rechallenge. Rechallenge is often omitted since it may result in anaphylaxis. If performed, rechallenge should be conducted in a hospital setting.

○ **At what age can children with milk protein allergy resume drinking cow's milk?**

Allergy to milk protein usually resolves between 9 months and 3 years of age.

○ **What is protein-induced proctitis/proctocolitis syndrome?**

This syndrome is characterized by erythema and erosion of the distal colon and rectum induced by protein ingested in breast milk or formula. This results in loose stools with blood and mucous presenting by 6 months, without diarrhea or failure to thrive. White cells are seen in stool samples, while biopsies demonstrate an eosinophilic inflammatory infiltrate with lymphoid hyperplasia.

○   **How is the protein-induced proctitis/proctocolitis syndrome treated?**

Elimination of the offending allergen results in resolution of bloody stools within days. In breast-fed infants this often requires elimination of cow's milk from the maternal diet.

○   **True/False: Patients with the protein-induced proctitis/proctocolitis syndrome are more likely to develop IBD in adolescence?**

False.

○   **What is food protein-induced enterocolitis syndrome (FPIES)?**

This syndrome is characterized by malabsorption and failure to thrive due to small bowel and colonic inflammation induced by food protein. Infants generally present with nausea, vomiting, and bloody diarrhea. Crypt abscesses and a plasma cell predominant inflammatory infiltrate are hallmark features seen in colonic biopsies.

○   **How is FPIES treated?**

Treatment of this condition involves complete dietary avoidance of the causal protein and administration of formula with hydrolyzed protein.

○   **Which laxatives are associated with melanosis coli?**

Anthraquinones, including cascara sagrada, aloe, rhubarb, senna, and frangula.

○   **How soon does melanosis coli appear and how quickly does it resolve?**

Melanosis coli can develop within 4 months of starting a laxative and resolve within approximately 9 months of its discontinuation.

○   **Name the pigment that is deposited in the mucosa in melanosis coli.**

The true identity of the pigment is unknown. It has been found to bear some biochemical similarity to lipofuscin, melanin, and the hepatic pigment of Dubin–Johnson syndrome.

○   **Describe the location and endoscopic appearance of the solitary rectal ulcer syndrome (SRUS).**

Endoscopy reveals a lesion on the anterior rectal wall between 6 and 10 cm from the anal verge. The lesion itself is variable and may appear as a single ulcer, a cluster of ulcers, a polypoid lesion, or an area of erythema.

○   **What are the typical histologic features of the SRUS?**

Fibromuscular obliteration of the lamina propria. As this term suggests, the lamina propria is replaced with fibroblasts, smooth muscle, and collagen. The muscularis mucosa is hypertrophied and disorganized.

○   **How does the SRUS usually present?**

Patients with SRUS most commonly present with rectal bleeding (up to 50%), straining (30%), or the sense of incomplete emptying (25%). Many are asymptomatic.

○ **What are the endoscopic and histologic features of melanosis coli?**

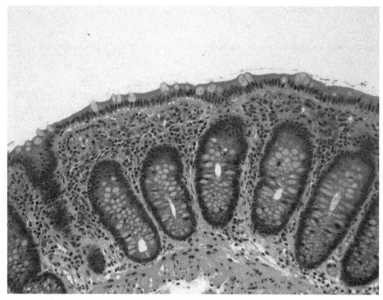

Figure 27-3 See also color plate. (Figure used with permission of Dr J. Radhi, McMaster University, Hamilton ON, Canada.)

Endoscopically, melanosis coli appears as a dark brown coloration of the colon, particularly affecting the rectosigmoid segment and with pale patches thought to overlie lymphoid follicles. Histologically, brown pigment is seen within macrophages of the lamina propria (see Figure 27-3).

○ **Describe hypotheses regarding the pathogenesis of SRUS.**

Self-digitation has been suggested as the cause of SRUS and is documented in up to 50% of patients. An alternate hypothesis is that SRUS results from prolapse and ischemia of the rectal mucosa in the setting of a high fecal voiding pressure. The latter may result from inadequate relaxation of the puborectalis during defecation.

○ **Which conditions can mimic SRUS?**

Diagnoses whose presentations overlap that of SRUS include IBD, ischemic colitis, malignancy, infection (eg, TB, amebiasis, CMV, lymphogranuloma venereum), autoimmune disorders (eg, Behcet's syndrome), nonsteroidal anti-inflammatory drug (NSAID) colopathy, and trauma.

○ **How is SRUS treated?**

Initial conservative therapy with bulk laxatives, avoidance of straining, and reassurance is recommended. Pelvic floor retraining (ie, biofeedback therapy) may be helpful in those with pelvic floor dyssynergia. Topical anti-inflammatory medication is generally ineffective. For refractory cases, the surgical procedure of choice is an abdominal rectopexy.

○ **What complications of NSAIDs have been described in the colon?**

Acute colitis, ischemic colitis, perforation of colonic diverticula, and diaphragmlike strictures have been reported after NSAID ingestion. NSAIDs may also exacerbate or trigger relapse of Crohn's disease and ulcerative colitis.

○ **Which disease-modifying anti-rheumatic drug has been associated with an acute colitis?**

Gold salts may induce an acute colitis characterized by ulceration and friability of the rectosigmoid mucosa. Symptoms typically resolve within 2 weeks of drug withdrawal.

○ **Name five classes of drugs that have been associated with ischemic injury of the colon.**

NSAIDs, oral contraceptives, vasoconstrictors (eg, vasopressin, ergotamine, cocaine, dextroamphetamine), neuroleptics, and digitalis.

○ **What are the three forms of colitis associated with cancer chemotherapy?**

Neutropenic enterocolitis (aka, typhlitis), ischemic colitis, and *Clostridium difficile* colitis.

○ **What is typhlitis?**

The Greek word *typhlos* refers to a blind sac. Typhlitis is an acute necrotic inflammation of the cecum. It has also been called neutropenic enterocolitis and ileocecal syndrome.

○ **In what clinical setting does typhlitis occur?**

Typhlitis classically affects leukemic patients with severe neutropenia but has been described in a number of other immunosuppressed states.

○ **How does typhlitis present?**

Typical symptoms include fever, abdominal pain, distension, vomiting, and bloody diarrhea. An associated mucositis may involve the oropharynx. Plain films may reveal cecal thumbprinting or pneumatosis. Computed tomography and ultrasound demonstrate bowel wall thickening.

○ **Which conditions mimic typhlitis?**

Typhlitis should be differentiated from acute appendicitis, appendiceal abscess, *Clostridium difficile* colitis, ischemia, and colonic pseudo-obstruction.

○ **How is typhlitis treated?**

The primary management is supportive, with hydration, broad-spectrum antibiotics, and nasogastric decompression. Refractory cases may require a right hemicolectomy with mucous fistula.

○ **What is the mortality rate from acute typhlitis?**

Short-term mortality from acute typhlitis may be as high as 40%–50%.

○ **What is topical colitis?**

Topical colitis has been reported after glutaraldehyde and hydrogen peroxide contamination of colonoscope channels.

○ **Which segments of the colon most frequently develop ischemic colitis?**

The splenic flexure and rectosigmoid junction are supplied by terminal branches of the inferior mesenteric artery. These areas are most susceptible to ischemic damage.

○   **What are risk factor for the development of ischemic colitis?**

Reported risk factors for the development of ischemic colitis include age over 60, hypotension (from dehydration, sepsis, myocardial infarction, or hemorrhage), aortoiliac or cardiopulmonary surgery, cardioembolic disease, hemodialysis, drugs (including cocaine, amphetamine, ergot, vasopressin, alosetron, estrogen, digoxin, diuretics, simvastatin, and sumatriptan), extreme exercise, prothrombotic conditions, and diabetes.

○   **What is the mechanism of injury in ischemic colitis?**

Ischemic colitis most commonly results from nonocclusive ischemia due to decreased blood flow and/or vasospasm.

○   **How does ischemic colitis usually present?**

Patients often present with left-sided abdominal pain and hematochezia.

○   **What are the endoscopic features of ischemic colitis?**

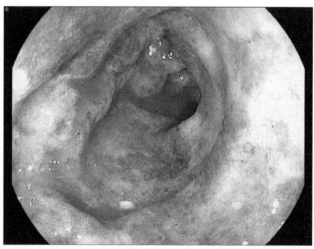

Figure 27-4 See also color plate.

Classically, the mucosa is pale with petechial hemorrhage. Submucosal hemorrhage and pseudomembranes may be noted. A single left-sided colonic ulcer, typically longer than 5 cm (the "single stripe sign"), may occur in mild disease states, whereas cyanosis with frank ulceration denotes severe disease (see Figure 27-4). These changes occur segmentally, often with rectal sparing.

○   **What are three complications of ischemic colitis?**

In the short term, ischemic colitis can progress to frank necrosis and gangrene. Over the longer term, ischemic colitis can lead to a chronic inflammatory state (persistent colitis) or stricture.

○   **How is ischemic colitis treated?**

Supportive measures including intravenous hydration and withdrawal of offending agents. Empiric antibiotics may be given in severe cases. A nasogastric tube may be placed if an ileus is present.

○   **Describe the gastrointestinal manifestations of acute intestinal graft versus host disease (GVHD).**

Acute GVHD occurs within 100 days of a stem cell transplant and results in profuse diarrhea and abdominal pain. Nausea, vomiting, and anorexia have also been described. Other systemic manifestations most commonly include skin rash and elevated liver tests.

○   **What are the histological features of acute GVHD?**

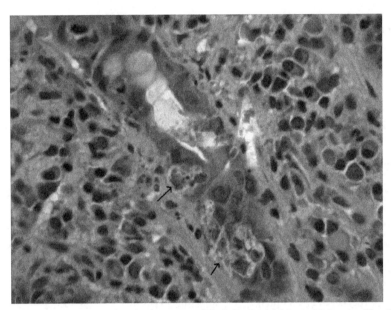

Figure 27-5 See also color plate. (Figure used with permission of Dr J. Radhi, McMaster University, Hamilton ON, Canada.)

Biopsies show a spectrum of findings including apoptosis, crypt necrosis (marked with black arrows in Figure 27-5), and ulceration with denuded epithelium in severe cases.

○   **In pneumatosis intestinalis, air-filled cysts are found in which layers of the colonic wall?**

The air-filled cavities of pneumatosis intestinalis are pseudocyts and can arise in the mucosa, submucosa, or subserosa. They are most commonly found in the submucosa. These appear endoscopically as blue polypoid lesions.

○   **How does pneumatosis intestinalis present?**

Most patients are asymptomatic; however, diarrhea, rectal bleeding, abdominal pain, bloating, and constipation have been reported.

○   **What are five complications of pneumatosis intestinalis?**

Bowel obstruction, hemorrhage, intussusception, volvulus, and pneumoperitoneum.

○   **How is symptomatic pneumatosis intestinalis treated?**

Mild symptoms have been treated with antibiotics, elemental diets, high-flow oxygen, hyperbaric oxygen, surgery, and endoscopic puncture with sclerotherapy. These treatments have not been validated by large clinical trials. Preliminary data suggest a high rate of recurrence (up to 40% within 18 months) after any therapy.

○   **What is diverticular colitis?**

Diverticular colitis is a segmental colitis associated with diverticular disease.

○   **True/False: Diverticular colitis and diverticulitis are synonymous.**

False.

○   **What are the endoscopic and histologic features of diverticular colitis?**

Mild disease is characterized by minimal inflammation with red spots surrounding diverticula ("Fawaz spots"). These red spots likely represent submucosal hemorrhage. Severe disease may be indistinguishable from IBD.

○   **What is the proposed pathogenesis of diverticular colitis?**

Proposed mechanisms include fecal stasis, bacterial overgrowth, and local ischemia.

○   **How does diverticular colitis usually present?**

This condition typically presents in the seventh decade of life with diarrhea, rectal bleeding, and abdominal pain.

○   **What is the treatment of diverticular colitis?**

A high-fiber diet is generally recommended. Small clinical trials demonstrate some efficacy for antibiotics, aminosalicylates, and probiotics; however, the long-term management remains controversial.

● ● ● **SUGGESTED READINGS** ● ● ●

Tursi A. Segmental Colitis Associated with Diverticulosis: Complication of Diverticular Disease or Autonomous Entity? *Dig Dis Sci.* 2011;56:27-34.

Feuerstadt P, Brandt LJ. Colon Ischemia: Recent Insight and Advances. *Curr Gastroenterol Rep.* 2010;12:383-390.

Yen EF, Pardi DS. Review article: microscopic colitis—lymphocytic, collagenous and "mast cell" colitis. *Aliment Pharmacol Ther.* 2011;34:21-32.

CHAPTER 28 Large Intestinal Tumors

Hemant K. Roy, MD and Amir Patel, MD

○ **True/False: A patient whose parents have familial adenomatous polyposis (FAP) has a normal flexible sigmoidoscopy at age 12. He is unlikely to develop FAP.**

False. Fifty percent of patients with FAP will develop polyps by age 15. In general, screening is accomplished by flexible sigmoidoscopy starting after puberty. For early diagnosis, gene testing is available if a proband is positive. The upper age for screening is unclear given that most patients will develop full-blown FAP by their 30s. Of note, the discovery of attenuated FAP syndromes, which can present later in life, has complicated this approach. Furthermore, attenuated FAP (mutations in the 5′ or 3′ end of the gene) has a predilection for involving the right side of the colon.

○ **What are recommended screening options for a patient with a family history of FAP? Of hereditary nonpolyposis colorectal cancer (HNPCC)?**

FAP: genetic counseling and consider genetic testing. A negative test result rules out FAP only if an affected family member has an identified mutation. Gene carriers or indeterminate cases should be offered flexible sigmoidoscopy every 12 months beginning at puberty and, if polyposis is identified, offered colectomy.

HNPCC: genetic counseling and consider genetic testing. They should undergo a colonoscopic examination every 1 to 2 years starting between the ages of 20 and 30 and yearly after age 40. Female patients should be counseled on their risks for endometrial and ovarian cancer and their screening options.

○ **What is the recommended for surveillance interval in patients with an adenomatous polyp?**

According to recent guidelines, patients with large or multiple adenomatous polyps should have repeat colonoscopy 3 years after the initial exam. If this exam is normal or shows only a small tubular adenoma, follow-up colonoscopy can be performed in 5 years. In special circumstances (eg, polyps with invasive cancer, large sessile adenomas, or numerous adenomas), follow-up colonoscopy may be done sooner.

○ **True/False: A 28-year-old woman with no significant family history is found to have thousands of colonic polyps. Based on this, she is given the diagnosis of FAP and undergoes colectomy. Genetic testing is negative. The patient's 2-year-old son is also tested for the adenomatous polyposis coli (APC) gene mutation and is negative. No further surveillance is necessary for the child.**

False. Approximately 20% of patients with APC gene mutations will not have a family history of FAP. The in vitro synthesized protein (IVSP) assay that is commercially available only has 80% sensitivity for APC gene mutations. Therefore, a negative test is not interpretable if no one else in the family is known to be positive for gene mutations by this assay.

○ **True/False: Gastric polyps in patients with FAP occur in the proximal stomach.**

True. Gastric polyposis typically occurs in half the patients with FAP. They generally consist of fundic gland polyps and are most common in the proximal stomach. Rarely, adenomatous polyps can be found in the antrum (5%).

○ **True/False: Gastric cancer is the next most common cause of mortality in patients with FAP following colectomy.**

False. The next most common cause of mortality is from periampullary duodenal carcinomas (lifetime risk 4%). Periodic screening with a side-viewing endoscope is probably cost-effective and is generally offered starting at the age of 25 to 30 years.

○ **True/False: Retinoblastomas are common in patients with FAP.**

False. Congenital hypertrophy of the retinal pigmented epithelium (CHRPE) may occur.

○ **What is the earliest histological abnormality that occurs during colon carcinogenesis?**

Aberrant crypt foci (ACF). ACF are clonal lesions present on macroscopically normal mucosa. They are often seen by examining, under magnification, colons stained with methylene blue. Recent studies have shown that these may be detectable by utilization of a magnifying colonoscope. These lesions typically demonstrate K-*ras* mutations with dysplastic ACF having APC mutations.

○ **True/False: Juvenile polyps have no malignant potential.**

False. Juvenile polyps are hamartomas characterized by distended mucus-filled glands. They typically occur in children and usually slough off or regress but occasionally may be found in adults. When single they have no malignant potential; however, when part of familial juvenile polyposis syndrome, they are associated with mixed juvenile-adenomatous polyps and have malignant potential.

○ **What is the inheritance pattern of juvenile polyposis?**

The genetics are unknown. It is thought to be an autosomal dominant condition with incomplete penetrance. Research in juvenile polyposis syndrome families has identified two specific gene changes causing disruption of the transforming growth factor beta: SMAD4 and BMPR1A. Recent data suggest that mutations may occur in stromal cells leading to a "landscaper" defect. The gene that has been implicated is PTEN (phosphatase and tensin homologue) on the deleted part of chromosome 10q.

○ **A 27-year-old man with mucocutaneous pigmentation presents with abdominal pain. What malignancies are associated with this syndrome?**

Peutz–Jeghers polyps are hamartomas that, not uncommonly, cause intussusception. These patients are at higher risk for carcinomas of the colon, duodenum, jejunum, and ileum. Ovarian sex cord tumors and testicular cancers have also been described. Breast and pancreatic cancers have been known to occur at a young age. Approximately half of the patients with this syndrome will develop cancer. The gene, recently discovered (STK11 also known as LKB1), is a serine-threonine kinase.

○ **True/False: K-*ras* is responsible for FAP in patients that are APC wild-type.**

False. MYH has been noted to cause FAP in a significant proportion of APC-negative FAP. MYH is autosomal recessive. K-*ras* is believed to initiate most ACF but the relationship to polyps is unclear.

○ **A 56-year-old woman is noted to have a sessile serrated adenoma. What is the most appropriate management strategy?**

Currently, sessile serrated adenomas are treated like conventional adenomas. There is some evidence that they may be more aggressive. Molecularly, they are more likely to be microsatellite unstable and frequently have B-raf involvement.

○ **True/False: A 62-year-old woman is found to have a 1.5-cm flat lesion in her cecum on colonoscopy. The malignancy risk is lower in this case than if she had a more raised lesion.**

False. Typically flat and depressed lesions have a higher risk of malignancy compared with more raised polypoid lesions and are more difficult to endoscopically visualize. Techniques such as chromoendoscopy and narrowband imaging may improve detection.

○ **In what segment of the colon are colon polyps most likely to remain undetected (ie, missed)?**

The emerging data suggests that right-sided lesions are less likely to be detected. There is emerging evidence that colonoscopy is suboptimally protective in the right colon. Procedural characteristics such as withdrawal time and, possibly, use of adjunctive approaches such as high-definition colonoscopes and chromoendoscopy may be involved. Microsatellite stability (three- to fourfold higher incidence in missed lesions), unsuccessful cecal intubation, and poor preparation in the proximal colon may also play a role.

○ **A 50-year-old man presents with diffuse gastrointestinal polyposis, dystrophic changes in the fingernails, alopecia, cutaneous hyperpigmentation, diarrhea, weight loss, abdominal pain, and complications of malnutrition. Do his children need to be screened?**

No. Cronkite–Canada syndrome is an acquired, nonfamilial syndrome. The polyps are juvenile-type but may have adenomatous epithelium. Carcinomas are quite rare. The malabsorption syndrome is progressive and portends a poor prognosis.

○ **Which is the best estimate for the risk of colorectal cancer in 1–2 cm tubular adenomatous polyps—3%, 10%, or 25%?**

10%. With adenomas <1 cm, the risk is about 1.3%, while the risk for those >2 cm is 46%. These rates are higher in villous compared to tubular adenomas. With regard to high-grade dysplasia, it may be found in 1.1% of polyps <0.5 cm, 4.6% of polyps between 0.5 and 0.9 cm and 20.6% of those >1.0 cm.

○ **True/False: The earliest mutation in colon carcinogenesis is K-*ras*.**

False. In the multistage colon cancer genetic model, the APC tumor suppressor gene is mutated in >80% in histologically normal mucosa followed by K-*ras* at the small adenoma stage, deleted in colon cancer (DCC) at the large adenoma stage and p53 at the malignancy stage. Often, if APC is not mutated, its downstream effector—β-catenin—is altered.

○ **True/False: Microsatellite instability is seen only in patients with HNPCC.**

False. Microsatellite instability is seen in 15% of all colorectal cancers. Fewer than 20% will have germline mutations in the mismatch repair enzymes. Recently, the analysis of BRAF mutations has been shown to be helpful in discriminating between sporadic and HNPCC-related colorectal cancers.

○ **HNPCC is associated with what genes?**

Lynch syndrome is a hereditary cancer syndrome that is inherited in an autosomal dominant manner. It is caused by germline mutations in the mismatch repair genes MLH1, MSH2, MSH6, and PMS2. MLH1 and MSH2 mutations account for the majority of mutations (approximately 30% are due to MLH1 and 40% due to MSH2).

○ **For Lynch syndrome (ie, HNPCC), does the gene involved result in any clinical significant difference in outcome?**

Yes. Typically the colorectal cancer risk is highest for MLH1 and lowest for MSH6. In contrast, MSH6 has a high risk for endometrial cancer.

○ **True/False: Tumors with microsatellite instability have a worse prognosis than standard colon cancers.**

False. While tumors with microsatellite instability are typically less differentiated and mucinous, they tend to have a significantly better prognosis than standard tumors. These tumors, whether sporadic or part of HNPCC, tend to be flat, right-sided and have lymphocyte infiltration. The general recommendations for screening for microsatellite instability in colon cancer (Bethesda criteria) include young patients, right-sided mucinous tumors, and family history of colon cancer.

○ **What genetic marker has prognostic implications for Dukes B2 colon cancer?**

DCC status. Adjuvant chemotherapy has not been shown to have a survival advantage for Dukes B2 colon cancer; however, recent evidence suggests that if this tumor suppressor gene is mutated, B2 tumors "behave" more like a C1 tumor. Adjuvant chemotherapy has been shown to provide a survival advantage for Dukes C tumors.

○ **True/False: Nonsteroidal anti-inflammatory drugs (NSAIDs) are helpful in preventing polyp formation in FAP but not sporadic colon cancer.**

False. Epidemiological and experimental studies have demonstrated responsiveness to NSAIDs in both of these conditions. Both conditions are characterized by upregulation of cyclooxygenase-2 early in carcinogenesis.

○ **What types of gastrointestinal polyps are associated with the basal cell nevus syndrome?**

Multiple gastric hamartomatous polyps.

○ **True/False: Colon cancer is common in Cowden's syndrome.**

False. The hallmark of Cowden's syndrome is facial trichilemmomas. It is characterized by multiple oral and dermatological hamartomas, breast disease (both fibrocystic and cancer), thyroid disease (nontoxic goiter and cancer), as well as hamartomatous polyps of the stomach, small bowel, and colon. The colorectal polyps have disorganization and proliferation of the muscularis mucosa with normal overlying colonic epithelium. These rarely cause symptoms or degenerate into colon cancer.

○ **What are the major extracolonic manifestations of Gardner's syndrome?**

Gardner's syndrome is a variant of FAP with a germline mutation in the APC gene. It is characterized by bone disease, especially osteomas of the long bones, skull, and mandible. Dental abnormalities including supernumerary teeth, impacted teeth, and mandibular cysts have been seen. CHRPE is commonly seen. Soft tissue tumors including fibromas, lipomas, and epidermoid cysts can be seen. Extracolonic malignancies are similar to classic FAP (peri-ampullary and gastric); however, papillary carcinoma of the thyroid and adrenals and tumors of the liver and biliary tree have also been reported.

○ **What tumors are commonly associated with HNPCC?**

Endometrial, ovarian, gastric, pancreatic, hepatobiliary, small intestinal and transitional cell carcinomas of the ureter, and renal pelvis.

○ **True/False: Bone cancer is the second leading cause of death in patients with Gardner's syndrome.**

False. Desmoid tumors have been reported in 8%–13% of patients and are second only to metastatic colon cancer as a cause of death. This diffuse mesenteric fibromatosis is often a reaction to a laparotomy but may appear spontaneously. The progressive growth of mesenteric fibroblasts can cause gastrointestinal obstruction, vascular compromise, and ureteral obstruction. While responsive to radiation therapy, this is often impractical because of concerns over mesenteric injury. NSAIDs and anti-estrogens may have some effect.

○ **True/False: Duodenal polyposis is rare in FAP.**

False. Sixty to ninety percent of patients have duodenal polyposis and 50%–85% have adenomatous changes of the papilla of Vater. Four to 12% of these patients develop duodenal/periampullary malignancies.

○ **True/False: Turcot's syndrome is associated with HNPCC and FAP.**

True, partially. The brain tumors that occur in FAP with Turcot's syndrome are generally medulloblastomas while gliomas are generally found with the HNPCC variant.

○ **True/False: Neurofibromatosis predisposes to colon cancer.**

False. Neurofibromas may be seen throughout the gut. Malignant tumors can be seen, often from degeneration of neurofibromas; however, colorectal adenocarcinomas are rare.

○ **True/False: Liver metastases from colorectal cancer are best treated with intra-arterial 5-FU or floxuridine (FUDR).**

False. This therapy remains investigational and is complicated by the development of a sclerosing cholangitis-like picture. If there is no evidence of extrahepatic disease and the tumor(s) involve either one lobe of the liver or are focal and surgically accessible in both lobes, surgical resection should be contemplated. After successful surgery, the 5-year survival rate is 20%–34%. Unfortunately, only 5%–6% of patients are considered surgical candidates. Recent data suggest that intra-arterial chemotherapy in combination with surgery is superior to surgery alone.

○ **True/False: Adjuvant chemotherapy has not been shown to have a survival benefit for Dukes B2 rectal cancer.**

False. Dukes B2 rectal cancer should be treated with either preoperative or postoperative chemotherapy accompanied by radiation therapy in order to enhance local therapy. This differs for colon cancer *per se*.

○ **True/False: The use of the carcinoembryonic antigen (CEA) level, abdominal CT scan, and chest x-ray in addition to colonoscopy as surveillance methods after curative resection for colon cancer has been shown to improve survival.**

False. Neither routine CT scanning nor chest x-rays have been shown to improve survival. Obtaining CEA levels annually may have a role, although its cost-effectiveness has been controversial.

○ **True/False: Patients with a family history of adenomatous polyps are at a higher risk for colorectal cancer.**

True. If diagnosed under age 55, there is a markedly increased risk of colorectal cancer.

○ **True/False: Most patients with a positive fecal occult blood test (FOBT) will have a colon cancer or polyp.**

False. While the sensitivity of FOBT is approximately 80%, the positive predictive value is only about 10%–20%.

○ **True/False: The risk of colon cancer in patients with inflammatory bowel disease may be affected by certain extraintestinal manifestations.**

True. While the predominant risk factors include the amount of bowel involved and duration of the disease, coexisting sclerosing cholangitis is also a significant risk factor.

○ **What endocrine disorder carries a higher risk of colonic neoplasia?**

Acromegaly. Although the studies are retrospective, the estimates of the prevalence of adenomatous polyps and colon cancer range from 6.3% to 25% and 14% to 35%, respectively. The risk may be higher in younger patients, those with a family history of colon cancer, and those with multiple skin tags (acrochordons). While the mechanism is unclear, it is not simply growth hormone-related since the risk of neoplasia may be greater in cured acromegalics than those with active disease.

○ **What organisms responsible for bacteremia are associated with the presence of colorectal neoplasia?**

Streptococcus bovis bacteremia has been associated with the presence of colorectal adenomas and carcinomas. *Clostridium septicum* bacteremia has also been associated with the colonic neoplasia. Finally, endocarditis associated with *Streptococcus agalactiae* has been reported in several patients with rectal villous adenomas containing small foci of carcinoma.

○ **True/False: Patients with breast cancer have an increased risk of colon cancer.**

False. There is no evidence in case-control studies that having a personal history of breast cancer is a risk factor for colon cancer. However, patients with familial breast cancer associated with mutations in BRCA 1 or 2 have a 3- to 6-fold increased incidence of colon cancer.

○ **What are potential mechanisms in colonic neoplasm-induced diarrhea?**

A syndrome of large-volume secretory diarrhea has been observed with large villous adenomas in the rectum and rectosigmoid colon and is associated with dehydration and electrolyte abnormalities, especially hypokalemia. The mechanisms are unclear. Some data suggest that prostaglandins are involved.

○ **How common are adenomatous polyps in the general population?**

Clinical studies indicate that adenomatous polyps occur in 25% of patients 50 years old and increase with age. By the late 70s, 50% of people have polyps. Autopsy studies suggest an even higher rate with approximately 60% of men and 40% of women having adenomatous polyps at age 50. They are found more commonly in men than in women. While data on large polyps (> 1 cm) is limited, one autopsy series suggested that 4.6% of the population at age 54 and 15.6% at age 75 had large polyps.

○ **True/False: The risk of colon cancer is lower in patients with Crohn's disease compared to those with ulcerative colitis.**

False. Crohn's colitis has the same risk as ulcerative colitis when matched for extent, duration, and age of onset of the disease. The cumulative risk for developing colorectal cancer with pancolitis is 30% after 35 years. Surveillance colonoscopy every 1–2 years is recommended after 8 years in those with pancolitis and after 15 years in those with left-sided colitis.

○ **A 63-year-old man had a 2-cm pedunculated polyp, which contained a focus of malignancy, removed from the sigmoid colon. What surveillance is recommended?**

If invasive carcinoma is found and poor prognostic features exist (eg, malignancy incompletely excised, less than a 2-mm margin from polypectomy, a relatively undifferentiated tumor or lymphatic or venous invasion), then hemicolectomy is recommended. Sessile polyps are also considered to have a worse prognosis. If no poor prognostic features exist, as in this patient, it would be reasonable to consider that the polypectomy is the definitive therapy. Colonoscopy is often recommended within 3 months of polypectomy and then 1 year later to ensure that there is no residual malignant tissue.

○ **A 10-year-old girl presents with hematochezia and is found to have two juvenile colonic polyps. Her family history is unremarkable. What is the recommended follow-up?**

This patient does not meet the criteria for juvenile polyposis which includes the presence of 10 or more juvenile polyps, juvenile polyps throughout the gastrointestinal tract, or juvenile polyps in a patient with a family history of polyposis. These nonneoplastic hamartomatous colonic polyps are extremely common occurring in 1%–2% of all children, usually between the ages of 4 and 14. A solitary polyp is seen in 70% of patients but 30% will have 2 or 3. If a polyposis syndrome is not identified, no other evaluation is necessary.

○ **A 28-year-old patient with Gardner's syndrome is noted to have nodular lymphoid hyperplasia of the terminal ileum. What therapy is necessary?**

Nodular lymphoid hyperplasia is a rare lymphoproliferative disorder associated with a variety of disorders including Gardner's. It is also present in 20% of patients with common variable immunodeficiency and is rarely associated with intestinal lymphoma. Of note, it has also been seen in otherwise healthy children. These hyperplastic lymphoid nodules are often found in the small bowel but may be seen in the stomach and colon. These nodules range in size from 3 to 6 mm. No therapy is required for nodular lymphoid hyperplasia.

○ **What agents are FDA-approved for preventing colon neoplasia?**

While NSAIDs as a class protect against colon cancer, only celecoxib has been approved for this indication in patients with FAP. However, given the cardiotoxicity, this needs to be utilized with caution.

○ **What agents have been shown to inhibit colon cancer?**

Epidemiological studies in humans have demonstrated that NSAIDs, estrogens, calcium, and folate inhibit colon cancer. The effect of dietary fiber is controversial. Animal studies suggest that ursodeoxycholic acid, vitamin D analogues, polyethylene glycol, and fish oil may also be protective.

○ **What are the screening recommendations for a patient with a 53-year-old brother who just had an adenomatous polyp removed?**

According to current guidelines, any person with a first-degree relative with either colon cancer or an adenomatous polyp should be offered the same screening options as average-risk patients, except starting at age 40 or 10 years prior to diagnosis of the affected relative, whichever comes first. The guideline states that if the patient had colorectal cancer before 55 or adenomatous polyp before age 60, special efforts should be made to ensure that screening takes place.

○ **What are the screening recommendations for patients at an average-risk for colon cancer?**

Starting at age 50, colonoscopy every 10 years, CT colonography or double-contrast barium enema every 5 years, annual FOBT, flexible sigmoidoscopy every 5 years, or a combination of FOBT and flexible sigmoidoscopy.

○   **True/False: Lack of exercise and obesity are associated with colonic neoplasia.**

True. Epidemiological studies have demonstrated that these are independent risk factors for colon cancer.

○   **Hereditary hemorrhagic telangiectasia (HHT) is an autosomal dominant disease of vascular dysplasia (epistaxis, telangiectasia, and arteriovenous malformations) that is associated with what familial cancer syndrome?**

Juvenile polyposis syndrome. Identification of SMAD4 mutations in HHT patients without a prior diagnosis of juvenile polyposis syndrome has been demonstrated in a subset of patients. These patients are at risk of having JP-HHT and an increased risk of gastrointestinal cancer.

○   **A 37-year-old male seeks your advice after his 62-year-old mother was recently diagnosed with colon cancer. His maternal uncle was also diagnosed with colon cancer and his maternal grandmother had a history of endometrial cancer. What would be the best way to manage this patient?**

This patient's history is suspicious for HNPCC. He should be referred to a genetic counselor. The best approach to test for HNPCC in this case would be to obtain tumor tissue from the patient's mother to test for microsatellite instability. If the test is positive, a blood test can be done to identify a germline mutation in the mismatch repair genes. A negative blood test does not exclude the diagnosis and aggressive screening should still be pursued.

○   **On screening colonoscopy, a 50-year-old man is found to have multiple adenomas (3 total) with the largest measuring 2 cm. There is no family history of colorectal cancer. When should the patient have a repeat colonoscopy to check for metachronous adenomas?**

Three years. Patients at high risk of developing advanced adenomas should have a repeat colonoscopy 3 years after the primary finding. High-risk patients include patients with multiple adenomas (> 2 adenomas), large adenomas (> 1 cm), adenomas of villous histology or high-grade dysplasia, and/or patients with a family history of colorectal cancer. Patients at low risk of developing advanced adenomas can have repeat colonoscopy 5 years after.

○   **A 63-year-old woman is found to have a malignant polyp on colonoscopy. It is completely excised. On pathology, the cancer is not poorly differentiated and the margins of excision are not involved. There is no vascular or lymphatic involvement. What is the next step in managing this patient?**

No further treatment is indicated. The patient has favorable prognostic criteria and should have a follow-up colonoscopy in 3 months to check for residual abnormal tissue at the polypetctomy site. The risk of local recurrence or local lymph node metastasis from invasive carcinoma in a colonoscopically resected polyp is less than the risk for death from colonic surgery. Therefore, the American College of Gastroenterology (ACG) recommends no further treatment if the following criteria are fulfilled: The polyp is completely excised; the cancer is not poorly differentiated; there is no vascular or lymphatic involvement; and the pathology laboratory can confirm the depth of invasion, grade of differentiation, and completeness of excision.

○   **A 65-year-old woman is evaluated after undergoing left hemicolectomy for colon cancer 3 months previously. She was found to have stage IIA disease and has been doing well. She did not undergo full colonoscopy prior to surgical resection. What is the most appropriate endoscopic management for this patient?**

An immediate colonoscopy and then again in 1 year. Patients diagnosed with colon cancer require a complete survey of the colon. If it has not been done preoperatively, it should be done postoperatively to check for other lesions. Surveillance colonoscopy should then be performed at 1, 3, and 5 years.

• • • SUGGESTED READINGS • • •

Jasperson KW, Tuohy TM, Neklason DW, Burt RW. Hereditary and familial colon cancer. *Gastroenterology*. 2010 Jun;138(6): 2044-2058.

Smith KD, Rodriguez-Bigas MA. Role of surgery in familial adenomatous polyposis and hereditary nonpolyposis colorectal cancer (Lynch syndrome). *Surg Oncol Clin N Am*. 2009 Oct;18(4):705-715.

Tops CM, Wijnen JT, Hes FJ. Introduction to molecular and clinical genetics of colorectal cancer syndromes. *Best Pract Res Clin Gastroenterol*. 2009;23(2):127-146.

Levin B, Lieberman DA, McFarland B, et al. Screening and surveillance for the early detection of colorectal cancer and adenomatous polyps, 2008: a joint guideline from the American Cancer Society, the US Multi-Society Task Force on Colorectal Cancer, and the American College of Radiology. *Gastroenterology*. 2008;134:1570-1595.

CHAPTER 29

Disorders of the Pelvic Floor and Anorectum

Yehuda Ringel, MD

○ **True/False: Hemorrhoidal disease is more frequently associated with constipation than with diarrheal disorders.**

False. Studies suggest that hemorrhoidal disease is more frequently associated with diarrheal disorders.

○ **Describe the classification of internal hemorrhoids according to their clinical severity.**

Internal hemorrhoids are classified according to their degree of protrusion and prolapse as follows:

First degree — bulge into the anorectal lumen but do not protrude out of the anus

Second degree — prolapse out of the anus with straining or defecation and spontaneously reduce back to their normal position

Third degree — prolapse out of the anus with straining or defecation and require digital reduction

Fourth degree — irreducible prolapse

○ **Procidentia refers to complete prolapse of the rectum. What are other forms of rectal prolapse?**

Procidentia involves visible protrusion of all the rectal layers through the anus. Two other forms of rectal prolapse are mucosal prolapse in which only the distal rectal mucosa protrude through the anus and occult rectal prolapse, which refers to internal intussusception of rectal tissue without visible protrusion through the anus.

○ **A 62-year-old female patient complains of a mass that intermittently protrudes through her anus. What is the differential diagnosis?**

Prolapsing internal hemorrhoids, anorectal varices, mucosal prolapse, rectal prolapse, anal/rectal polyps, anal/rectal tumors, and hypertrophic anal papillae.

○ **True/False: Cirrhotic patients usually develop hemorrhoidal disease secondary to portal hypertension.**

False. Anorectal varices, not hemorrhoids, develop as a result of portal hypertension. They represent the communication between the portal circulation through the superior hemorrhoidal veins and the systemic circulation through the middle and inferior hemorrhoidal veins.

○ **True/False: The classic endoscopic appearance of solitary rectal ulcer syndrome is a shallow, discrete 1–4 cm ulcer located at the posterior wall of the rectum 4–15 cm from the anal verge.**

False. The name is a misnomer. The appearance in many patients with this condition includes multiple ulcers, hyperemic mucosa, or a polypoid lesion(s). In addition, although the lesion(s) may be found on the posterior wall of the rectum, they are more commonly located on the anterior wall of the rectum.

○ **What functional and morphological abnormalities can be associated with solitary rectal ulcer syndrome?**

Solitary rectal ulcer syndrome is associated with some form of rectal redundancy and prolapse or mucosal prolapse and thicker muscularis propria in the rectal wall. The condition is commonly associated with high anal sphincter pressure, failure of the puborectalis to relax during defecation, and persistent straining and delayed rectal evacuation. Biofeedback treatment may improve rectal blood flow and help ulcer healing.

○ **What conditions predict a favorable response to biofeedback (pelvic floor retraining) therapy for fecal incontinence?**

The ability to contract the external sphincter during squeezing, some degree of rectal sensation, cooperative patient (ie, no cognitive impairment, mental retardation, dementia, or psychosis), and no evidence of complete denervation on electromyography.

○ **True/False: Anal and rectal carcinomas are more common in men.**

False. Rectal carcinoma is more common in men, whereas anal canal tumors are nearly twice as common in women.

○ **True/False: Because of the anus' location at the very distal part of the gastrointestinal tract and its easy accessibility for digital examination, anal canal tumors produce symptoms early in the course of the disease and are usually diagnosed at an early stage.**

False. In about 60% of the patients with anal canal tumors, the tumor is discovered late. Indeed, 15%–30% of patients are found to have metastatic spread at presentation. The symptoms are usually mild and nonspecific. Approximately 25% of patients with anal canal tumors are symptom-free and the tumor is found incidentally during a routine examination.

○ **True/False: Adenocarcinoma is the most common malignant tumor of the anal canal.**

False. The most common tumor of the anal canal is squamous cell carcinoma (70%–80%). Adenocarcinoma is a rare tumor of the anal canal.

○ **True/False: Most benign, idiopathic anal fissures develop in the posterior midline of the anal orifice and often have a skin tag at the external edge and/or hypertrophied anal papilla at the internal edge.**

True. Benign, idiopathic anal fissures commonly develop in the posterior midline. Fissures in lateral or anterior position, presence of warning signs, and appearance in older age should raise concern and may require further evaluation.

○   **What is the rationale for the management and the treatment options for chronic anal fissure?**

Therapy aims to break the cycle of pain, spasm, and ischemia thought to be responsible for the development of the fissure. Goals of treatment include pain relief, relaxation of the internal anal sphincter, and institution of atraumatic passage of stool. Available treatment options include:

- Bulking agents and stool softeners.
- Warm Sitz baths two to three times a day.
- Conservative medical treatment includes topical nitroglycerin, topical nifedipine or diltiazem, and botulinum toxin injections. In one study, the injection of botulinum toxin into the internal anal sphincter was found to be more effective than topical application of 0.2% nitroglycerin ointment.
- Surgical treatment. Lateral internal sphincterotomy is reserved for fissures that have failed medical therapy. A meta-analysis of four randomized trials found superior fissure healing with surgery over topical nitroglycerin treatment.

○   **True/False: Pruritus ani is a relatively common symptom and a careful evaluation usually reveals the underlying etiology and leads to effective and successful treatment.**

False. The differential diagnosis of pruritus ani is relatively wide. The symptom may be secondary to a variety of local or dietary irritants, medications, and a wide range of disease conditions including anorectal diseases (eg, fistula, fissure, prolapse), diarrheal conditions (eg, Crohn's disease, ulcerative colitis, IBS), systemic disorders (eg, diabetes mellitus, Hodgkin's lymphoma), dermatologic conditions (eg, psoriasis, seborrhea, atopic dermatitis), infections (eg, pinworm, Candida, *Herpes simplex*, HIV), and neoplasms (eg, extramammary Paget's disease, squamous cell carcinoma, Bowen's disease). There are no guidelines regarding the optimal diagnostic approach and, in the majority of the patients, the cause of pruritus ani remains unknown.

○   **What is the prevalence of fecal incontinence?**

The prevalence of fecal incontinence in the Western Hemisphere is 2%–7% and increases with age. Surveys have shown prevalence rates of 18% in the older female population and 45%–47% in nursing home residents and hospitalized elderly patients.

○   **What information can be obtained from anorectal manometry?**

Anorectal manometry provides an objective measure of anal sphincter and rectal function at rest and during defecatory maneuvers. This includes measurements of anal sphincter tone (at rest, during squeezing and during increase in intra-abdominal pressure), rectal sensation thresholds, and rectal compliance. It also provides information about anorectal reflexes that are important in continence and defecation processes.

○   **What is the rectoanal inhibitory reflex (RAIR)? Why is it important and in which conditions is it typically absent?**

The RAIR refers to the decrease in internal anal sphincter resting pressure that occurs in response to rectal balloon distension that is performed during anorectal manometry. This reflex, mediated by the myenteric plexus, plays an important role in the sampling and discrimination of rectal contents. Rectal distension also induces a pelvic splanchnic and pudendal nerve-mediated contractile response for the external anal sphincter—the rectoanal contractile reflex (RACR)—that prevents release of rectal contents. Absence of the RAIR should raise suspicion of Hirschsprung's disease, megarectum, structural damage to internal anal sphincter, or a tonically contracted external anal sphincter.

○ **Describe the imaging techniques available for clinical use in the evaluation of anorectal disorders and the information that can be obtained from each test.**

- Endoscopic anal ultrasound is helpful in assessing the integrity of the anal sphincters. Endoanal ultrasound (EAU) is not helpful in the assessment of anal function.
- Evacuation proctography (defecography) is useful for assessing the defecation process. It can provide important information on functional parameters (eg, anorectal angle at rest and during straining, perineal descent, puborectalis contraction/relaxation, degree of rectal emptying, and retained stool) as well as abnormal anatomy (eg, pelvic organ prolapse, rectocele, and enterocele).
- Magnetic resonance imaging (MRI) with rapid sequences. Performed in specialized referral centers, this test can visualize both anal sphincter anatomy and global pelvic floor motion in real-time without radiation exposure. MRI can also identify atrophy of the external sphincter and puborectalis which may be found in some patients with fecal incontinence.

○ **What are the differences between the internal and external anal sphincters and their role in maintaining continence?**

The internal anal sphincter is composed of smooth muscle and is under the control of the enteric nervous system. Its main function is to maintain the resting tone of the anal sphincter. The external anal sphincter is composed of striated muscle innervated by the pudendal nerve (sacral branches S2 to S4) and is under voluntary control. The main role of the external anal sphincter is to contract voluntarily in response to a sudden increase in rectal or abdominal pressure so as to prevent inappropriate defecation.

○ **What is the relative contribution of the internal and external anal sphincter muscles to the resting anal tone?**

About 70% of the anal canal resting tone is derived from the internal anal sphincter and the remainder by the external anal sphincter muscle.

○ **A manometric evaluation in a patient with fecal incontinence reveals a failure to increase anal sphincter pressure when asked to squeeze but a normal increase in pressure in response to coughing. Besides poor motivation or comprehension, what is the most probable explanation?**

An increase in external anal sphincter pressure in response to an abrupt increase in intra-abdominal pressure is triggered by receptors in the pelvic floor and mediated through a spinal reflex arc. Lesions of the cauda equina or sacral plexus will result in loss of both the reflex response and the voluntary squeeze. Higher spinal cord lesions may result in the findings described in the question.

○ **What are the treatment options for patients with fecal incontinence?**

- Conservative measures including diet changes, skin care, and occasionally, antidiarrheal medications.
- Biofeedback therapy using a rectal balloon with anal manometry or a surface electromyography device. Patients are taught to contract the external anal sphincter when they perceive balloon distention. Patients can also be trained to increase their perception of rectal distention.
- Sacral nerve stimulation, a recent FDA-approved implantable device for treating urinary, and fecal incontinence. This is a staged procedure that involves a trial of temporary external stimulation for 3 weeks followed by permanent implantation of the device subcutaneously if improvement is noted during the temporary stimulation.
- Surgical options for patients with anal sphincter defects not responding to conservative management include anal sphincteroplasty, artificial anal sphincter, and dynamic graciloplasty. Diverting colostomy may be considered in patients who have failed all other options.

○ **What are typical findings on physical examination and anorectal manometry in patients with proctalgia fugax?**

Proctalgia fugax is one of the functional disorders of the anorectum. The diagnosis is based on symptoms alone. There are no specific findings on physical examination or anorectal manometry testing.

○ **A 40-year-old female complains of recurrent episodes of dull "pressure-like" pain in the rectum that last for hours and are often brought on by sitting or lying down. Posterior traction of the puborectalis on rectal examination produces tenderness and pain. What is the diagnosis?**

The description is typical of levator ani syndrome. This syndrome is one of the functional disorders of the anorectum. The diagnosis is based on the presence of characteristic symptoms and tenderness and discomfort on puborectalis palpation during rectal examination. Evaluation is often required to exclude alternative diseases.

○ **True/False: Levator ani syndrome and proctalgia fugax frequently coexist.**

True. Although the two disorders can be distinguished on the basis of duration, frequency, and quality of pain, they coexist more often than expected by chance.

○ **What are functional defecation disorders? Name two recognized subtypes of these disorders.**

Functional defecation disorders describe important etiologic subtypes of functional constipation that involve delayed or obstructed defecation that may coexist with slow colonic transit. The multinational working team (Rome Committee) defines two subtypes of functional defecation disorders: *Dyssynergic defecation* characterized by paradoxical contraction or inadequate relaxation of the pelvic floor muscles during attempted defecation and *inadequate defecatory propulsion* characterized by inadequate rectal propulsive forces during attempted defecation.

○ **True/False: The multinational working team (Rome Committee) recommends that the diagnosis of functional defecation disorders be based on symptoms of constipation and abnormal diagnostic anorectal physiological tests including manometric, electromyographic, and/or radiologic evidence of failure of the pelvic floor to relax when attempting to defecate.**

True. The rationale for these diagnostic criteria is based on the recognition that symptoms alone do not consistently distinguish patients with functional defecation disorders from those without. Thus, to meet the diagnostic criteria for functional defecation disorders, patients must satisfy diagnostic criteria for functional constipation and have at least two of the following:
- Evidence of impaired evacuation, based on balloon expulsion test or imaging.
- Inappropriate contraction of the pelvic floor muscles or less than 20% relaxation of basal resting sphincter pressure by manometry, imaging, or EMG.
- Inadequate propulsive forces assessed by manometry or imaging.

○ **True/False: Digital rectal examination is a reliable way to identify dyssynergic defecation in patients with chronic constipation.**

True. Studies have shown that digital rectal examination is a reliable tool (75% sensitivity, 87% specificity, and 97% positive predictive value) for identifying dyssynergia in patients with chronic constipation. It can also detect normal, but not abnormal, sphincter tone. Digital rectal examination may be useful to direct the selection of appropriate patients for further physiologic testing and treatment.

○ **True/False: The majority of patients with pelvic floor dyssynergia will benefit from biofeedback (pelvic floor retraining) treatment.**

True, when performed in experienced centers. Approximately two-thirds of these patients can learn to relax the external anal sphincter and puborectalis muscles with biofeedback training and report associated decreases in both straining during defecation and the feeling of incomplete evacuation.

○ **True/False: Rectocele and mucosal intussusception are commonly present in healthy, asymptomatic individuals.**

True. Rectocele, mucosal prolapse, and rectal intussusception have been commonly reported in healthy asymptomatic subjects. Therefore, these findings should be interpreted with caution since they may not necessarily suggest a causal relationship with defecation disorders.

○ **True/False: Pelvic floor descent can be evaluated on physical examination.**

True. With the patient in the left lateral decubitus position, the level of the perineum relative to the ischial tuberosities is observed. With the patient straining, the perineum should not descend beyond the outlet of the bony pelvis.

○ **True/False: Fecal impaction can be definitively excluded by digital rectal examination.**

False. Digital rectal examination can miss 30% of fecal impactions in the elderly because a large amount of feces can accumulate above the reach of the examining finger.

○ **What are the indications for evacuation proctography (defecography) in the evaluation of anorectal and pelvic floor disorders?**

The American Gastroenterological Association Medical Position Statement on anorectal testing techniques suggests the use of evacuation proctography in patients with constipation in whom functional defecation disorders, enterocele or anterior rectocele, are suspected as the cause of impaired defecation. There is no support for the use of this technique for other purposes.

○ **What are the clinical findings of anorectal syphilis?**

Anal chancres in the skin around the anus, anal or rectal ulceration, and rectal lesions resembling carcinoma have all been described. Enlarged and tender inguinal lymph nodes are often present. Serologic tests for syphilis should be performed prior to surgery for any atypical rectal lesion.

○ **True/False: Vesicles on the perianal region and within the anal canal are commonly seen in anorectal herpes infections.**

False. Although perianal vesicles are a characteristic finding in anorectal herpes infection, they are uncommon within the anal canal. Ulcerations of the anal canal are more commonly seen in anorectal herpes infection.

○ **True/False: The intersphincteric space is the most common anatomic location of anorectal abscesses.**

False. Perianal abscesses located just beneath the perianal skin are most common.

○ **True/False: In at least one-half of ulcerative anal lesions in HIV-positive patients, no specific cause is found.**

True. Diagnostic considerations include syphilis, tuberculosis, *Mycobacterium avium-intracellulare*, herpes simplex, cytomegalovirus, fungi, and neoplasm.

○ **True/False: Anogenital condylomata acuminata caused by human papillomavirus (HPV) is associated with adenocarcinoma of the anus.**

False. HPV (types 16 and 18) is associated with squamous cell carcinoma of the anus as well as the cervix and vulva. Condylomata acuminata and anal cancer may coexist; thus, it is advisable to obtain biopsies from suspected lesions and examine the anal canal before beginning treatment.

○ **What is anal sampling and how is it related to the continence mechanism?**

The anal canal is highly innervated and sensitive to pain, touch, and temperature. This allows differentiation between gas, solids, and liquids and allows for selective passage of rectal contents or voluntary contraction of the external anal sphincter to maintain continence. Loss of this anal sampling function may contribute to the development of fecal incontinence.

○ **True/False: The most common cause of primary anorectal abscess and anorectal fistula is Crohn's disease.**

False. The most common cause of primary anorectal abscess and fistula is primary infection of anal cryptoglandular tissue. Other conditions that can be associated with anorectal abscesses and fistulae include Crohn's disease, proctitis, and anorectal cancer.

○ **What is the most common type/location of an anorectal fistula?**

Intersphincteric fistula.

○ **True/False: EAU and MRI are the most useful tests to diagnose an anorectal fistula.**

True. EAU and MRI have been shown to be highly accurate in identifying a fistula and describing its anatomy. EAU is more easily performed and less expensive than MRI; however, it is also more difficult to perform in patients with severe anal pain. The modality of choice depends on local expertise, cost, and patient convenience.

○ **True/False: A broad-spectrum antibiotic is the treatment of choice for an anorectal abscess.**

False. The primary treatment of an anorectal abscess is surgical incision and drainage. Except in patients with diabetes mellitus, leukemia, and valvular heart disease, antibiotics are usually not required.

○ **True/False: Up to 30% of women will have an anal sphincter defect on endoanal ultrasonography after their first vaginal delivery.**

True. In addition, about 10% will complain of urgency or incontinence.

● ● ● SUGGESTED READINGS ● ● ●

Bharucha AE, Wald A, Enck P, Rao SS. Functional anorectal disorders. *Gastroenterology.* 2006;130:1510-1518.

Whitehead WE, Bharucha AE. Diagnosis and treatment of pelvic floor disorders: what's new and what to do. *Gastroenterology.* 2010;138:1231-1235.

Rao SS. Advances in diagnostic assessment of fecal incontinence and dyssynergic defecation. *Clin Gastroenterol Hepatol.* 2010;8: 910-919.

Camilleri M, Bharucha AE, Di Lorenzo C, et al. American Neurogastroenterology and Motility Society consensus statement on intraluminal measurement of gastrointestinal and colonic motility in clinical practice. *Neurogastroenterol Motil.* 2008;20:1269-1282.

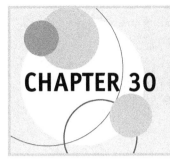

CHAPTER 30

Inflammatory Bowel Disease

Renee L. Young, MD

○ **True/False: Oral aphthous ulcerations may be seen in patients with Crohn's disease or ulcerative colitis.**

True. Oral aphthae occur in at least 10% of patients with active ulcerative colitis and typically resolve when this disease goes into remission. Aphthous ulcerations occur more commonly in Crohn's disease.

○ **Kidney stones develop with increased frequency in Crohn's disease. What types of stones may be seen?**

Oxalate kidney stones are seen in 5%–10% of Crohn's disease patients. Steatorrhea promotes excess colonic absorption of oxalate, which leads to the development of oxalate kidney stones. Urate stones are seen less frequently and are often associated with the presence of an ileostomy and/or dehydration.

○ **True/False: Crohn's disease patients are predisposed to gallstone formation.**

True. Fifteen percent to 30% of patients with small bowel Crohn's disease develop gallstones. Ileal dysfunction or resection leads to alterations in the bile salt pool.

○ **Which patients with Crohn's disease are most at risk for the development of amyloidosis?**

Those with long-standing suppurative or fistulous complications.

○ **Amyloidosis is an unusual but life-threatening complication of inflammatory bowel disease (IBD). What is the most common presentation of this rare complication?**

Nephrotic syndrome. Amyloid may also be diffusely deposited in bowel, spleen, liver, heart, and thyroid.

○ **True/False: Primary sclerosing cholangitis is associated with both ulcerative colitis and Crohn's disease.**

True. Primary sclerosing cholangitis is seen less frequently in Crohn's disease. With either disease, it can be complicated by the development of cholangiocarcinoma.

○ **In what trimester of pregnancy are relapses most frequently seen in women with Crohn's disease?**

First trimester. Approximately 75% of women in remission remain so throughout pregnancy, while only one-third of women with active Crohn's disease at the time of conception will achieve remission during pregnancy.

○   **True/False: Crohn's disease almost always flares after delivery in recently pregnant women.**

False. The activity of the disease at conception generally reflects disease activity at term.

○   **On the basis of radiologic and endoscopic findings, most patients with Crohn's disease can be subdivided into three anatomic groups. Name those groups and the approximate percentage of each.**

Colon alone   - 15%–25%

Small intestine and colon   - 40%–55%

Small intestine alone   - 30%–40%

○   **What percentage of Crohn's colitis involves the entire colon, exclusive of small bowel disease?**

Twenty-five percent. Crohn's disease involving the colon alone has more frequent involvement of the distal colon than those patients with ileocolitis. Only one-fourth of patients with Crohn's colitis exhibit skip lesions.

○   **True/False: "Skip" areas are characteristic of Crohn's disease. These areas appear normal grossly, radiologically, endoscopically, and histologically.**

False. "Skip" areas of the intestine may have normal or abnormal histology.

○   **True/False: Involvement of the rectum in a patient with colitis rules out Crohn's disease.**

False. Although rectal sparing is characteristic of Crohn's disease and helps distinguish it from ulcerative colitis, the rectum can be involved.

○   **True/False: The siblings of a Crohn's disease patient are more likely to develop Crohn's disease.**

True. They are about 17 to 35 times more likely to develop Crohn's disease than the general population.

○   **True/False: The incidence of Crohn's disease is declining.**

False. Most recent studies throughout the world show a rising incidence of Crohn's disease and a declining incidence of ulcerative colitis.

○   **True/False: Smoking cessation has been associated with an increased relative risk of the occurrence of Crohn's disease.**

False. Smoking is associated with an increased relative risk for the occurrence of Crohn's disease by a factor of 2 to 5. Smoking cessation has been associated with an increased relative risk of the occurrence of ulcerative colitis, however.

○   **Granulomas are a pathognomonic feature of Crohn's disease. Do these granulomas most resemble those seen in tuberculosis or sarcoidosis?**

Sarcoidosis. The granulomas found in sarcoid and Crohn's disease lack central caseation.

○   **Describe the earliest endoscopic features of inflammation in Crohn's disease.**

Mild mucosal hyperemia and edema are the earliest findings followed by aphthae or discrete ulcerations in more advanced cases.

○ **Describe how the mucosal surface acquires the "cobblestone" appearance frequently seen in Crohn's disease.**

Longitudinal and transverse serpiginous ulcerations form and the intervening edematous mucosa swells.

○ **Crohn's disease consists of transmural involvement of the intestinal tract. The bowel wall becomes thickened and the lumen narrows. Surgeons describe "creeping fat" in Crohn's disease. What is "creeping fat"?**

In Crohn's disease, the mesentery becomes thickened, edematous, hypervascular, and fatty. Finger-like projections of this inflamed mucosa "creep" along the serosal surface of the intestine and encase the involved segment of the intestine.

○ **True/False: Sulfasalazine has been proven to maintain remission in Crohn's disease.**

False. Sulfasalazine has been shown to be a remission-maintaining drug in ulcerative colitis only, not in Crohn's disease.

○ **The gastrointestinal presentation of Crohn's disease in children and adolescents is similar to adults. Children, however, have prominent systemic complaints that often precede their gastrointestinal complaints by months to years. Name some systemic manifestations of Crohn's disease in children and adolescents.**

Arthralgias and arthritis are seen in approximately 15%. Weight loss, failure to thrive, growth failure, fever, and anemia are all manifestations of Crohn's disease in children, particularly when the small bowel is involved.

○ **Small bowel barium x-ray in Crohn's disease may demonstrate separation of barium-filled loops of small bowel. Why does this occur?**

Edema of the bowel wall, especially the deeper layers of the bowel, produces this separation.

○ **When differentiating gastrointestinal tuberculosis from Crohn's disease, which of the following can be seen in both: fistulae, granulomas, and/or normal chest x-ray?**

All may be seen in both conditions. Fistulization occurs less frequently in tuberculosis. Granulomas can be seen in mesenteric lymph nodes in tuberculosis when there are no granulomas of the bowel. Crohn's disease, however, only produces granulomas of the lymph nodes when they are also present in the bowel wall.

○ **True/False: 6-Mercaptopurine (6-MP) and azathioprine are efficacious in treating Crohn's disease and maintaining remission; however, acute pancreatitits develops in about 1%–3% of patients. Patients who develop pancreatitis while on one of these drugs could be challenged with the other drug.**

False. Pancreatitis is reversible on withdrawing the drug but recurs upon rechallenge with 6-MP or azathioprine. Pancreatitis secondary to one drug is an absolute contraindication to use of either drug.

○ **What is the phenomenon called when a child develops IBD at an earlier age than his/her parent?**

Genetic anticipation.

○ **True/False: Ulcerative colitis is more common in nonsmokers than smokers.**

True. The relative risk of developing ulcerative colitis in nonsmokers compared with smokers is 2.6. The risk is particularly high in former smokers and especially former heavy smokers.

○ **True/False: There is an association between ulcerative colitis and autoimmune disorders.**

True. There is an increased incidence of thyroid disease, pernicious anemia, and diabetes.

○ **What percentage of ulcerative colitis patients are perinuclear antineutrophilic cytoplasmic antibody (p-ANCA) positive?**

p-ANCA occurs in 60%–80% of ulcerative colitis patients and 20%–30% of patients with Crohn's disease. This antibody is of the IgG type and its titer does not change with disease activity. However, the titers have been reported to decline after colectomy for greater than 10 years or after very long-standing disease remission.

○ **Which is more common in patients with ulcerative colitis—pancolitis or distal colitis?**

Distal colitis. The disease is limited to rectosigmoid in 40%–50%, is pancolonic in 20%, and is left-sided in 30%–40%.

○ **True/False: The rectum is always involved in ulcerative colitis.**

False. There are rare exceptions when, in severe acute disease, the proximal colon is more severely involved than the rectum. Another etiology of apparent rectal sparing is in patients being treated with topical agents.

○ **True/False: The shortening and narrowing of the colon in patients with history of recurrent attacks of ulcerative colitis is due to fibrosis.**

False. Fibrosis is uncommon in ulcerative colitis unlike Crohn's disease. The foreshortened colon is a result of abnormalities in the muscle layer.

○ **Inflammation is predominantly confined to the mucosa in ulcerative colitis. What specific area of the epithelium do the neutrophils attack?**

The crypts, giving rise to cryptitis.

○ **True/False: Pseudopolyps spare the rectum.**

True. The reason for this is unknown.

○ **True/False: Active ulcerative colitis with diarrhea is almost always associated with macroscopic blood.**

True. If blood is not present, the diagnosis should be questioned.

○ **Why will patients with proctitis or proctosigmoiditis sometimes complain of constipation instead of bloody diarrhea?**

Colonic motility is altered by inflammation. In distal proctitis, there is slowing of proximal colon transit and prolonged transit in the small bowel. Distal transit remains rapid.

○ **A 62-year-old woman presents with diarrhea and, during her evaluation, a flexible sigmoidoscopy is performed. The mucosa is unremarkable. Biopsies show a thick subepithelial collagen band. What is the diagnosis?**

Collagenous colitis usually reveals a normal appearing mucosa on endoscopic exam; however, it can cause friable and granular mucosa. It can be differentiated from ulcerative colitis and infectious colitis by the thickened subepithelial collagen band. A normal collagen layer is 3- to 6.9-μm thick. In collagenous colitis, the layer is 7- to 93-μm thick. The diagnosis of collagenous colitis is usually not made unless the collagen layer is at least 10-μm thick. Of note, the disease can be patchy and more prominent in the colon than the rectum.

○ **A 20-year-old woman presents with rectal pain and pus coming from her rectum. Proctoscopic exam reveals granular rectal mucosa and a biopsy shows an intense neutrophil infiltration and Gram-positive cocci. What is the diagnosis?**

Gonococcal proctitis, included in the differential of ulcerative colitis, rarely presents with diarrhea but instead with rectal pain. Biopsy confirms the diagnosis.

○ **A patient with active ulcerative colitis was hospitalized and treated with intravenous steroids. All symptoms subsided and the patient was discharged on mesalamine and oral steroids. The patient returned in 3 months with no GI symptoms but erythema nodosum over her lower extremities. Flexible sigmoidoscopy showed no active colitis. What do you suspect is the etiology of her erythema nodosum?**

Erythema nodosum is usually associated with active colitis and presents as multiple tender and inflamed nodules usually over the shins. It occurs in 2%–4% of cases of active colitis. Erythema nodosum can also occur as a reaction to sulfasalazine or mesalamine.

○ **What haplotype is most often associated with primary sclerosing cholangitis?**

HLA-DR3 B8.

○ **Which of the following IBD patient-types is most often associated with primary sclerosing cholangitis: fulminant colitis requiring colectomy, proctitis, or mild pancolitis?**

Mild pancolitis. In fact, the IBD may remain undiagnosed until after the diagnosis of liver disease. Colectomy is not protective against future development of primary sclerosing cholangitis.

○ **True/False: Pseudopolyps or inflammatory polyps are a premalignant condition.**

False.

○ **When should colonoscopic surveillance for dysplasia begin for patients with chronic IBD?**

In patients with colitis, after 8–10 years of disease. Repeat surveillance, if no dysplasia is found, should be undertaken every 1 to 2 years.

○ **True/False: The incidence of pyoderma gangrenosum is higher in ulcerative colitis compared to Crohn's disease.**

True. The incidence, while higher in ulcerative colitis, is only 1%–5%. It is most often associated with extensive disease of long-standing duration. One-half to one-third of patients with pyoderma have IBD.

○ **True/False: Pericholangitis is the most common hepatic complication of IBD.**

True, with a prevalence as high as 50%–80%. These patients usually present with asymptomatic elevations of alkaline phosphatase.

○ **True/False: The development of calcium oxalate stones in Crohn's disease occurs most often in patients with ileostomies.**

False. The presence of an ileostomy in a Crohn's patient predisposes to the development of urate stones resulting from decreased urine volumes related to high ostomy outputs. Calcium oxalate stones require an intact colon. With an absent or diseased ileum, fat malabsorption leads to unabsorbed fatty acids in the gut lumen. Calcium binds to the fatty acids instead of oxalate. Oxalate then binds to sodium (instead of calcium) and forms sodium oxalate, which is absorbed in the colon.

○ **Granulomas in Crohn's disease occur more commonly in the mucosa or submucosa?**

Submucosa. This explains why granulomas are found more commonly in surgical specimens than endoscopic specimens.

○ **True/False: Perforation of the colon occurs most often during the first acute attack of ulcerative colitis.**

True. Free perforation can occur without toxic megacolon and occurs most frequently in the left colon.

○ **A dermatologist refers you a patient with pyoderma gangrenosum. The patient has no gastrointestinal symptoms. What should you do?**

Evaluate for the presence of IBD. At least one-third of patients with pyoderma have IBD.

○ **True/False: Sacroileitis is symptomatic only when patients have active IBD.**

False. Of the extraintestinal manifestations of IBD, sacroileitis is not one that follows the course of the bowel disease activity.

○ **True/False: Patients with ulcerative colitis and p-ANCA positivity often have a more aggressive course.**

True. These p-ANCA-positive patients may have a more treatment-resistant (5-ASA products) disease and are more likely to develop chronic pouchitis after ileal pouch anal anastomosis.

○ **What effect does sulfasalazine have on fertility in males?**

Sulfasalazine may reduce the total sperm count and sperm motility. These effects are reversible with discontinuation of the drug.

○ **True/False: Fertility problems occur commonly in women with Crohn's disease.**

True. Fertility is normal in ulcerative colitis but impaired in Crohn's disease. The exact explanation is yet unknown but contributing factors include impaired ovulation, fallopian tube blockage, dyspareunia, and avoidance of pregnancy on medical advice or fear of becoming pregnant and passing disease to children. Nevertheless, many women with IBD become pregnant without difficulty and deliver healthy babies.

○ **Describe the clinical presentation of gastroduodenal Crohn's disease.**

Nearly all cases of gastroduodenal Crohn's disease present with symptoms of peptic ulcer disease. Most cases are associated with more distal small bowel involvement.

○ **True/False: All IBD medications should be stopped if a woman with the disease becomes pregnant or desires to become pregnant.**

False. A flare of IBD during pregnancy is associated with higher infant mortality; thus, it is desirable to continue the medications. Patients with quiescent disease at conception tend to have well-controlled disease during pregnancy, as long as medications are continued. Many of the drugs used to treat IBD have not been extensively studied in pregnancy. The 5-ASA preparations are considered safe to use during pregnancy. There is data on azathioprine in pregnant renal transplant patients that suggests this drug is safe in pregnancy. Methotrexate is contraindicated during pregnancy. Extensive counseling should take place with each patient concerning the risks, benefits, and alternatives of medication use during and after pregnancy.

○ **True/False: Olsalazine frequently causes watery diarrhea.**

True. Sixteen percent of patients on olsalazine develop watery diarrhea. Gradual titration of the dose and the administration of olsalazine with meals may reduce the incidence of diarrhea.

○ **In patients with ulcerative colitis requiring colectomy, which patients should not be considered for ileoanal pouch construction?**

Women with multiple pregnancies, women with difficult deliveries, older patients, and patients with diminished anal sphincter tone. The most important contraindication to the ileoanal pouch anastomosis is poor anal sphincter function. The patient groups listed are all at risk for anal sphincter dysfunction.

○ **Crohn's disease patients that develop short fibrotic symptomatic strictures should be sent for surgical intervention and stricturoplasty. List contraindications to stricturoplasty.**

Sepsis, perforation, phlegmon, fistula (enteroenteric or enterocutaneous—in the area of the stricturoplasty), multiple strictures in a short segment that might lend itself better to a single resection, gross ulceration and fragile mucosa at the site, colonic stricture, and carcinoma.

○ **A 41-year-old man with a 15-year history of pancolonic ulcerative colitis that is currently in remission undergoes surveillance colonoscopy. A single biopsy shows definite high-grade dysplasia (confirmed by a second expert pathologist). What should you recommend to the patient?**

Colectomy should be performed when high-grade dysplasia is found either in flat mucosa or a mass lesion (dysplasia-associated lesion or mass [DALM]).

○ **True/False: Adenomatous polyps occur in patients with and without IBD. The management of adenomas in patients with ulcerative colitis differs from that in patients without colitis.**

True. Colitis-associated cancer typically arises from flat mucosa or a DALM. A polyp should be presumed to represent a DALM if it occurs in involved mucosa. Pedunculated or sessile polyps that occur in uninvolved mucosa in patients who do not have pancolitis should be managed as they would in a patient without colitis. If a sessile adenoma is found within involved bowel, a colectomy may be considered. When a pedunculated adenoma arises in involved bowel, the bowel around the polyp should be sampled after performing a polypectomy. If there is no evidence of dysplasia in the surrounding mucosa or elsewhere, a colectomy is not necessary.

○ **True/False: Prophylactic use of mesalamine or metronidazole has been proven to prevent postoperative recurrence of Crohn's disease.**

False.

○ **True/False: Calcium supplements will increase the risk of formation of oxalate kidney stones in the patient with Crohn's disease who has had a terminal ileal resection.**

False. Calcium supplements can actually decrease the formation of oxalate stones by binding with the oxalate to keep it in the gut and not in the kidney.

○ **Considering the mucosal adaptive immune system, which interleukin involved in the Th17 pathway is likely involved in both ulcerative colitis and Crohn's disease?**

IL-23 in the newly recognized T helper 17 subset of T cell immune phenotypes has been shown to have a central role in inflammation of the colon.

○ **True/False: The patient with colitis who is found to have positive markers for both IgG and IgA anti-Saccharomyces antibody (ASCA) is more likely to have ulcerative colitis than Crohn's disease.**

False. The so-called double ASCA-positive Crohn's patient is more likely to have fibrostenosing and internal penetrating disease behavior.

○ **In a female patient who is undergoing proctocolectomy for ulcerative colitis with planned ileal anal pouch anastomosis, what effect will this operation have on her fertility?**

Any surgery in the pelvis, as in a proctocolectomy, can decrease fertility, generally as a result of scarring of the Fallopian tubes. Preoperative discussion should include this risk. Most of these patients have normal uterine function and may require in vitro fertilization for a successful pregnancy.

○ **True/False: Jewish people of Ashkenazi descent are 2–3 times more likely to develop IBD, either Crohn's disease or ulcerative colitis, than non-Jews.**

True, especially Crohn's disease.

○ **What are risk factors for the development of colorectal cancer in the patient with ulcerative colitis?**

Extent of disease (pancolitis higher risk than left-sided colitis), family history of colon cancer (first-degree relative), concomitant primary sclerosing cholangitis, and long duration of disease (increasing incidence of colorectal cancer [CRC] after 8–10 years of disease).

○ **Compare the risk of proctocolectomy and ileal pouch anal anastomosis in a patient who has p-ANCA-positive ulcerative colitis to the patient who has p-ANCA-negative ulcerative colitis.**

The complications of proctocolectomy and ileal pouch anal anastomosis include pouchitis, fistula, infertility, sepsis, and other surgical complications. The risk of pouchitis is much higher in the p-ANCA-positive patient.

○ **A 34-year-old man with Crohn's disease is admitted with acute epigastric abdominal pain. He has both small and large bowel involvement and has a history of a perianal fistula. His admission medications include mesalamine and azathioprine, and he just had his first infusion of infliximab last week. Lab studies are most remarkable for an elevated lipase. He does not drink alcohol and is on no other medications, has no family history of pancreatitis, and has never had pancreatitis. What is the only drug not associated with pancreatitis on his list of medications?**

Infliximab has not been associated with pancreatitis. Pancreatitis can be secondary to azathioprine or 6-MP and is considered idiosyncratic. These medications should not be tried again, if there is a history of pancreatitis from either agent as pancreatitis will likely recur. More unusual and less well recognized is the occurrence of pancreatitis from mesalamine use.

○ **A 50-year-old woman comes to your office with fever to 38.7°C and diffuse myalgias that started 10 days after her last infusion of infliximab. She has been treated with infliximab for fistulizing Crohn's disease for the last 3 months. She was not treated with concomitant azathioprine as she developed pancreatitis 5 years ago when azathioprine was tried. She is on infliximab as a single agent and has had great results with healing of fistula. She had been treated approximately 10 years ago with a single infusion of infliximab in a clinical trial. She went to her primary care provider (PCP) initially and chest x-ray and blood and urine cultures are negative. What is the most likely cause of her fever and myalgias.**

Delayed hypersensitivity reaction to infliximab. Fever and myalgias (and sometimes a rash) occurring 2–12 days post infliximab infusion in a patient that was previously exposed to infliximab and then a long period of time without infliximab is most often a delayed hypersensitivity reaction to infliximab.

○ **What radiologic imaging test of the small bowel exposes the patient to the least amount of radiation?**

Magnetic resonance enterography (MRE). In past years, small bowel barium studies were used to image the small intestine. More recently, computerized tomography enterography (CTE) and MRE have generally replaced the barium study to image the small bowel. MRE exposes the patient to less radiation than does CTE. Capsule endoscopy and small bowel enteroscopy are also used to examine the small bowel in certain instances.

○ **True/False: Active uveitis predicts active IBD.**

False. Although uveitis is an extraintestinal manifestation of IBD, it does not predict active bowel disease. Episcleritis parallels the disease activity, however.

○ **Pyoderma gangrenosum can be seen as an extraintestinal manifestation of IBD and occurs in 1%–4% of IBD patients. Is it more common in ulcerative colitis or Crohn's disease?**

Pyoderma gangrenosum can be seen in either but seems to be slightly more common in ulcerative colitis. The ulcerative variant of pyoderma is the most common type and is the classic type seen in IBD patients.

○ **True/False: Prednisone is the only etiology of osteopenia in patients with IBD.**

False. Prednisone does contribute to bone loss in IBD patients but inflammatory cytokines also contribute. In particular, Crohn's patients can have osteopenia or osteoporosis without any exposure to prednisone. Nutritional and other factors may also play a role.

○ **Natalizumab is a humanized monoclonal antibody targeted against what cellular adhesion molecule?**

Alpha 4-integrin.

○ **Certolizumab pegol is a monoclonal antibody targeted against what?**

Tumor necrosis factor alpha. Certolizumab is a PEGylated Fab' fragment of a humanized TNF inhibitor monoclonal antibody.

○ **Explain the most likely etiology of fecaluria occurring in a patient with fistulizing Crohn's disease.**

Fecaluria is generally a manifestation of a fistula to the bladder (ie, enterovesicular fistula). Patients present with stool (fecaluria) and/or air (pneumaturia) with urination and frequently develop polymicrobial bladder infections.

○ **What drugs have been associated with definite increased risk of congenital malformation when used during pregnancy for treating IBD?**

Methotrexate and thalidomide.

○ **A 25-year-old woman with ulcerative colitis refractory to medical management is contemplating surgery but wants your input in selecting the type of operation. Her top priority is to have a child within the next few years. What is the surgical option with the least risk of infertility?**

Subtotal colectomy with ileostomy and Hartmann's pouch may be the best choice to optimize her chances of normal fertility. The ostomy can be taken down at a later date when she is done with conception. Pelvic dissection increases the risk of infertility. Total proctocolectomy with ileal pouch-anal anastomosis and total proctocolectomy with end ileostomy are procedures that require pelvic dissection to remove the rectum with increased risk of adhesions and subsequent infertility. Patients should be advised of the reduction of fertility when undergoing these surgeries. In the female patient who has undergone proctocolectomy and ileal pouch-anal anastomosis and is unable to conceive, in vitro fertilization may be an option.

● ● ● SUGGESTED READINGS ● ● ●

Inflammatory bowel disease: an update on fundamental biology and clinical management. *Gastroenterology.* 2011;140(Suppl): 1701-1846.

Lichtenstein GR, Hanauer SB, Sandborn WJ; The practice parameters committee of the American College of Gastroenterology. Management of Crohn's Disease in Adults. *Am J Gastroenterol.* 2009;104:465-483.

An evidence-based systematic review on medical therapies for inflammatory bowel diseases. *Am J Gastroenterol.* 2011;106(Suppl 1): S1-S25.

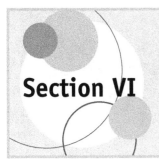

Section VI

GALLBLADDER, BILE DUCTS, AND PANCREAS

CHAPTER 31

Gallbladder, Bile Duct, and Pancreatic Congenital and Structural Abnormalities

Linda S. Lee, MD and
Darwin L. Conwell, MD, MS

○ **Define biliary atresia.**

Obliteration of the intra- or extrahepatic bile ducts. There is some evidence to suggest that the ducts originally were present but were destroyed by an unknown process.

○ **True/False: The gallbladder is usually also involved in extrahepatic biliary atresia.**

True. Usually, only a fibrous remnant of the gallbladder and entire extrahepatic bile duct remains.

○ **True/False: It is usually apparent at birth when biliary atresia is present.**

False. It usually does not become evident until several weeks after birth.

○ **How is biliary atresia diagnosed?**

Hepatobiliary iminodiacetic acid (HIDA) scan which is 100% sensitive and 94% specific.

○ **What is the treatment for biliary atresia and the success rate?**

Kasai procedure (hepatic portoenterostomy) with one-third good long-term results, one-third requiring immediate liver transplantation, and one-third eventually needing transplantation due to progressive liver failure.

○ **True/False: Regardless of an anomalous position of a gallbladder (eg, left-sided, intrahepatic, floating, etc), the cystic duct usually joins the common bile duct in a relatively normal position.**

True. In general, the cystic duct joins the common hepatic duct in the usual position to form the common bile duct. The cystic duct may rarely join the right hepatic duct.

○ **Define accessory and aberrant ducts.**

Accessory ducts offer a second drainage route from the liver, whereas aberrant ducts are the only drainage routes for a specific region of the liver, but run along an unusual extrahepatic course rather than the normal intrahepatic route.

○ **In which part of the liver are accessory and aberrant ducts usually found?**

Accessory ducts are more common in the right side of the liver. Aberrant ducts almost exclusively drain the right anterior liver.

○ **True/False: Choledochal cysts more commonly occur in men.**

False. These cysts are about four times more common in women. There is also a higher incidence among Asians.

○ **Describe the five types of choledochal cysts.**

Type I	– fusiform dilation of the common bile duct
Type II	– diverticula of the common bile duct
Type III (choledochocele)	– cystic dilation of intraduodenal segment of common bile duct
Type IV	– multiple extrahepatic or both intra- and extrahepatic cysts
Type V (Caroli's disease)	– only intrahepatic cysts

○ **Which type of choledochal cyst is most common?**

Type I.

○ **What are two theories of pathogenesis of choledochal cysts?**

1) Pancreatic reflux and 2) distal common bile duct obstruction (presumably, failure of recanalization of the distal bile duct during intrauterine development leads to narrowing of the distal bile duct with proximal dilation).

○ **What is anomalous pancreaticobiliary junction (APBJ)?**

This congenital anomaly is defined as the junction of the common bile duct and pancreatic duct located outside the duodenal wall with a long common channel.

○ **How often is APBJ associated with choledochal cysts?**

70% of the time.

○ **What is the significance of the presence of APBJ?**

APBJ increases the risk of malignancy in the choledochal cyst when present and gallbladder in patients without biliary cysts.

○ **What are potential risks of choledochal cysts if left unattended?**

Severe cholangitis and adenocarcinoma (about 10%). Surgical excision is the usual treatment of these cysts, which may become massive in size.

○   **True/False: A cholangiogram is useful to diagnose a choledochocele.**

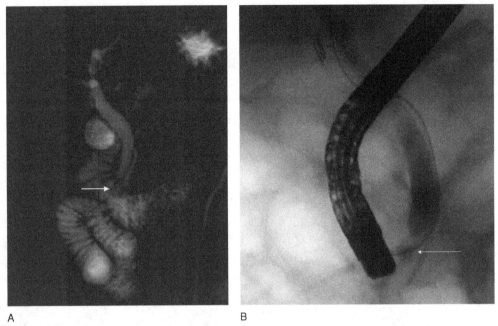

A

B

Figure 31-1A, B

True.

○   **How are symptomatic choledochoceles treated?**

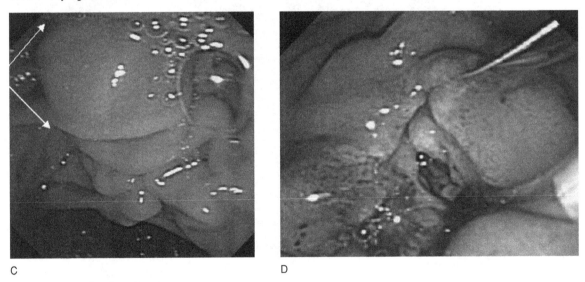

C

D

Figure 31-1C, D See also color plate.

Endoscopic sphincterotomy. Because the risk of malignant degeneration is very low, surgical resection is not required.

See Figure 31-1A for a magnetic resonance cholangiopancreatography (MRCP) of choledochocele. The arrow points to choledochocele. Figure 31-1B shows endoscopic retrograde cholangiopancreatography (ERCP) of choledochocele. The arrow points to choledochocele. See Figure 31-1C for an endoscopic view of choledochocele. Figure 31-1D shows choledochocele s/p sphincterotomy.

○   **What is a Phrygian cap?**

A congenital deformity of the gallbladder of no clinical significance whereby the fundus of the gallbladder is kinked.

○   **Air in the gallbladder in the setting of acute cholecystitis suggests the development of what clinical entity?**

Cholecystoenteric fistula due to necrosis of the gallbladder wall.

○   **What gallstone-related syndrome produces obstruction via external compression of the common bile duct?**

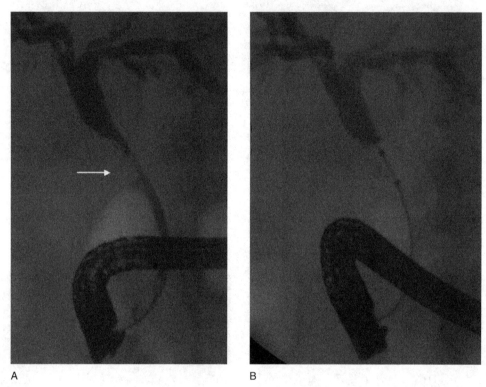

A   B

Figure 31-2

In Mirizzi's syndrome, a gallstone impacted in the cystic duct leads to compression and obstruction of the bile duct. See Figure 31-2A for cholangiogram of Mirizzi's syndrome. The arrow points to a stone in cystic duct. Figure 31-2B shows cholangiogram of Mirizzi's syndrome with stone extraction balloon sliding by stone in cystic duct.

○   **What are the crescent-shaped folds of the cystic duct mucosa that may block passage of stones into the common bile duct?**

Spiral valves of Heister.

○   **What are the two main developmental abnormalities of morphology that account for most pancreatic congenital anomalies?**

Abnormalities of rotation and fusion.

○ **At about what week of gestation does the embryological development of the pancreas first appear?**

About the fourth week of gestation, the pancreas first appears as two diverticula arising from the primitive foregut just distal to the stomach.

○ **What are the names given to the pancreatic ducts that arise from the ventral and dorsal pancreatic buds?**

The ventral duct joins with the dorsal duct to form the main pancreatic duct of Wirsung. The dorsal bud arises directly from the duodenal wall and undergoes varying degrees of atrophy to remain as the accessory duct of Santorini.

○ **True/False: The pancreas lies within the peritoneal cavity.**

False. The pancreas is a retroperitoneal organ.

○ **What percentage of the population has normal pancreatic ductal anatomy?**

Approximately 60%–70%.

○ **True/False: Pancreas divisum is the most common congenital anomaly of the pancreas.**

True.

○ **What is the embryological cause of pancreas divisum?**

Pancreas divisum results from incomplete fusion of the dorsal and ventral pancreatic ductal systems.

○ **What percentage of autopsies is found to have pancreas divisum?**

Pancreas divisum has been reported in up to 5%–10% in autopsy series. The prevalence may be even higher in patients undergoing ERCP for investigations of idiopathic pancreatitis.

○ **What is the most common clinical presentation of patients with symptomatic pancreas divisum?**

Most patients with pancreas divisum are asymptomatic with incidental detection of the anomaly. Those patients that are symptomatic have symptoms suggestive of acute pancreatitis that is thought to occur secondary to a combination of the anomaly and stenosis of the minor duodenal papilla.

○ **At what age do patients with symptomatic pancreas divisum usually present?**

The age of presentation varies widely but is most common between the third and forth decades of life.

○ **What should be the initial therapeutic management of patients with symptomatic recurrent pancreatitis from pancreas divisum?**

Although surgical minor papilla sphincteroplasty has traditionally been the treatment of choice, in experienced hands, endoscopic minor papilla dilation or sphincterotomy with temporary stenting has been shown to decrease the frequency of recurrent attacks of pancreatitis in pancreas divisum.

○   **What test is most useful in diagnosing pancreas divisum?**

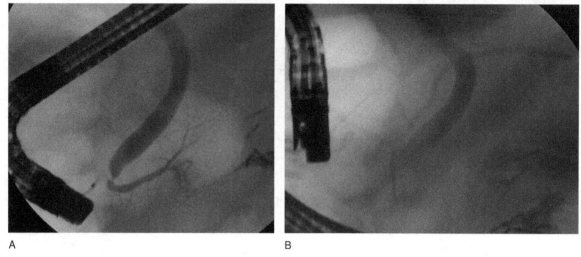

A   B

Figure 31-3

ERCP with injection of the main and minor pancreatic ducts demonstrates incomplete fusion of the dorsal and ventral pancreatic ductal systems. See Figure 31-3A for pancreatogram of complete pancreas divisum with injection into ventral pancreatic duct. Figure 31-3B shows pancreatogram of pancreas divisum with injection into the dorsal pancreatic duct.

○   **What ectopic tissue is being demonstrated in the figure below?**

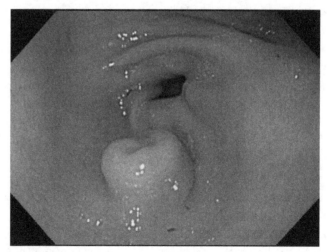

Figure 31-4 See also color plate.

A heterotopic pancreas also known as ectopic or aberrant pancreas (or pancreatic rest) is defined as the presence of pancreatic tissue that lacks anatomic and vascular continuity with the main body of the pancreas. Ectopic pancreas appears as a well-defined dome-shaped subepithelial nodule with central umbilication.

○ **Where are the most common locations for ectopic pancreatic tissue?**

Seventy percent of the ectopic pancreatic tissue is found in the upper gastrointestinal tract, including the stomach, duodenal, and jejunum. However, it has been seen in many other abdominal locations. The most common location is the preplyoric antrum along the greater curvature.

○ **What is the most common presentation of patients with heterotopic pancreas?**

Most cases of heterotopic pancreas are asymptomatic and the condition is generally discovered incidentally during the endoscopic evaluation of other gastrointestinal disorders.

○ **What are the histologic findings on endoscopic biopsy of the nodule seen in heterotopic pancreas?**

Endoscopic biopsy of the nodule yields only normal gastric mucosa because the pancreatic tissue is submucosal or subserosal in origin.

○ **True/False: Any pathologic change in the normal pancreas such as malignancy, cyst formation, or islet cell tumors can occur in pancreatic rests.**

True. While pancreatic rests are usually asymptomatic, symptoms may occur due to pathologic change of the ectopic pancreatic tissue and also due to the location of the pancreatic rest.

○ **What treatment is recommended for heterotopic pancreatic tissue when discovered?**

Incidental lesions should be left alone since long-term follow-up has not established a relationship between ectopic tissue and symptoms in most patients.

○ **What is an annular pancreas?**

An annular pancreas is a band of pancreatic tissue completely encircling the second portion of the duodenum.

○ **What is the usual clinical presentation of annular pancreas in the pediatric and adult populations?**

In the newborn, the lesion is associated with polyhydramnios and typically presents with inability to tolerate feedings. In adults, obstructive symptoms such as nausea and vomiting occur, particularly postprandially along with abdominal pain and bloating. Upper GI bleeding and duodenal ulcers occur in one-third of adults. Pancreatitis may also occur.

○ **How is a diagnosis of annular pancreas established?**

In neonates, a plain abdominal x-ray may reveal a classic "double-bubble," which is diagnostic of duodenal obstruction. In adults and older children, plain x-ray films are unhelpful and other studies such as ERCP, magnetic resonance cholangiopancreatography, and/or abdominal CT scan are necessary to make the diagnosis.

○ **What is the management of an annular pancreas?**

In both newborns and adults, the management is surgical bypass of the obstructing lesion.

○ **What congenital anomalies are associated with annular pancreas?**

Duodenal atresia, Down's syndrome, Meckel's diverticulum, malrotation of intestine, intestinal webs, tracheoesophageal fistula, and imperforate anus.

○ **What conditions are associated with multiple congenital cysts of the pancreas?**

Multiple congenital cysts are associated with polycystic disease, cystic fibrosis, and Von Hippel–Lindau syndrome.

○ **What is the management of a congenital cyst of the pancreas?**

Surgical resection or drainage may be required for some patients with symptomatic solitary cysts; however, surgery is not usually necessary or advisable for patients with multiple cysts.

○ **What is hypoplasia of the pancreas?**

A congenital disease of the exocrine pancreas characterized by fatty replacement of acinar cells.

○ **What is another name for hypoplasia of the pancreas?**

Lipomatous pseudohypertrophy of the pancreas.

○ **What is the usual clinical presentation of hypoplasia of the pancreas?**

Severe pancreatic exocrine insufficiency

● ● ● **SUGGESTED READINGS** ● ● ●

DiMagno MJ, Wamsteker EJ. Pancreas divisum. *Curr Gastroenterol Rep.* 2011;13:150-156.

Kamisawa T, Takuma K, Anjiki H, et al. Pancreaticobiliary maljunction. *Clin Gastroenterol Hepatol.* 2009;7:S84-S88.

Simeone DM, Mulholland MW. Pancreas: anatomy and structural anomalies. In: Yamada T, ed. *Textbook of Gastroenterology.* Philadelphia: Lippincott Williams & Wilkins; 2003:2013-2025.

Simeone DM. Gallbladder and biliary tract: anatomy and structural anomalies. In: Yamada T, ed. *Textbook of Gastroneterology.* Philadelphia: Lippincott Williams & Wilkins; 2003:2166-2176.

CHAPTER 32

Gallbladder, Bile Duct, and Pancreatic Infectious Disorders

David W. McFadden, MD, MBA and Denise McCormack, MD

○ **What organism is most commonly associated with recurrent pyogenic cholangitis?**

Clonorchis sinensis.

○ **What parasite can predispose to intrahepatic gallstones?**

Ascaris lumbricoides.

○ **What is the intermediate host for *Fasciola hepatica*?**

Lymnaeca trunculata—snail. Patients are infected by eating infected watercress.

○ **Eosinophilia, elevated alkaline phosphatase, and cholangiography findings of filamentous filling defects with blunted tips in the bile duct suggest what infection?**

C. sinensis, the Chinese liver fluke, or *F. hepatica*, the common or sheep liver fluke.

○ **When is surgical treatment indicated for patients with infestation of the biliary tract by *C. sinensis* (Chinese liver fluke)?**

Surgical treatment is reserved for complications, such as biliary obstruction, due not only to the parasites themselves but also to secondary formation of stones and acute cholangitis. Some patients present with pancreatitis, presumably caused by passage of the stones or the worms. In addition to cholecystectomy and clearing the bile ducts of stones and flukes, improved biliary drainage by choledochoduodenostomy, hepaticojejunostomy, or transduodenal sphincteroplasty is thought to reduce the rate of recurrent biliary obstruction, which otherwise exceeds 40%.

○ **What class of antibiotic has been shown to achieve therapeutic concentrations in bile and is useful in treating cholangitis?**

Fluoroquinolones.

○ **What antibiotic may lead to the development of biliary sludge?**

Ceftriaxone precipitates a calcium salt that has the ultrasonic appearance of biliary sludge.

○ **Which of the following primary duct stones has the highest positive culture rate for bacteria—black, brown, or cholesterol?**

Brown.

○ **What factors are associated with the development of black pigment stones?**

Chronic hemolysis, as can occur in hereditary spherocytosis, thalassemia and the presence of mechanical heart valves, cirrhosis, total parenteral nutrition, and advanced age.

○ **What bacterial infection and anatomical deformity play a role in the formation of brown pigment stones?**

Escherichia coli and a juxtapapillary duodenal diverticulum.

○ **What bacterial enzyme is responsible for hydrolysis of conjugated bilirubin and may play a role in the development of pigment stones?**

Bacterial beta-galactosidase, which is homologous to human beta-glucuronidase.

○ **What bacterium may cause acute cholecystitis and also be nonpathogenic in a carrier state?**

Salmonella.

○ **Name two nonbacterial infectious entities that predispose to acute cholecystitis in an immunocompromised host.**

Cytomegalovirus (CMV) and *Cryptosporidium.*

○ **What are the three most common organisms isolated from blood cultures in patients with acute ascending cholangitis?**

E. coli, Klebsiella, and *Pseudomonas.* Anaerobes are isolated in approximately 15%.

○ **What is the mechanism of biliary obstruction in tuberculosis?**

Obstructive jaundice is a rare complication of tuberculosis. The obstruction is caused by tuberculous infection involving lymph nodes in the porta hepatis or the retroduodenal area that compresses the bile duct.

○ **Charcot's triad plus what other two clinical features define Reynold's pentad?**

Hypotension and altered mental status.

○ **In Oriental cholangitis, which side of the hepatic ductal system most commonly develops strictures and intrahepatic stones?**

The left hepatic ductal system, presumably due to its more acute angle at the bifurcation.

○ **Bacillary angiomatosis with peliosis is caused by what organism?**

Bartonella henselae or *Bartonella quintana.*

○ **What is the treatment of bacillary angiomatosis with peliosis in a patient with fever, abdominal pain, and elevated liver tests?**

Antibiotic therapy with erythromycin or doxycycline.

○   **What species of *Microsporidia* is responsible for causing AIDS cholangiopathy?**

Enterocytozoon bieneusi.

○   **True/False: The signs and symptoms of an acute pancreatic infection differ from those that occur with acute pancreatitis.**

False. Epigastric pain, fever, nausea, and/or vomiting are frequent symptoms. Signs include leukocytosis and elevations in serum amylase and lipase.

○   **What are the most common viral infections of the pancreas?**

Mumps, rubella, coxsackievirus B, Epstein–Barr virus (EBV), CMV, herpes simplex virus (HSV), HIV, and hepatitis A , B, and C.

○   **What virus is the most common cause of infection-related pancreatitis in children?**

Mumps.

○   **What fungal infections can involve the pancreas and/or cause pancreatitis?**

Candida species, *Torulopsis glabrata*, and *Cryptococcus* are the most common. *Aspergillus fumigatus*, *Coccidioides immitis*, *Paracoccidioides brasiliensis*, *Histoplasma capsulatum*, and *Pneumocystis jiroveci* may also be involved.

○   **What appears to be the most effective treatment for fungal infections involving the pancreas?**

Amphotericin B. Drainage and debridement of infected necrosis are also important.

○   **What is the most common type of parasitic infection of the pancreas?**

A. lumbricoides, the giant roundworm. Other parasitic infections include *Echinococcus granulosis*, *Giardia lamblia*, *Plasmodium falciparum*, *C. sinensis* and *Strongyloides stercoralis*.

○   **True/False: The most common bacteria that cause pancreatic infections are Gram-negative enteric organisms.**

True. Gram-negative enteric bacteria, anaerobes, and *Candida* species are most common pathogens; however, *Staphylococcus aureus* is also frequently isolated.

○   **True/False: Pancreatic abscess is a frequent complication of acute pancreatitis.**

False. Pancreatic abscess complicates about 5% of cases of acute pancreatitis and occurs about 2 to 6 weeks after the initial attack.

○   **What is the treatment of pancreatic abscess?**

External (percutaneous) catheter drainage and broad-spectrum antibiotics. If this fails, surgical debridement is usually needed.

○   **Describe the pathogenesis of infected pancreatic necrosis in a patient with acute necrotizing pancreatitis.**

Infected pancreatic necrosis develops as a result of transmural, transductal, lymphatic, or hematogenous spread of infectious organisms to necrotic regions of the pancreas. It usually occurs less than four weeks after the initial onset of pancreatitis.

○   **What is the gold standard for establishing a diagnosis of infected pancreatic necrosis?**

CT-guided percutaneous aspiration with Gram stain and culture is indicated in patients who exhibit signs and symptoms suggestive of infected pancreatic necrosis.

○   **A visiting shepherd from South America is transferred to your service with fever, weight loss, and diarrhea. A CT scan of the abdomen reveals a large calcified cyst with fenestrations in the pancreas and several smaller cysts nearby. What is your diagnosis?**

Hydatid cysts of the pancreas.

○   **What organism is responsible for hydatid cyst disease?**

Echinococcus granulosus, or occasionally *E. multilocularis*, a parasitic worm that normally resides in the intestine of dogs.

○   **What are the intermediate hosts in hydatid disease?**

Man, sheep, and cattle.

○   **How is the diagnosis of hydatid disease made?**

Diagnosis is based on history of exposure from endemic areas and characteristic radiographic findings including evidence of daughter cysts within larger primary cysts. A negative serologic test does not necessarily exclude the diagnosis.

○   **What is the treatment of hydatid cysts of the pancreas?**

Surgical excision, if technically possible without major pancreatic resection, or infusion of scolicidal agents (eg, 95% ethanol and hypertonic saline) and high-dose mebendazole or albendazole are the mainstays of treatment.

○   **How does the HIV affect the pancreas?**

Indirectly through secondary infections, infiltrative processes (lymphoma, Kaposi's sarcoma), or drugs used in its treatment (eg, 2′,3′ dideoxyinosine).

○   **What is the most common opportunistic infection of the pancreas in AIDS patients?**

CMV. Others include *Cryptococcus*, *Toxoplasma gondii*, *Cryptosporidium*, *M. tuberculosis* and *M. avium* complex.

● ● ● **SUGGESTED READINGS** ● ● ●

Trikudanathan G, Navaneethan U, Vege SS. Intra-abdominal fungal infections complicating acute pancreatitis: a review. *Am J Gastroenterol*. 2011;106:1188-1192.

Behrman SW, Bahr MH, Dickson PV, Zarzaur BL. The microbiology of secondary and postoperative pancreatic infections: implications for antimicrobial management. *Arch Surg*. 2011 May;146(5):613-619.

Devarbhavi H, Sebastian T, Seetharamu SM, Karanth D. HIV/AIDS cholangiopathy: clinical spectrum, cholangiographic features and outcome in 30 patients. *J Gastroenterol Hepatol*. 2010 Oct;25(10):1656-1660.

Julka K, Ko CW. Infectious diseases and the gallbladder. *Infect Dis Clin North Am*. 2010 Dec;24(4):885-898.

CHAPTER 33 Gallbladder and Biliary Motility Disorders

Stephanie L. Hansel, MD, MS

○ **True/False: The gallbladder empties during fasting.**

True. During fasting, 25% of gallbladder contents empty approximately every 120 minutes. This coincides with the phase III component of the migrating motor complex seen in the intestine.

○ **What happens to the gallbladder in the fed state?**

Eating initiates gallbladder contraction through both neural (cephalic and local gastroduodenal reflexes) and hormonal (cholecystokinin) influences. This results in the emptying of over 75% of the gallbladder contents.

○ **What are the phases of gallbladder emptying?**

Gallbladder emptying after meals consists of three phases: 1) Cephalic phase—stimulated by sham feeding; 2) gastric phase—stimulated by distension of the stomach and the gastroduodenal reflex; and 3) intestinal phase—stimulated by hormones. The bulk of the contractions occur during the gastric and intestinal phases.

○ **True/False: Fat, protein, and carbohydrate lead to gallbladder contraction.**

True. Meal composition determines cholecystokinin release and, hence, gallbladder contraction. Protein and fat result in gallbladder contraction via cholecystokinin release, while carbohydrate also causes gallbladder contraction but via an unknown mechanism.

○ **How does motilin affect the gallbladder?**

Motilin induces gallbladder contraction indirectly via cholinergic nerves.

○ **True/False: Patients with gallstones have reduced gallbladder emptying.**

True. This impairment results from depression of gallbladder contractility and not the gallstones themselves.

○ **What are the Rome III criteria for diagnosis of functional gallbladder disorder (aka, gallbladder dyskinesia)?**

- Episodic pain in the right upper quadrant or epigastrium.
- Episodes last ≥ 30 minutes.
- Symptoms recur at different intervals (not daily).
- Pain builds up to a steady level and is of moderate to severe intensity to the point of interrupting daily activities or prompting a visit to the emergency room.
- Pain not relieved by bowel movements, postural changes, or antacids.
- Other structural diseases to explain the symptoms have been excluded.
- The pain may be associated with nausea and vomiting, radiation to the back and/or right subscapular region, or nocturnal awakening.
- Gallbladder is present.
- Normal liver and pancreatic enzymes.

○ **What is the prevalence of gallbladder dyskinesia?**

The estimated prevalence is 8% in men and 21% in women.

○ **True/False: The pathophysiology of gallbladder dyskinesia is well established?**

False. The pathogenesis is poorly understood. Multiple theories have been proposed including cholesterolosis, microlithiasis, biliary sludge, chronic cholecystitis, gallbladder dysmotility, narrowed cystic duct, cystic duct spasm, and visceral hypersensitivity.

○ **What test should be ordered to support the diagnosis of gallbladder dyskinesia?**

Cholecystokinin-cholescintigraphy (CCK-CS), commonly referred to as a "CCK-HIDA scan" since the test utilizes both CCK and ^{99m}technicium-labeled hepatoiminodiacetic acid (HIDA). HIDA is a radioisotope that is taken up by the liver and excreted into the biliary system, where it accumulates in the gallbladder, thus allowing for calculation of the gallbladder ejection fraction after stimulating gallbladder emptying.

○ **True/False: The reproduction of the patient's characteristic pain and/or other symptoms during a CCK-HIDA scan reliably predicts which patients will respond best to cholecystectomy.**

False. Pain reproduction with CCK infusion is generally considered to be poorly predictive of outcome following cholecystectomy.

○ **Why is cholecystokinin used?**

Cholecystokinin is the most potent stimulus of gallbladder emptying and, in addition, causes relaxation of the sphincter of Oddi via inhibitory nerves.

○ **What is the gallbladder ejection fraction?**

It is a quantitative measurement of gallbladder emptying. The cut-off value of an abnormal gallbladder ejection fraction remains unclear due to differences in CCK-CS technique; however, a recent study using a state-of-the-art 60-minute CCK infusion methodology suggests that a value less than 38% should be considered abnormal.

○ **What drugs cause impaired gallbladder emptying?**

The most common drugs that cause impaired gallbladder emptying are narcotics and anticholinergic agents.

○ **What is the treatment for gallbladder dyskinesia?**

Cholecystectomy.

○ **True/False: Patients with suspected gallbladder dyskinesia who have primarily atypical symptoms such as bloating and epigastric fullness respond to cholecystectomy as well as patients with only the classical symptoms of episodic epigastric or right upper quadrant pain.**

False.

○ **What are the three components of the sphincter of Oddi?**

The three components are the sphincter choledochus, sphincter pancreaticus, and sphincter ampulla, which surround the distal common bile duct, duct of Wirsung, and common channel, respectively.

○ **What is the role of the sphincter of Oddi?**

It regulates flow of pancreatic and biliary secretions into the duodenum by its basal pressure and prevents the reflux of material from the duodenum into the duct by its phasic contractions.

○ **What is the normal basal sphincter of Oddi pressure?**

The normal mean basal sphincter of Oddi pressure is less than 35 mmHg.

○ **What are the features of the normal phasic contractions of the sphincter of Oddi?**

The phasic contractions consist of three components: amplitude, duration, and frequency. The amplitude is less than 220 mmHg with a duration less than 8 seconds and a frequency of less than 10 per minute.

○ **What drugs relax the sphincter of Oddi?**

Anticholinergics, nitrates, calcium channel blockers, and glucagon.

○ **What is the gold standard for the diagnosis of functional sphincter of Oddi disorder (aka, sphincter of Oddi dysfunction [SOD])?**

Sphincter of Oddi manometry.

○ **What manometric findings are typical in patients with SOD?**

Manometric criteria include: 1) elevated basal sphincter pressure, 2) increased frequency of phasic contractions, 3) increased proportion of phasic contractions propagated in the retrograde direction, and 4) paradoxical sphincter response to CCK-OP (cholecystokinin-octapeptide) injection. In clinical practice, a basal sphincter pressure >40 mmHg is the single most useful parameter in which to make this diagnosis.

○ **What type of catheter is most commonly used in biliary manometry?**

A triple-lumen, water-perfused catheter. The use of one lumen for aspiration may reduce the risk of procedure-related pancreatitis. The use of a solid-state, nonperfused catheter is available; however, further studies are needed before its routine use can be recommended.

○ **True/False: Glucagon affects sphincter of Oddi manometry.**

True. Glucagon causes a relatively brief period of relaxation of the sphincter and so a waiting period of 8–10 minutes is suggested before measuring the basal sphincter pressure if glucagon was used to aid in cannulation.

○ **True/False: Benzodiazepines affect sphincter of Oddi manometry.**

False. Benzodiazepines do not affect the sphincter and can be used as a sedative for patients undergoing sphincter of Oddi manometry.

○ **True/False: Anticholinergics affect sphincter of Oddi manometry.**

True. Anticholinergics should be avoided as they inhibit sphincter of Oddi motor activity.

○ **True/False: The use of meperidine should be avoided during sphincter of Oddi manometry.**

False. Meperidine at a dose of <1 mg/kg does not alter basal sphincter pressure although it does influence phasic activity.

○ **What are the indications for sphincter of Oddi manometry?**

Patients with idiopathic pancreatitis and patients with unexplained pancreaticobiliary pain with or without abnormal liver or pancreatic enzymes.

○ **What are the four clinical criteria for the diagnosis of SOD type I?**

1) Typical biliary-type pain, 2) elevated aspartate aminotransferase or alkaline phosphatase >2 times normal and measured on more than two occasions, 3) delayed drainage of contrast more than 45 minutes at the time of ERCP, and 4) dilated common bile duct more than 12 mm. The third criterion is seldom used in routine clinical practice.

○ **What is SOD type II?**

Patients with typical biliary-type pain and one or two of the previously mentioned criteria.

○ **What is SOD type III?**

Patients with typical biliary-type pain and no other abnormalities. The clinical relevance of this category remains controversial.

○ **True/False: Sphincter of Oddi manometry is always indicated in type I SOD.**

False. It is not necessary before endoscopic sphincterotomy since these patients appear to benefit from sphincterotomy regardless of findings on manometry.

○ **True/False: Sphincter of Oddi manometry is always indicated in type II or III SOD.**

True. Sphincter of Oddi manometry is mandatory in these patients to confirm the presence of SOD and to predict the subset that will benefit from sphincterotomy. Those with elevated basal pressures more predictably experience improvement of pain after sphincterotomy.

○ **How does SOD cause pain?**

It is postulated that, by impeding the flow of pancreatic and biliary secretions, there is a resulting increase in the ductal pressure (ductal hypertension), causing pain.

○ **What is the estimated frequency of SOD in patients with biliary-type pain following cholecystectomy?**

9%–11%.

○ **What is the best predictor of pain relief in patients with SOD after sphincterotomy?**

Elevated basal sphincter pressure (>40 mmHg).

○   **What are the indications for surgical sphincter of Oddi ablation?**

1) Recurrent stenoses after repeated endoscopic sphincterotomies, 2) when an experienced therapeutic endoscopist is not available, and 3) when endoscopic sphincterotomy is not technically feasible.

○   **What pharmacological agents have been used in the treatment of SOD?**

Nitrates and nifedipine. There has also been recent interest in the use of botulinum toxin injections into the sphincter of Oddi.

○   **What is the Nardi test?**

A positive result occurs when the injection of morphine, 10 mg subcutaneously, or neostigmine, 1 mg subcutaneously, causes typical biliary-type pain with an associated fourfold increase in aminotransferases, alkaline phosphatase, amylase, or lipase. A positive test may occur in patients with SOD; however, it can also occur in patients with choledocholithiasis. This test is neither sensitive nor specific. Morphine causes sphincter of Oddi contraction, whereas neostigmine increases the pancreatic flow of secretions.

○   **What is a positive secretin stimulation test?**

A positive result occurs when secretin administration leads to dilatation of the common bile duct and main pancreatic duct, as detected by ultrasound or magnetic resonance imaging. This may occur when the sphincter of Oddi is dysfunctional causing obstruction. Secretin normally results in sphincter of Oddi relaxation.

○   **What is the role of magnetic resonance cholangiopancreatography (MRCP) in the diagnosis of SOD?**

MRCP can be used instead of ERCP to noninvasively assess for alternative etiologies of the patient's symptoms such as biliary stone disease or pancreatic disease. The use of a provocative MRCP (eg, secretin-stimulated MRCP) to stimulate bile flow and measure ductal diameter changes with MRCP is available but remains poorly validated in the setting of SOD and the clinical utility remains uncertain.

○   **What is a positive hepatobiliary scintigraphy test?**

This test assesses bile flow through the biliary tract and into the duodenum. A positive test is defined as a duodenal arrival time greater than 20 minutes and a hilum to duodenal time greater than 10 minutes. This test is not widely performed and remains of uncertain clinical utility in the diagnosis of SOD.

● ● ● SUGGESTED READINGS ● ● ●

Hansel SL, DiBaise JK. Functional gallbladder disorder: gallbladder dyskinesia. *Gastroenterology Clinics of North America*. 2010 Jun;39(2):369-379.

Petersen BT. Functional gall-bladder and sphincter of Oddi disorders. In: Talley NJ, Lindor KD, Vargas HE, eds. *Practical gastroenterology and hepatology. Liver and biliary disease.* Chichester, Hoboken: Wiley-Blackwell; 2010:365-373.

CHAPTER 34 Gallbladder and Bile Duct Miscellaneous Inflammatory Diseases

Isaac Raijman, MD

○ **What biliary tract disease is associated with the acquired immunodeficiency syndrome (AIDS)?**

AIDS can produce a sclerosing cholangitis-like picture associated with upper abdominal pain and elevated liver function tests, especially alkaline phosphatase. The cholangitis may be associated with the AIDS virus alone or with other infections such as cytomegalovirus (CMV), *Cryptosporidium*, or *Microsporidia*. A causative organism is found in about 60% of cases.

○ **What infections may cause acalculous cholecystitis in patients with AIDS?**

Most frequently CMV, but also *Cryptosporidia*, *Microsporidia*, and *Isospora belli*.

○ **True/False: The most common infection of the bile duct in patients with AIDS is cytomegalovirus infestation.**

False. The most common organism is *Cryptosporidium parvum*. In about 20%–40% of patients, no causative organism is found.

○ **At what T lymphocyte count is AIDS cholangiopathy more likely to occur?**

When the helper T-cell count is < 200.

○ **What is the most likely diagnosis in a patient with AIDS who complains of severe abdominal pain and has an elevated alkaline phosphatase?**

Papillary stenosis. AIDS may produce severe abdominal pain associated with elevated alkaline phosphatase due to papillary stenosis. The pain may improve dramatically after endoscopic sphincterotomy.

○ **True/False: AIDS cholangiopathy adversely affects the overall outcome of AIDS patients.**

False. AIDS cholangiopathy does not appear to have any influence on the progression of the underlying disease.

○ **What patient group is at high risk for infectious and parasitic cholangiopathies?**

Patients from Southeast Asia are particularly at risk for parasite-related bile duct disease.

○ **What are the most common parasites implicated in biliary obstruction?**

Clonorchis sinensis and *Ascaris lumbricoides* are the most frequently found parasites causing biliary disease. More frequent than stricturing is the presence of undulating and elongated filling defects of the bile ducts. Certain organisms are more specific to certain geographic areas. *C. sinensis* is more common in China, Japan, Vietnam, and Korea. *Opistorchis felineus* occurs not only in Southeast Asia but also in Siberia. *Fasciola hepatica* can occur anywhere in the world while *F. gigantica* is more common in the tropics.

○ **What is Oriental cholangitis?**

Oriental cholangitis is characterized by the development of pigmented stones, diffuse biliary strictures, and chronic, recurrent episodes of cholangitis. This is particularly common in people from Southeast Asia.

○ **What is autoimmune cholangitis?**

The clinical expression of autoimmune cholangitis is very similar to that of primary biliary cirrhosis except it is not associated with antimitochondrial antibodies.

○ **What type of cholangiographic injury has been associated with intra-arterial infusion of 5-fluorodeoxyuridine?**

An intrahepatic sclerosing cholangitis-type picture.

○ **What conditions are associated with the development of bile duct disease causing stricture formation?**

- Surgical trauma
- Anastomotic arterial strictures
- Hepatic artery thrombosis
- Biliary infections
- Biliary stenting, especially if prolonged
- Choledocholithiasis
- Bile duct ischemia
- Neoplasia

○ **Jaundice occurs in what percentage of patients with acute cholecystitis without evidence of cystic duct or common bile duct obstruction?**

Fifteen percent. This may be due to inflammation and swelling of the cystic duct.

○ **Name five causes of secondary sclerosing cholangitis.**

Operative trauma and ischemia, chronic choledocholithiasis, cholangiocarcinoma, chronic pancreatitis, and toxins such as absolute alcohol and formaldehyde.

○ **Besides inflammatory bowel disease, name five chronic systemic diseases associated with sclerosing cholangitis.**

Recurrent pancreatitis, diabetes mellitus, celiac disease, rheumatoid arthritis, and sarcoidosis.

○ **In primary sclerosing cholangitis (PSC), how often is the pancreatic duct involved?**

10%–15%.

○ **Name two conditions that can mimic PSC.**

Extrahepatic portal venous obstruction and metastatic cancer of the liver.

○ **Describe two possible causes of obstructive jaundice in a patient with annular pancreas.**

1) Recurrent pancreatitis in the head of the gland, causing edema or fibrosis that constricts the bile duct within the pancreas, and 2) fibrosis of the duodenal wall, through which the terminal portion of the bile duct passes.

○ **How frequently do patients with hepatic artery aneurysms present with jaundice?**

Hepatic artery aneurysms, which are situated close to the bile ducts, present with jaundice in 50% of cases.

○ **Cholangitis is found in what percentage of patients with malignant strictures?**

10%–15%.

○ **What is the preferred treatment for lymphoma patients who present with obstructive jaundice?**

Chemotherapy is the preferred treatment. Local irradiation of the hilus of the liver may be used adjunctively.

○ **True/False: Bacterial involvement of the gallbladder is a primary event in the development of acute calculous cholecystitis.**

False. Bacterial inflammation is considered a secondary event and is found in as many as 80% of patients with acute calculous cholecystitis undergoing cholecystectomy.

○ **True/False: The presence of bacteria is uncommon in gallstone disease.**

False. Approximately 70% of patients with gallstones have evidence of bacteria in the bile. *Escherichia coli* is the most common Gram-negative organism, whereas *Enterococcus* is the most common Gram-positive organism.

○ **True/False: Jaundice occurs more commonly in adults with acute calculous cholecystitis compared to those with acalculous cholecystitis.**

False. Approximately 20%–25% of patients with acalculous cholecystitis can have obstructive jaundice due to common bile duct obstruction from inflammatory changes. Jaundice occurs in approximately 10% of patients with calculous cholecystitis.

○ **True/False: In patients with a rapidly rising bilirubin and no evidence of biliary obstruction, gallbladder perforation with secondary increased absorption of bilirubin through the peritoneal cavity should be considered.**

True.

○ **True/False: The most common complication of acute cholecystitis is gallbladder perforation.**

False. The most common complication of acute cholecystitis is gallbladder gangrene, which can occur in about 20% of the cases. Perforation occurs in approximately 2% of the patients.

○ **What is the most common location of a gallbladder perforation?**

The fundus of the gallbladder due to its larger diameter and thus greater tension.

○   **True/False: Hepatobiliary scanning of the gallbladder is useful in diagnosing acute acalculous cholecystitis.**

True. A positive test occurs when there is no filling of the gallbladder, usually within 1 hour. However, in some normal patients, it may take up to 4 hours for the gallbladder to fill. Causes of false positives include parenteral nutrition, prolonged (>24 hours) or limited (<2 hours) fasting, and alcoholism.

○   **What percentage of patients with acute acalculous cholecystitis develop complications?**

- Gallbladder empyema (2%–12%)
- Perforation (3%–15%)
- Gangrenous cholecystitis (<2%)
- Bleeding or hemoperitoneum (very rare)
- Emphysematous cholecystitis (usually due to *Clostridium* species) occurs rarely. The incidence of gangrenous gallbladder in these patients is as high as 75%.
- Septic metastases (rare)

○   **What percentage of all cases of acute cholecystitis is due to acalculous disease?**

Acute acalculous cholecystitis accounts for approximately 6%–17%.

○   **What factors are involved in the development of acute acalculous cholecystitis?**

Obstruction of the cystic duct by sludge, inspissation of bile with associated reduced flow, mechanical obstruction of the cystic duct by other diseases such as tumors or nodes, decreased gallbladder motility, systemic volume depletion, ischemia, and possibly infectious agents.

○   **True/False: Infections may cause acute acalculous cholecystitis.**

True. Infections are particularly important in patients with AIDS, where cytomegalovirus and *Cryptosporidium* play an important role. Typhoid fever is also associated with acalculous cholecystitis.

○   **Acute acalculous cholecystitis may occur in those with serious injury or illness and after major complicated surgeries, particularly in the elderly. What is the cause of acute acalculous cholecystitis?**

The etiology of acalculous cholecystitis is unknown but possibilities include biliary/gallbladder stasis resulting from long-standing fasting, alterations in gallbladder flow, especially in elderly patients with peripheral vascular disease, prostaglandins, and endotoxins. Gangrene, empyema, and perforation of gallbladder more commonly complicate the course of acalculous cholecystitis than acute calculous cholecystitis.

○   **Acalculous cholecystitis accounts for what percentage of gallbladder perforations?**

40%.

○   **What diseases are associated with the development of acute acalculous cholecystitis?**

Diseases associated with mesenteric vascular compromise (vasculitis), sepsis, prolonged use of total parenteral nutrition, severe burns, and intra-abdominal surgery.

○   **What patient group is more commonly associated with acute acalculous cholecystitis?**

Contrary to calculous disease, acalculous cholecystitis is more common in men, especially the elderly.

○ **What is the overall mortality in acute acalculous cholecystitis?**

Approximately 50%.

○ **What is the most common cholangiographic pattern of PSC?**

While it may affect both intra- and extrahepatic ducts, PSC more commonly presents as multiple short strictures found throughout the liver with characteristic beading and pruning and isolated dilations of the intrahepatic ducts.

○ **True/False: Endobiliary stents are the nonsurgical treatment of choice for PSC-related bile duct strictures.**

False.

○ **True/False: Cholangiocarcinoma is usually easily detected in the setting of PSC.**

False.

○ **What is the most common cause of acute suppurative cholangitis?**

Intrahepatic or extrahepatic stones are the cause of almost all cases. Patients with a biliary endoprosthesis and/or previous biliary manipulation are also at risk.

○ **What is the treatment of choice in acute suppurative cholangitis?**

Endoscopic decompression along with systemic antibiotics.

● ● ● **SUGGESTED READINGS** ● ● ●

Barie PS, Eachempati SR. Acute acalculous cholecystitis. *Gastroenterol Clin North Am.* 2010;39(2):343-357.

Alderlieste YA, van den Elzen BD, Rauws EA, Beuers U. Immunoglobulin G4-associated cholangitis: one variant of immunoglobulin G4-related systemic disease. *Digestion.* 2009;79(4):220-228.

CHAPTER 35 **Pancreatic Miscellaneous Inflammatory Diseases**

Denise McCormack, MD and David W. McFadden, MD

○ **True/False: An elevated amylase is always indicative of acute pancreatitis in the setting of acute calculous cholecystitis.**

False. Hyperamylasemia may reflect a gangrenous gallbladder. Additionally, minor (<2–3 times normal) elevations may be seen in acute cholecystitis without gangrene.

○ **What connective tissue diseases and vasculitides may have pancreatic involvement?**

Systemic lupus erythematosus, rheumatoid arthritis, polyarteritis nodosa, Henoch–Schönlein purpura, Wegener's granulomatosis, and Behçet's syndrome.

○ **True/False: Autoimmune pancreatitis involvement of the pancreas may be either diffuse or focal.**

True. Autoimmune pancreatitis is a fibroinflammatory pancreatic disease that may present with either focal or diffuse involvement. The focal form requires careful evaluation, since it may be confused with pancreatic cancer.

○ **What are the four main criteria used in the diagnosis of autoimmune pancreatitis?**

Pancreatic histology, radiologic features, other organ involvement, and clinical response to steroid treatment. Serum IgG4 and positive IgG4 plasma cells in pancreatic biopsies may also support its diagnosis.

○ **True/False: Elevated levels of IgG4 antibodies correlate with disease severity in autoimmune pancreatitis.**

True. The median serum IgG4 concentration in autoimmune pancreatitis is approximately 600 mg/dL. Elevated serum IgG4 levels may help to distinguish autoimmune pancreatitis from other conditions of the pancreas or biliary tree.

○ **True/False: Treatment with corticosteroids has been shown in well-controlled clinical trials to result in rapid improvement of autoimmune pancreatitis.**

False. Although treatment with steroids is a diagnostic criterion and steroid use may result in rapid improvement, there are no prospective, randomized, placebo-controlled trials of any treatment in autoimmune pancreatitis. The effect of steroids on the natural history of autoimmune pancreatitis is unclear.

○ **True/False: Extrapancreatic disease occurs in about 15%–20% of patients with autoimmune pancreatitis.**

False. Extrapancreatitic disease occurs in 40%–90% of cases. Biliary disease is one of the most common extrapancreatic manifestations; however, organs distant from the pancreas can be involved.

○ **Describe the difference between type 1 and type 2 autoimmune pancreatitis.**

Type 1 is characterized by pancreas involvement as one part of a systemic IgG4-positive disease, whereas type 2 is characterized by pancreas involvement without systemic involvement or IgG4 positivity.

○ **What are the HISORt criteria?**

HISORt refers to diagnostic criteria for autoimmune pancreatitis and stands for *H*istology, *I*maging, *S*erology, other *O*rgan involvement, and *R*esponse to steroids.

○ **What is the name of the uncommon condition characterized by fibrotic inflammation affecting the anatomical area between the head of the pancreas, the duodenum, and the common bile duct?**

Groove pancreatitis.

○ **True/False: Groove pancreatitis is often misdiagnosed as pancreatic malignancy or autoimmune pancreatitis because of its "pseudotumor" formation.**

True.

○ **Describe the inheritance pattern of hereditary pancreatitis.**

Hereditary pancreatitis is usually caused by a mutation in the cationic trypsinogen gene and accounts for 2% of all cases of chronic pancreatitis. The disease has an autosomal dominant inheritance pattern with 80% penetrance.

○ **True/False: The clinical presentation of hereditary pancreatitis is similar to other forms of chronic pancreatitis.**

True. However, individuals usually present with recurrent acute pancreatitis in childhood, chronic pancreatitis as adolescents or young adults, and a markedly increased risk of pancreatic cancer in their fifth decade of life.

○ **True/False: Mortality in hereditary pancreatitis without pancreatic cancer is the same as the general population.**

True. However, mortality is significantly increased in those who develop pancreatic cancer.

○ **What is the most common hereditary disease involving the exocrine pancreas?**

Cystic fibrosis (CF), which affects 1 in every 2000 live births.

○ **Describe the inheritance pattern of CF.**

Autosomal recessive with a gene frequency of approximately 5% among Caucasians.

○ **What are pancreatic manifestations of CF?**

In the early stages, the pancreas may appear normal or there may be a deposition of eosinophilic concretions within ductules. Larger ductular involvement may lead to dilatation and acinar disruption. Later on, the pancreas may appear indistinguishable from chronic pancreatitis as cyst development may occur, and fat and scar may replace pancreatic lobules.

○ **True/False: Pancreatic exocrine insufficiency is a common complication of CF.**

False. Only about 15% of CF patients show clinical evidence of pancreatic exocrine insufficiency resulting from pancreatic duct obstruction.

○ **What percentage of patients with CF has diabetes mellitus?**

Cystic fibrosis–related diabetes (CFRD) occurs in approximately 20% of adolescents and 40%–50% of adults.

○ **Describe the pathophysiology of pancreatic endocrine insufficiency that may occur in CF.**

Replacement of pancreatic tissue with fibrosis and fat in severe disease leads to disruption of normal islets by autodigestion and diminution of the number of islets.

○ **True/False: Gallstones are more common in CF and can lead to acute inflammatory exacerbations.**

True. Cholelithiasis, sludge, and gallbladder wall thickening occur in 12%–24% of patients with CF.

○ **True/False: Laparoscopic cholecystectomy should be considered for CF patients with asymptomatic gallstones detected during screening radiography.**

False.

○ **True/False: Pancreatitis is a rare manifestation of CF.**

True. Patients with CF may develop chronic pancreatic insufficiency; however, acute pancreatitis is seen in less than 1%.

○ **True/False: Microscopic pancreatic involvement is seen in the majority of patients with sarcoidosis.**

False. Pancreatic involvement occurs in only 1%–6% of all affected individuals and is rarely seen before the diagnosis is made from the upper aerodigestive tract.

○ **True/False: Microscopic gastrointestinal involvement is seen in the majority of patients with sarcoidosis.**

True. Granulomas are seen in nearly 100% of patients with known sarcoidosis, although symptoms are described in less than 1%.

○ **Briefly describe the pathophysiology of sarcoidosis.**

Noncaseating granulomata occur in sarcoidosis. Enlarged lymph nodes may cause pressure-related symptoms and granulomatous infiltration may cause dysfunction or dysmotility in the gastrointestinal tract.

○ **True/False: Involvement of the pancreas in Crohn's disease is not seen in the absence of duodenal involvement.**

False.

○ **What are potential mechanisms underlying Crohn's disease involvement of the pancreas?**

There are four suggested mechanisms: ampullary involvement, cholelithiasis secondary to ileal disease, immunologic injury, and drug therapy.

○ **Name the usual, albeit rare, manifestation of Wegener's granulomatosis involving the pancreas.**

Pancreatic mass.

○ **What is the classic triad of Wegener's granulomatosis?**

Focal glomerulonephritis, vasculitis, and necrotizing granulomata.

○ **Classically, Wegener's granulomatosis affects what part of the alimentary tract?**

The intestine. The associated vasculitis can lead to intestinal or colonic bleeding, ischemia, or perforation.

○ **What is the most common cause of pancreatitis in childhood?**

Trauma (child abuse must be considered). Systemic disease, drugs, and infection are the other major causes in children.

○ **What is Shwachman's syndrome (aka, Shwachman–Diamond syndrome)?**

A disorder of pancreatic exocrine insufficiency, hematologic abnormalities, and growth retardation with normal sweat electrolytes. This autosomal recessive disorder is the second most common cause of pancreatic insufficiency in children.

○ **A patient recovering from gallstone pancreatitis develops multiple painful, erythematous subcutaneous nodules. What is the diagnosis?**

Pancreatic panniculitis. Subcutaneous fat necrosis occurs in 2%–3% of patients with acute pancreatitis or pancreatic cancer. The lesions may resemble erythema nodosum.

○ **What are the effects of end-stage renal disease on the pancreas?**

Morphologically, multiple abnormalities (acinar dilation, interlobular fibrosis) may be seen. Functionally, an elevated trypsin with a normal output of lipase and impaired bicarbonate secretion may be seen. Hyperamylasemia and hyperlipasemia may be seen due to a lack of renal clearance, even in the absence of pancreatic inflammation. Clinically, the frequency of acute pancreatitis may be increased in these patients, but the mechanisms are unclear.

○ **What are the pancreatic effects of hereditary hemochromatosis?**

Selective accumulation of excess iron in islet beta-cells results in a loss of endocrine granules and subsequent glucose intolerance or frank diabetes.

○ **True/False: Diabetics have an increased risk of exocrine pancreatic insufficiency.**

True. Nearly 40% of diabetics will have impaired pancreatic secretion. This is thought to be due to the inhibitory effects of excess glucagon and lack of stimulatory effects of insulin on the pancreas, vagal neuropathy, and nutritional wasting.

● ● ● SUGGESTED READINGS ● ● ●

Detlefsen S, Löhr JM, Drewes AM, Frøkjær JB, Klöppel G. Current concepts in the diagnosis and treatment of type 1 and type 2 autoimmune pancreatitis. *Recent Pat Inflamm Allergy Drug Discov.* 2011 May;5(2):136-149.

Lal A, Lal DR. Hereditary pancreatitis. *Pediatr Surg Int.* 2010 Dec;26(12):1193-1199.

CHAPTER 36 Gallbladder and Bile Duct Tumors

Jana G. Hashash, MD and Randall E. Brand, MD

○ **What is the most common cancer involving the hepatobiliary tree?**

Gallbladder adenocarcinoma. Gallbladder carcinoma is the fifth most common cancer of the gastrointestinal tract and is responsible for 2%–4% of all gastrointestinal malignancies and about half of all biliary tract tumors. It occurs most frequently in the sixth and seventh decades of life and is more common in women and Native Americans.

○ **Identify two risk factors for the development of gallbladder carcinoma.**

Gallstones larger than 2.5 cm and calcified or "porcelain" gallbladder. Other risk factors include gallbladder polyps (> 1 cm), obesity, anomalous pancreaticobiliary duct junction or choledochal cysts, and carcinogens such as nitrosamines and azotoluene.

○ **Which chronic infections are associated with gallbladder cancer?**

Salmonella typhi carrier state is an independent risk factor for gallbladder cancer (six-fold risk). There are reports that *Helicobacter* colonization of the biliary epithelium may be associated with gallbladder cancer.

○ **What are the most common routes of gallbladder carcinoma metastasis?**

Lymphatic spread and direct invasion.

○ **True/False: The most common benign neoplasm of the gallbladder is an adenoma.**

True. The most common benign, nonneoplastic gallbladder lesion is the cholesterol "polyp," also known as cholesterosis followed by adenomyomas and inflammatory polyps.

○ **What size of benign adenomas of the gallbladder is at an increased risk for gallbladder carcinoma?**

Adenomas greater than 10 mm have been observed to have malignant foci.

○ **True/False: Gallbladder polyps of any size require surgical removal.**

False. Gallbladder polyps <5 mm are usually benign and represent cholesterolosis, whereas lesions >10 mm should be considered to possibly harbor malignancy. Lesions between 5 and 10 mm may be either benign or malignant. Serial imaging is recommended to determine stability of size. Lesions that increase in size should undergo cholecystectomy.

○ **Name two carcinogens associated with the development of gallbladder carcinoma.**

Dimethylnitrosamine and petroleum products.

○ **Name the biliary tree cancer that a patient with anomalous pancreaticobiliary duct junction and no biliary cysts is prone to develop.**

Gallbladder cancer. In those patients, a prophylactic cholecystectomy is recommended.

○ **Name three clinical entities associated with extrahepatic bile duct tumors.**

1) Choledochal cysts or polycystic liver disease; 2) primary sclerosing cholangitis; and 3) chronic infection with *Clonorchis sinensis*, *Ascaris lumbricoides*, and *Opisthorcis viverrini* (worldwide the most common cause). Other clinical entities are ulcerative colitis, hepatolithiasis, Caroli syndrome, and obesity.

○ **What contrast agent can predispose to cholangiocarcinoma?**

Thorotrast.

○ **What is the second most common tumor of the biliary tract?**

Cholangiocarcinoma. Cholangiocarcinoma follows gallbladder carcinoma as the second most common tumor of the biliary tract. Over 70% of patients are over the age of 65.

○ **Patients with congenital biliary cysts are at an increased risk of developing which biliary tree cancer?**

Cholangiocarcinoma.

○ **Name two nonspecific tumor markers of the gastrointestinal tract that may be elevated in cholangiocarcinoma.**

CA 19-9 and carcinoembyonic antigen (CEA). Alpha fetoprotein is elevated in <5% of cases of cholangiocarcinoma.

○ **Name two physical exam findings occasionally seen with ampullary carcinoma besides jaundice and excoriations from pruritis.**

Hepatomegaly and Courvoisier's sign (a palpably enlarged, nontender gallbladder). These findings are found in 25%–40% of patients with ampullary carcinoma. Left supraclavicular lymphadenopathy (Virchow's node) or a palpable rectal shelf may be present in patients with widespread disease. The 5-year survival of ampullary carcinoma ranges from 20% to 40%.

○ **Alternating jaundice and gastrointestinal bleeding are suggestive of what biliary tumor?**

Ulcerating ampullary carcinoma.

○ **What histologic subtype of ampullary carcinoma has the best prognosis?**

Intestinal type has a better prognosis than pancreatobiliary type.

○ **Identify three risk factors for the development of ampullary carcinoma.**

Ampullary adenoma, familial adenomatous polyposis, and Gardner's syndrome.

○ **What hormone receptor may be found in cholangiocarcinomas?**

Somatostatin.

○ **Recent studies have reported an association between hepatitis C viral infection and which biliary tract cancer?**

Intrahepatic cholangiocarcinoma.

○ **Which side of the intrahepatic biliary tree, the right or left system, is preferentially drained by the presence of only one stent in the setting of a proximal intrahepatic bile duct tumor?**

The left hepatic ductal system can be drained with a single stent. The right hepatic duct bifurcates extensively proximal to the confluence with the left hepatic duct.

○ **Apart from CT/MRI of the abdomen, what other anatomical region of imaging is important for the staging of both gallbladder cancer and cholangiocarcinoma?**

Chest imaging.

○ **What is the current first-line chemotherapy for locally advanced and metastatic gallbladder and cholangiocarcinomas?**

Gemcitabine and cisplatin.

○ **What is the primary concern regarding an externally obtained (ie, percutaneously or via endoscopic ultrasound [EUS]) fine needle aspiration (FNA) or biopsy of a biliary tract cancer, in particular extrahepatic tumors?**

Tumor seeding. Most institutions will not perform FNA or biopsy of these lesions percutaneously due to concerns about tumor seeding. However, some institutions will do these procedures on distal common bile duct (CBD) lesions (intrapancreatic portions) if the FNA is done under EUS guidance since the tract would be removed at the time of surgical resection.

• • • **SUGGESTED READINGS** • • •

Heinrich S, Clavien PA. Ampullary cancer. *Curr Opin Gastroenterol.* 2010 May:26(3):280-285.

Charbel H, Al-Kawas FH. Cholangiocarcinoma: epidemiology, risk factors, pathogenesis, and diagnosis. *Curr Gastroenterol Rep.* 2011 Apr;13(2):182-187.

Rustagi T, Dasanu CA. Risk factors for gallbladder cancer and cholangiocarcinoma: similarities, differences and updates. *J Gastrointest Cancer.* 2011 May 20. [Epub ahead of print]

Gurusamy KS, Abu-Amara M, Farouk M, Davidson BR. Cholecystectomy for gallbladder polyp. *Cochrane Database Syst Rev.* 2009 Jan 21;(1):CD007052.

CHAPTER 37 Pancreatic Tumors

Jana G. Hashash, MD and
Randall E. Brand, MD

○ **The vast majority of primary malignant tumors of the pancreas are of what histological type?**

Ductal adenocarcinomas and its variants constitute approximately 90% of primary malignant tumors of the pancreas. About 5% of pancreatic tumors are of islet cell origin. The rarer types of primary pancreatic cancer include squamous cell carcinoma, giant cell carcinoma, carcinosarcoma, cystadenocarcinoma, acinar cell carcinoma, sarcoma, malignant fibrous histiocytoma, lymphoma, and pancreaticoblastoma.

○ **The majority of adenocarcinomas are derived from what part of the pancreas?**

Pancreatic ductal epithelium. Over half of tumors are found in the head of the pancreas.

○ **What are the three established precursor lesions for development of an adenocarcinoma?**

Pancreatic intraepithelial lesions (PanINs), mucinous cystadenomas (MCNs), and intraductal papillary mucinous neoplasms (IPMNs).

○ **Diabetes mellitus or impaired glucose intolerance occurs in what percentage of patients with pancreatic cancer?**

Sixty percent to 80% of patients with pancreatic cancer have diabetes mellitus or impaired glucose tolerance with the majority of patients found to be diabetic within 2 years of the diagnosis of pancreatic cancer. Glucose intolerance is noted to improve after pancreatic tumor resection.

○ **What hormone is felt to be responsible for the occurrence of diabetes in patients with pancreatic cancer?**

The overproduction of amylin (islet amyloid polypeptide) has been reported in patients with pancreatic cancer.

○ **What are some epidemiologic and etiologic factors that are associated with an increased risk for the development of pancreatic cancer?**

Cigarette smoking, animal fat-rich diet (reduced levels of lycopene), idiopathic chronic pancreatitis, alcoholic chronic pancreatitis, diabetes mellitus, and gallstones.

○   **True/False: Cigarette smoking is the most consistent environmental risk factor predisposing to pancreatic cancer.**

True. Cigarette smoking is the only risk factor consistently found in epidemiological studies to predispose to pancreatic cancer.

○   **Why does CA 19-9 only have a maximum sensitivity of 95% for the diagnosis of pancreatic cancer?**

The carbohydrate antigen, CA 19-9, is not expressed in the 5% of individuals who are sialylated Lewis[a] antigen negative.

○   **What are the more common presenting symptoms in patients with pancreatic cancer?**

Epigastric pain, weight loss, anorexia, and obstructive jaundice.

○   **What is the most common presentation in patients with resectable pancreatic carcinoma?**

Painless jaundice is seen in about 50% of patients with a resectable lesion.

○   **What is the most common genetic alteration detected in pancreatic carcinomas?**

A K-*ras* mutation is detected in 95% of cases.

○   **True/False: A mutation at codon 15 of K-*ras* is the most commonly identified gene abnormality in pancreatic cancer.**

False. Mutations of K-*ras* almost uniformly occur at codon 12 in pancreatic cancer.

○   **Approximately what percentage of pancreatic carcinoma cases are related to hereditary factors?**

A genetic predisposition for adenocarcinoma of the pancreas may account for up to 10% of cases. Such genetic predispositions include hereditary pancreatitis, Peutz–Jeghers syndrome and BRCA-2-positive individuals among others.

○   **True/False: The risk of pancreatic cancer is increased in all familial atypical multiple mole melanoma (FAMMM) syndrome kindreds.**

False. Only in those kindreds with a p16 germ-line mutation.

○   **What other disorders can lead to elevations in serum CA 19-9 levels?**

Most commonly, those disorders that cause biliary tract obstruction such as cholangitis, cholangiocarcinoma, gallbladder carcinoma, and benign biliary tract diseases. Additionally, elevations may be seen in acute and chronic pancreatitis and chronic liver disease.

○   **What imaging techniques can be used to assist in obtaining tissue to make the diagnosis of pancreatic cancer?**

Fine-needle aspiration can be performed under endoscopic ultrasound (EUS), CT, or transabdominal ultrasound guidance. In addition, brushings can be obtained during endoscopic retrograde cholangiopancreatography (ERCP).

○ **What imaging modality is generally considered to be the best initial study when evaluating patients presenting with symptoms that suggest pancreatic disease?**

A pancreatic-protocol multidetector CT scan is recommended since it can detect tumors in the pancreas, stage for resectability, and evaluate for liver metastases.

○ **What imaging study is most accurate in the detection of small (< 2 cm) pancreatic neoplasms?**

EUS has been found in several studies to be the most accurate imaging study available for the detection of small carcinomas.

○ **Which structures are technically difficult to assess via EUS?**

Superior mesenteric vessels. EUS is better at imaging the portal and splenic veins. EUS may lack accuracy in assessing vascular invasion at the level of the superior mesenteric vessels.

○ **What percentage of patients with adenocarcinoma of the pancreas are unresectable at the time of diagnosis?**

Due to the insidious nature of the disease, more than 80% of patients are unresectable at the time of diagnosis.

○ **What helical CT scanning criteria are used to define unresectability in pancreatic cancer?**

• Presence of extrapancreatic (metastatic) disease.
• Evidence of direct tumor extension to the celiac axis and/or superior mesenteric artery.

○ **What is the perioperative mortality rate of pancreaticoduodenectomy (Whipple procedure) when performed at experienced centers?**

Current perioperative mortality rates are less than 5% at experienced centers.

○ **True/False: Poorly differentiated pancreatic adenocarcinomas have significant cellular atypia, significant mitotic activity, and significant mucin production.**

False. Well-differentiated pancreatic adenocarcinoma cells produce a significant amount of mucin.

○ **How many long-term survivors of pancreatic cancer die of recurrent or metastatic disease?**

Unlike most other types of cancer, 5-year survival with this disease does not ensure that the patient has been cured of it. One study of long-term survivors (>5 years) reported that almost half of these patients died of recurrent or metastatic disease.

○ **What is the preferable method of nonoperative palliative biliary decompression?**

For reasons of less morbidity, it is preferable to place a stent by ERCP rather than percutaneously through a transhepatic approach.

○ **True/False: Preoperative stenting of the bile duct to relieve jaundice decreases perioperative morbidity and mortality.**

False. Recent studies do not support preoperative stenting of the bile duct except in cases of acute cholangitis. This seems to be due to an increased rate of complications in patients undergoing routine preoperative biliary stenting.

○   **What is the double-duct sign?**

This sign is caused by a mass in the head of the pancreas causing dilation of both the pancreatic and common bile duct. When this sign is present, the patient should be assumed to have pancreatic cancer until proven otherwise.

○   **What are the advantages of preoperative chemoradiation therapy compared to postoperative chemoradiation therapy in resectable patients?**

A recent study demonstrated no change in survival advantage; however, 24% of patients were unable to receive postoperative treatment as a result of delayed recovery after surgery. Additionally, there is a subset of patients that develop metastatic cancer while receiving preoperative therapy, thereby eliminating a group of patients that would not have benefited from a surgery (due to the presence of unrecognized pancreatic cancer).

○   **What options are available for treatment of gastric outlet obstruction caused by a pancreatic adenocarcinoma?**

The use of expandable metallic stents offers an endoscopic method for palliation of this complication. Prior to endoscopic palliation, the traditional management was a surgical bypass procedure such as a gastrojejunostomy. Depending upon the clinical scenario, the placement of a venting gastrostomy tube and/or a feeding jejunostomy is another option.

○   **What pathologic characteristics predict long-term survival following surgical resection for pancreatic cancer?**

Negative resection margins, negative nodal status, and tumor size < 1–2 cm are strong predictors of long-term survival.

○   **After a patient is initially diagnosed with pancreatic cancer, what are the next management decisions?**

There are three categories into which a newly diagnosed pancreatic cancer patient can be placed depending on spread of the disease: 1) metastatic and unresectable tumors will require chemotherapy +/− palliation, 2) locally advanced and border-line resectable tumors are candidates for chemotherapy or chemoradiation, and 3) resectable tumors are surgical candidates. The third group should receive either neoadjuvant or adjuvant therapy in addition to surgery.

○   **True/False: Total pancreatectomy and extensive retroperitoneal lymphadenopathy excision have shown survival benefits over pancreaticoduodenectomy in patients with pancreatic cancer.**

False. Whipple pancreaticoduodenectomy is the most common surgery for pancreatic cancer. Total pancreatectomy has not shown to improve survival compared to the Whipple operation and is associated with a higher rate of exocrine insufficiency and brittle diabetes. Also, extensive retroperitoneal lymphadenopathy excision, in addition to the Whipple surgery, has shown no significant survival benefit over the Whipple procedure alone.

○   **True/False: About 3% of cystic pancreatic tumors are neoplastic.**

False. About 15% are neoplastic. These cystic neoplasms include serous cystadenomas, IPMNs, cystic neuroendocrine tumors, and solid pseudopapillary tumors.

○   **True/False: Once a pancreatic cyst is discovered, the possibility of the lesion being a pseudocyst should be excluded.**

True. Patient evaluation should be directed toward exclusion of a pancreatic pseudocyst including inquiring about a history of acute pancreatitis. Pseudocysts lack the epithelial lining that true cysts have. Radiographically, pseudocysts tend to lack septae, loculations, solid components, or cyst wall calcifications.

○ **What elements present in pancreatic cysts have been evaluated in attempt to improve the diagnostic yield of cyst fluid aspiration?**

Fluid color and viscosity, cytology, amylase, and a variety of tumor markers including carcinoembryonic antigen (CEA), CA 19-9, CA 125, and CA 72-4. Genetic markers may also be checked but are generally reserved for cysts in which the cytology and CEA testing yields indeterminate premalignant or malignant findings.

○ **What is the single most clinically useful test done on a pancreatic cyst fluid aspirate in the evaluation of a cystic lesion of the pancreatic tail?**

A CEA level is the most informative test to discriminate between a mucinous and nonmucinous cystic lesion with an accuracy of about 80%.

○ **True/False: A serous cystadenoma occurs more commonly in females than males.**

True.

○ **True/False: A serous cystadenoma is most commonly diagnosed in patients before the age of 40.**

False. These neoplasms are most commonly detected in the sixth decade of a patient's life.

○ **What are the most common presenting symptoms of a serous cystadenoma?**

Abdominal pain (50%), asymptomatic abdominal mass (33%), and weight loss (20%).

○ **What is the typical ultrasonographic appearance of a serous cystadenoma?**

It appears as a complex echo-lucent cystic structure with septae, similar to a honeycomb structure. The individual cysts are usually small.

○ **What is the classic calcification pattern of a serous cystadenoma seen on abdominal plain films?**

Central calcification known as a "sunburst" pattern.

○ **How does a serous cystadenoma usually appear on CT scan?**

A multiloculated cystic mass ranging in size from 4 to 6 cm. A central stellate calcification may be present. The neoplasm can occur anywhere within the pancreas but is found most commonly in the body or tail.

○ **True/False: Serous cystadenomas are generally benign.**

True.

○ **True/False: MCNs are more common in women and occur around the age of 50.**

True.

○ **What is the usual appearance of a mucinous cystadenoma on either ultrasonography or CT scan?**

A loculated cystic mass that does not communicate with the main pancreatic duct and is located in the body or tail of the pancreas. Malignant lesions tend to be larger (8–11 cm) and often have rim calcifications within the wall identified on CT scan.

○ **What is the treatment of choice for a mucinous cystic neoplasm?**

Surgical resection is the treatment of choice due to difficulties in differentiating a benign versus malignant lesion by biopsy of the cyst wall or by fine needle aspiration of the cyst contents.

○ **How are IPMNs classified?**

IPMNs can be classified as main duct, side-branch (either single or multifocal), or mixed main duct-side-branch on the basis of their appearance of imaging studies.

○ **What are the classic characteristics of a main duct intraductal papillary mucinous tumor of the pancreas as seen during ERCP?**

A dilated and irregular main pancreatic duct with filling defects and extrusion of mucin through the major papilla.

○ **True/False: Surgical resection is recommended for all main duct and mixed variant IPMNs regardless of whether symptomatic.**

True. Resection is also recommended for symptomatic side-branch IPMNs in surgically fit patients with reasonable life expectancy.

○ **Which pancreatic tumors are associated with peripheral fat necrosis?**

A minority of patients with acinar cell carcinoma present with lipase hypersecretion syndrome, which results in peripheral fat necrosis.

○ **Which is the most likely type of pancreatic tumor being demonstrated in the following figure?**

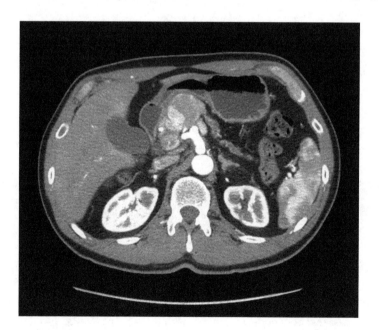

Figure 37-1

The hypervascular, necrotic nature of the pancreatic head mass is most suggestive of a neuroendocrine tumor.

○ **What neuroendocrine tumor is associated with a syndrome of large volume diarrhea, achlorhydria, and hypokalemia?**

VIPoma. This syndrome, caused by overproduction of vasoactive intestinal peptide, is characterized by the acronym WDHA (watery diarrhea, hypokalemia, and achlorhydria).

○ **What neuroendocrine tumor is associated with a dermatitis, glucose intolerance, weight loss, and anemia?**

Glucagonoma. Up to 90% of cases will present with characteristic skin lesions and glucose intolerance.

○ **What is the characteristic skin rash that may be seen in patients with glucagonoma?**

Necrolytic migratory erythema. This rash may wax and wane and occurs in 64%–90% of cases.

○ **Deficiencies of amino acids are a common occurrence in what pancreatic neuroendocrine tumor?**

Glucagonoma. The severity of the deficiency is correlated with the intensity of the disease.

○ **A 55-year-old white man with a history of diabetes and steatorrhea underwent an emergent cholecystectomy for acute cholecystitis. Intraoperatively, he is found to have a small tumor in the head of the pancreas. The patient most likely has what neuroendocrine tumor?**

Somatostatinoma. Diabetes occurs in 95%, gallstone disease in 94%, and steatorrhea is found in 83% of cases of pancreatic somatostatinomas.

○ **The majority of gastrinomas are found in what anatomic area?**

The gastrinoma triangle, which is bordered superiorly by the confluence of the common bile duct (CBD), inferiorly by the junction of the second and third portions of the duodenum, and medially by the junction of the neck and body of the pancreas.

○ **Gastrinomas are classically associated with what syndrome?**

Multiple endocrine neoplasia (MEN) type 1 is reported in approximately 25% of gastrinoma patients.

○ **Describe Whipple's triad?**

Whipple's triad consists of hypoglycemic symptoms, blood glucose levels of less than 50 mg/dL, and symptom relief after glucose ingestion. It may be seen in patients with an insulinoma.

○ **Besides a CT scan of the abdomen, what is the best imaging study to evaluate for metastatic gastrinoma?**

An octreotide scan (somatostatin receptor scintigraphy). In most series, it assists in the localization of gastrinomas more than 90% of the time.

○ **Where is the most common extrapancreatic site for a gastrinoma?**

The duodenal wall.

○ **What is the neuroendocrine tumor with the lowest rate of metastasis?**

Insulinoma, with a rate of < 10%.

○ **True/False: Both EUS and somatostatin receptor scintigraphy are useful in the localization of insulinomas and gastrinomas.**

False. Although both modalities are useful in the evaluation of gastrinomas, only 10% of insulinomas are detected with an octreotide scan.

○ **What type of lymphoma may affect the pancreas?**

Non-Hodgkin's lymphoma accounts for 1%–2% of all pancreatic neoplasms. About 1% of non-Hodgkin lymphomas appear to arise from the pancreas. At autopsy, about one-third of all patients with non-Hodgkin's lymphoma will have some microscopic involvement of the pancreas.

○ **What is a typical presentation of pancreatic lymphoma?**

Weight loss and jaundice. Some patients may also have night sweats.

○ **True/False: Surgical resection is usually required in cases of pancreatic lymphoma.**

False. Combination chemotherapy and radiation therapy results in a cure rate of 30%. Surgery may occasionally be performed either for tissue diagnosis or for resection of small, localized tumors.

● ● ● **SUGGESTED READINGS** ● ● ●

Costello E, Neoptolemos JP. Pancreatic cancer in 2010: new insights for early intervention and detection. *Nat Rev Gastroenterol Hepatol.* 2011;8(2):71-73.

Al-haddad M, Schmidt MC, Sandrasegaran K, Dewitt J. Diagnosis and treatment of cystic pancreatic tumors. *Clin Gastroenterol Hepatol.* 2011;9:635-648.

Matthaei H, Schulick RD, Hruban RH, Maitra A. Cystic precursors to invasive pancreatic cancer. *Nat Rev Gastroenterol Hepatol.* 2011;8(3):141-150.

Batcher E, Madaj P, Gianoukakis AG. Pancreatic neuroendocrine tumors. *Endocr Res.* 2011;36(1):35-43.

CHAPTER 38

Acute and Chronic Pancreatitis

Enrique Molina, MD and
Jamie S. Barkin, MD, MACP, MACG

○ **What are the most common causes of acute pancreatitis?**

Gallstones and alcohol. Idiopathic acute pancreatitis accounts for 8%–25% of cases; however, up to two-thirds of these patients may have microlithiasis or sphincter of Oddi dysfunction identified by inspection of bile and sphincter of Oddi manometry, respectively. Other causes include hypertriglyceridemia, hypercalcemia, trauma, iatrogenic trauma (eg, post endoscopic retrograde cholangiopancreatography [ERCP]), autoimmune pancreatitis, pancreatic tumors (both primary and metastatic), medications, vasculitis, and certain viral and bacterial infections. Pancreas divisum has been suggested as a cause of acute pancreatitis, although this remains controversial.

○ **True/False: The most important therapy of acute pancreatitis is volume resuscitation.**

True. Appropriate and timely fluid resuscitation in acute pancreatitis is critical as it is associated with reduced morbidity and mortality, including a reduced incidence of systemic inflammatory response syndrome (SIRS) and organ failure. Appropriate early resuscitation requires at least 250–300 mL/hour of IV fluids for the first 48 hours of hospitalization; however, patients with severe volume depletion may require up to 500–1000 mL/hour of IV hydration. Crystalloids are the preferred parenteral fluid in most cases.

○ **True/False: Patients with coexisting alcohol dependence and cholelithiasis should undergo prophylactic cholecystectomy in order to prevent an episode of acute pancreatitis.**

False. Cholecystectomy has not been shown to prevent recurrent episodes of pancreatitis in patients with coexisting alcohol dependence. The pancreatitis nearly always follows the course of alcohol-related pancreatitis.

○ **What is the mortality rate of gallstone-associated pancreatitis?**

Approximately 12% during the first attack; however, it varies depending on the severity of the attack. Mortality tends to decrease with subsequent attacks.

○ **What is the role of shock wave lithotripsy in acute pancreatitis caused by obstructive pancreatic stones?**

Extracorporeal shock wave lithotripsy of obstructive pancreatic duct stones may prevent further attacks in patients with recurrent episodes of acute pancreatitis.

○   **True/False: Prophylactic pancreatic stent placement during ERCP reduces the risk of post-ERCP pancreatitis.**

True.

○   **What etiology of acute pancreatitis documented by CT scan should be suspected in patients without measurable elevation in serum amylase levels?**

Severe hypertriglyceridemia may result in false-negative serum values of amylase and lipase. While measured serum amylase activity is frequently normal, urinary amylase concentration is markedly elevated. Recurrences may be prevented by treatment aimed at avoiding elevations in serum triglycerides greater than 1000 mg/dL.

○   **Which of the following etiologies of pancreatitis is most likely to result in the eventual development of chronic pancreatitis: biliary pancreatitis, hypercalcemia-induced pancreatitis, or post-ERCP pancreatitis?**

Hypercalcemia often leads to the development of chronic pancreatitis (with an estimated incidence of 0.1%–3.3%).

○   **What is the cause of the increased incidence of acute pancreatitis during pregnancy?**

Cholelithiasis or microlithiasis is present in about 90% of cases; however, nonbiliary sources should be sought as they are associated with worse outcomes. Hypercalcmeia of hyperparathyroidism may be falsely lowered due to hypoalbuminemia or magnesium tocolysis. Most episodes of biliary pancreatitis occur in the third trimester or in the early postpartum period. Elective cholecystectomy after the first trimester is generally recommended. The overall prognosis is good; however, the first trimester episodes of acute pancreatitis are associated with a high risk of fetal loss of about 20%.

○   **What percentage of acute pancreatitis is medication-related?**

5%. However, drug-induced pancreatitis is probably underestimated because of the difficulty in determining definitively the causative agent. Epidemiologic data suggest the risk of pancreatitis is highest for mesalamine and azathioprine. Other drugs that are definitely associated with acute pancreatitis include 6-mercaptopurine, sulfonamides, thiazide diuretics, furosemide, estrogens, tetracyclines, valproic acid, pentamidine, didanosine, intravenous lipid infusion, and L-asparaginase. Other drugs with a less certain association include chlorthalidone, ethacrynic acid, phenformin, nonsteroidal anti-inflammatory agents, nitrofurantoin, methyldopa, corticosteroids, angiotensin converting enzyme (ACE) inhibitors, cimetidine, ranitidine, acetaminophen, metronidazole, lamivudine, carbamazepine, rifampin, and salicylates.

○   **What compounds have a dose-related effect in drug- and poison-induced pancreatitis?**

Ethyl alcohol, organophosphorus insecticides, and intravenous lipid infusions.

○   **What percentage of patients with intraductal papillary mucinous neoplasms (IPMNs) develop acute pancreatitis?**

Acute pancreatitis occurs in up to 34% of patients with IPMNs, with branch duct IPMN being the most commonly associated with acute pancreatitis. Severe pancreatitis is uncommon but recurrent acute pancreatitis is common and should be considered in older patients.

○   **What etiologies must be considered in posttransplant patients with acute pancreatitis?**

Secondary hyperparathyroidism, hyperlipidemia, viral infections, vasculitis, and immunosuppressive therapy (particularly corticosteroids, azathioprine, and L-asparaginase). Posttransplant pancreatitis is associated with a high mortality.

○ **What infections may cause acute pancreatitis in immunocompetent hosts?**

Overall, infection-associated pancreatitis is uncommon; however, several viruses have been implicated and include mumps, coxsackie, and hepatitis A and B. Bacterial causes include *Mycoplasma*, *Salmonella*, and *Mycobacterium tuberculosis*. Intraductal parasitic infections, particularly ascaris, fasciola, and clonorchis, have also been described.

○ **What are the two most common causes of acute pancreatitis in AIDS patients?**

Drugs and infections. Drugs commonly implicated in these patients include pentamidine, trimethoprim-sulfamethoxazole, and didanosine. Cytomegalovirus accounts for the majority of infection-related cases. Other infectious agents implicated include *Cryptococcus neoformans*, *M. tuberculosis*, and herpes simplex virus. Disseminated infections with *M. avium* complex, *Toxoplasma gondii*, *Pneumocystis carinii*, *Leishmania* species, and *Candida* species may involve the pancreas but rarely cause clinical symptoms.

○ **What is the most common cause of acute pancreatitis in children?**

Trauma is the most common cause of acute pancreatitis in children, often resulting from bicycle handle bar injury and steering wheel injury (in older children). A not uncommon sequela of trauma includes pancreatic duct stricture, which may result in recurrent and chronic pancreatitis. Blunt, rather than penetrating, trauma may induce pancreatitis and usually involves compression of the body of the pancreas against the spine. In adults, this frequently results from seat belt injury and may result in a pancreatic body stricture causing acute recurrent pancreatitis.

○ **True/False: A patient with so-called "idiopathic" acute pancreatitis should undergo pancreatic duct imaging.**

True. This is done primarily to evaluate for ultrasound-negative choledocholithiasis and cholelithiasis (microlithiasis); choledochoceles; obstruction of pancreatic duct by calculi, strictures, small pseudocysts, annular pancreas, or carcinoma; ampullary tumors; sphincter of Oddi dysfunction; and (more controversial) pancreas divisum. Magnetic resonance cholangiopancreatography (MRCP) is a noninvasive imaging modality which also allows direct visualization of the pancreaticobiliary system without intrapancreatic ductal contrast medium injection and thus avoids the most frequent complication of ERCP—acute pancreatitis. Its diagnostic accuracy in centers with sufficient expertise rivals that of ERCP.

○ **What clinical prognostic scoring criteria are used to assess the severity of patients with acute pancreatitis?**

Ranson's criteria and APACHE-II grading systems are used to assess the degree of severity of patients' pancreatitis. The CT severity index (CTSI) uses CT scan features of acute pancreatitis and pancreatic necrosis to calculate severity; however, this is based on local complications and does not reflect the SIRS found in patients with acute pancreatitis. A new prognostic scoring system, the bedside index for severity in acute pancreatitis (BISAP), has been validated and is as accurate as the APACHE-II and Ranson's criteria for prognosis and uses five criteria: blood urea nitrogen (BUN), mental status, age, presence of SIRS, and presence of pleural effusions.

○ **Describe Ranson's criteria.**

Ranson's criteria, used in assessing the severity and prognosis of ethanol-associated pancreatitis, can only be applied at 48 hours after hospitalization, and this is the major drawback to its use. Fewer than three positive signs indicate mild disease with a mortality rate near zero. The mortality rate increases to 10%–20% when three to five signs are present and is >50% with six or more signs. A variant of these criteria is utilized to assess the severity of non-alcohol-related pancreatitis.

○   **Describe the APACHE-II scoring system as used for acute pancreatitis.**

The APACHE-II scoring system can be calculated at the time of hospital admission and is based on a point system depending on the patient's age, chronic illness, and a number of physiologic variables. It is, however, a cumbersome and clinically less practical system. A score of >8 suggests the presence of severe pancreatitis.

○   **True/False: The magnitude of hyperamylasemia correlates with the severity of pancreatitis.**

False. The serum amylase level typically rises 2–12 hours after onset of symptoms and slowly declines over 3–5 days. Conversely, elevations of serum lipase levels tend to rise later and persist longer. The magnitude of hyperamylasemia has no prognostic value in acute pancreatitis; levels may remain normal in up to 10% of cases of fatal pancreatitis.

○   **What are nonpancreatic sources of hyperamylasemia and hyperlipasemia?**

Diseases of the salivary glands, lungs, fallopian tubes, ovarian cysts, gallbladder, and small bowel may result in elevations of serum amylase as may tumors of the colon, lung, and ovary. Any condition associated with increased small bowel permeability (perforation, infarction, or obstruction) or renal disease resulting in diminished renal clearance of pancreatic enzymes may cause elevations in both amylase and lipase in the absence of clinical pancreatitis. Patients with chronic hepatitis C infection, diabetic ketoacidosis, and inflammatory bowel disease (IBD) may also present with increased enzymes of nonpancreatic origin. Macroamylasemia and macrolipasemia may also result in elevations of serum pancreatic enzymes.

○   **What are macroamylasemia and macrolipasemia?**

These are conditions in which amylase or lipase complexes with immunoglobulin (IgA, IgG) and/or polysaccharides. These large molecules do not undergo glomerular filtration; therefore, serum amylase/lipase levels are increased but urinary amylase levels and the amylase-creatinine clearance ratio are low. Diagnosis can be established by measuring the molecular weight of amylase and lipase, or by immunologic assays. These conditions have been associated with celiac disease, HIV, cirrhosis, rheumatoid arthritis, ulcerative colitis, monoclonal gammopathy, and non-Hodgkin's lymphoma.

○   **What pulmonary manifestations may be found in patients with acute pancreatitis?**

Approximately 10%–20% of patients with acute pancreatitis will have pleural effusions. They are usually left-sided and are exudative with high fluid amylase levels. Early arterial hypoxemia may also occur and results from right-to-left shunting due to microthrombi of the pulmonary vasculature. Finally, adult respiratory distress syndrome occurs in up to 20% of patients with severe acute pancreatitis.

○   **True/False: All acute peripancreatic fluid collections that develop in the course of acute pancreatitis should be drained.**

False. More than half of all peripancreatic fluid collections associated with acute pancreatitis will resolve spontaneously within 6 weeks. They may occur as a result of sympathetic effusion or extravasated pancreatic exocrine secretions secondary to duct rupture. Intervention may be considered when the collection persists beyond 6 weeks after the onset of pancreatitis and results in symptoms or complications resulting from mass effect or infection.

○   **True/False: All pancreatic pseudocysts developing after an episode of acute pancreatitis should undergo drainage.**

False. Pancreatic pseudocyst occurs in approximately 15% of patients after acute pancreatitis. Pseudocysts do not have a true epithelial lining but are instead surrounded by granulation tissue and collagen. Eighty-five percent are located in the body or tail and 15% in the head of the pancreas. Pseudocysts that are asymptomatic and not increasing in size should be observed. Those that are expanding in size, usually above 6 cm, and are symptomatic should be considered for drainage.

○ **True/False: A CT scan should always be obtained in a patient with acute pancreatitis.**

False. A CT scan with rapid bolus intravenous contrast should be obtained in patients with acute pancreatitis who: 1) fail to improve clinically, 2) have evidence of organ failure, or 3) are suspected of having infected pancreatic necrosis. Sterile necrosis may be distinguished from infected necrosis by needle aspiration of fluid. A CT scan should not be performed early in the course of acute pancreatitis in patients with volume depletion and/or renal impairment.

○ **What is the significance of pancreatic necrosis identified by an IV contrast-enhanced abdominal CT scan?**

The presence of pancreatic necrosis portends a more unfavorable outcome. Areas of pancreatic necrosis fail to enhance during CT scanning after rapid bolus injection of contrast material. The diagnosis of pancreatic necrosis is established when there are focal or diffuse zones of nonenhanced pancreatic parenchyma > 3 cm or involving > 30% of the pancreas. Patients with pancreatic necrosis have a 30%–50% chance of developing infection of the necrosis; the extent of the necrosis correlates with worsening prognosis. CT scan findings are generally not helpful in differentiating sterile from infected necrosis, although the presence of gas bubbles is suggestive of infected necrosis. CT-guided needle aspiration with Gram stain and culture of the aspirate allows diagnosis of suspected infected necrosis.

○ **What are the causes of early mortality in acute pancreatitis?**

The most common cause of early mortality in acute pancreatitis is SIRS, defined as body temperature < 36°C or > 38°C, heart rate > 90 beats per minute, tachypnea, leukopenia, or leukocytosis; SIRS can be complicated by acute lung injury, acute kidney injury, shock, and multiple organ failure. When acute renal failure occurs in the setting of prolonged hypovolemia and shock, acute tubular necrosis ensues and the mortality rate approaches 50%. In addition, adult respiratory distress syndrome, intraabdominal hemorrhage, and acute cholangitis can account for early mortality in acute pancreatitis.

○ **What are the causes of late mortality in acute pancreatitis?**

Septic complications, particularly infected pancreatic necrosis and abscess formation, and pneumonitis tend to occur after the first week of illness.

○ **True/False: The mortality rate of patients with pancreatitis who develop infected pancreatic necrosis is increased fourfold compared with patients with similar extent of sterile necrosis.**

True. The mortality rate is increased considerably in patients with infected necrosis (38% compared with 9% of patients with sterile necrosis). Blood cultures are neither sensitive for isolation of responsible microorganisms nor specific for site of infection. Sonographic or CT-guided percutaneous aspirates of suspected areas of necrosis are the procedures of choice when infected necrosis is suspected.

○ **What is the most common organism isolated in infected pancreatic necrosis?**

Escherichia coli is isolated in about 50% of percutaneous aspirates. Gram stain or culture of these pancreatic aspirates may identify a single microorganism or a polymicrobial infection. Other common organisms include *Enterococcus* (19%), *Staphylococcus* (18%), *Proteus* (10%), *Klebsiella* (10%), *Pseudomonas* (10%), *Streptococcus faecalis* (7%), and *Bacteroides* (6%) species. These organisms likely reach the pancreas by translocation across the colonic wall followed by local lymphatic, rather than hematogenous, spread.

○   **True/False: Patients with infected pancreatic necrosis who are stable should undergo immediate surgical drainage.**

False. Treatment with antibiotics is still the initial treatment of choice if the condition of the patient is stable, since over 75% of patients are able to avoid surgery. However, if there is no response to antibiotics, then therapeutic intervention by either percutaneous, endoscopic, laparoscopic, or open surgical approach should be pursued. The preferred surgical intervention is necrosectomy; however, it should be performed as late as possible (approximately 1 month after diagnosis of acute pancreatitis). For patients with a pancreatic abscess, drainage is recommended.

○   **True/False: The role for prophylactic antibiotics in patients with acute necrotizing pancreatitis has been conclusively defined.**

False. Indiscriminate use of antibiotics is neither advocated nor supported by the preponderance of the scientific evidence in the effort to prevent pancreatic infection.

○   **What other organ system complications outside the abdomen may be affected by acute pancreatitis?**

Polyserositis of articular synovium, pleura, or pericardium may also occur. Subcutaneous fat necrosis may cause a skin rash resembling erythema nodosum. Fat necrosis adjacent to synovium may result in arthritis revealing synovial fluid with many leukocytes and high lipase concentration. Evidence of distant fat necrosis, while clinically evident in only 1% of cases of acute pancreatitis, may be seen in up to 10% of patients on autopsy. Purtscher's retinopathy is a rare complication of acute pancreatitis and is manifested by sudden blindness due to occlusion of the posterior retinal artery with aggregated granulocytes.

○   **What are the potential causes of acute pancreatitis in patients with IBD?**

The increased incidence of acute pancreatitis in Crohn's disease can be explained on the basis of the high predisposition to cholesterol and pigment stones as a result of ileal disease, anatomic abnormalities of the duodenum (with obstructive pancreatitis), immunologic disturbances associated with IBD, and primary sclerosing cholangitis with associated biliary stones. Medications including sulfasalazine, 5-aminosalicylic acid, azathioprine, and 6-mercaptopurine, used in the treatment of Crohn's disease and ulcerative colitis, can cause acute pancreatitis.

○   **What complications of acute pancreatitis may result in acute upper gastrointestinal bleeding?**

Gastric variceal hemorrhage and hemosuccus pancreaticus. Isolated gastric varices resulting from splenic vein thrombosis may complicate acute pancreatitis, so-called left-sided portal hypertension. Splenectomy with gastric devascularization is curative. Usually, hemosuccus pancreaticus refers to bleeding in the pancreas into the pancreatic duct and then into the duodenum. It typically arises from erosion of a pseudocyst into adjacent vasculature. Selective mesenteric arteriography during active bleeding distinguishes hemosuccus pancreaticus from hemobilia, identifies the source of arterial or venous bleeding, and determines if the blood traverses a pancreatic pseudocyst or abscess prior to drainage into the pancreatic duct. Selective arterial embolization during angiography may control bleeding.

○   **What clinical findings are suggestive of intrapseudocyst hemorrhage?**

Abdominal pain associated with a sudden increase in the size of the pseudocyst, a localized bruit over the pseudocyst, and a sudden decrease in hemoglobin and hematocrit without obvious external blood loss.

○   **True/False: Pancreas divisum is associated with an increased incidence of acute recurrent pancreatitis.**

False, although controversial. Pancreas divisum is a congenital failure of fusion of the ventral and dorsal pancreatic anlagen resulting in drainage of the dorsal duct draining via the minor ampulla and the ventral duct via the major ampulla. It is the most common congenital anatomic variant (5%–10%) of the human pancreas. The majority of patients are not predisposed to develop pancreatitis; however, it is believed that the combination of pancreas divisum with a small accessory ampullary orifice may lead to pancreatitis. Clues to pancreatic divisum as a cause of pancreatitis include a dilated dorsal pancreatic duct and stones within the dorsal duct.

○ **What is the most common cause of chronic pancreatitis in adults?**

Chronic alcohol abuse accounts for 70%–80% of chronic pancreatitis. The type of alcohol and pattern of drinking have no influence on the risk of developing chronic pancreatitis. It may be influenced by genetic predisposition in the host.

○ **True/False: Alcohol consumption and cigarette smoking are independent risk factors for chronic pancreatitis.**

True.

○ **What is tropical pancreatitis?**

It is a nutritional pancreatitis seen in African and Asian countries resulting from severe protein-calorie malnutrition. It is characterized by hypoalbuminemia, marked emaciation, bilateral parotid gland enlargement, and hair and skin changes resembling kwashiorkor. The pathophysiology of this form of chronic pancreatitis is felt to be due to nutritional antioxidant deficiencies (zinc, copper, selenium). Severe chronic calcific pancreatitis with large intraductal stones may develop and diabetes typically occurs several years after the onset of abdominal pain. Nutritional repletion may lead to a return to normal pancreatic exocrine function if instituted before extensive atrophy and fibrosis of the gland occurs.

○ **What genetic factors influence the development of chronic pancreatitis?**

Hereditary pancreatitis, inherited through an autosomal dominant gene of incomplete penetrance, has been described in different areas of the world (New Zealand, United States, Ireland, France). It affects both sexes equally and typically presents as episodes of acute pancreatitis in childhood by age 10 to 12. These patients progress from episodes of acute pancreatitis to chronic pancreatitis and have an increased incidence of pancreatic carcinoma. Mutations of the cystic fibrosis transmembrane conductance regulator (CFTR) gene, the cationic trypsinogen gene (PRSS1), and pancreatic secretory trypsin inhibitor (PSTI), otherwise known as SPINK1, can lead to the development of chronic pancreatitis. Concomitant mutation of both CFTR and SPINK1 enhances the risk of pancreatitis above that of CFTR mutations alone (600-fold versus 40-fold).

○ **Which serologic marker is elevated in autoimmune pancreatitis?**

Serum IgG4 is usually elevated more than two times the upper limit of normal (>140 mg/dL). Only about 1% of patients with pancreatic cancer have a serum IgG4 above 280 mg/dL.

○ **What are the diagnostic criteria of autoimmune pancreatitis?**

The "HISORt" criteria proposed by the Mayo Clinic are commonly used, and include the presence of one or more of the following: Diagnostic histology (see below), pancreatic imaging (diffusely enlarged pancreas with featureless borders and delayed enhancement with or without a capsule-like rim; narrowed main and dorsal pancreatic duct), serology (elevated IgG4), other organ involvement (biliary strictures, parotid/lacrimal gland involvement, mediastinal lymphadenopathy, retroperitoneal fibrosis), and response to steroid treatment.

○   **What are the histologic features of autoimmune pancreatitis?**

Type 1 autoimmune pancreatitis is characterized by a lymphoplasmacytic sclerosing pancreatitis or >10 IgG4 positive cells with at least two of the following: periductal lymphoplasmacytic infiltrate, obliterative phlebitis, and acinar fibrosis. Type 2 autoimmune pancreatitis is characterized by idiopathic duct centric pancreatitis or a granulocytic epithelial lesion in the pancreatic duct with minimal IgG4 positive cells in the pancreatic parenchyma.

○   **What is the long-term prognosis of autoimmune pancreatitis?**

There is a recurrence rate of approximately 41%.

○   **True/False: The diagnosis of chronic pancreatitis may be excluded in patients without abdominal pain.**

False. Although pain is the most common presenting symptom of patients with chronic pancreatitis, it may be absent in up to 15% of patients with alcohol-related chronic pancreatitis and in up to 23% of patients with nonalcoholic chronic pancreatitis.

○   **What specialized test directly measures pancreatic exocrine function?**

In chronic pancreatitis, exocrine secretion is decreased. The secretin stimulation test measures the volume of secretion and the concentration of bicarbonate (collected via aspiration of duodenal contents) in response to injection of secretin. Bicarbonate levels <50 mEq/L are consistent with the diagnosis of chronic pancreatitis. This test is invasive, requiring duodenal tube insertion for collection of secretions, and has a reported sensitivity of approximately 80%–90%.

○   **True/False: Steatorrhea is an early symptom of chronic pancreatitis.**

False. Ninety percent of exocrine function is typically lost before steatorrhea develops. A secretin test may be abnormal when 60% of the exocrine function is lost. Patients with so-called early chronic pancreatitis can have symptoms of bloating, abdominal discomfort, abdominal pain, or change in bowel habits when 60%–90% of the pancreatic function is lost. Thus, early chronic pancreatitis can mimic a wide variety of gastrointestinal disorders.

○   **What indirect tests of pancreatic secretory function are available?**

Serum trypsinogen, fecal chymotrypsin, fecal elastase, and 72-hour quantitative fecal fat determination. They all lack sensitivity except in patients with advanced chronic pancreatitis, when patients typically have already developed steatorrhea. Furthermore, these tests do not influence management in most cases.

○   **True/False: Plain abdominal radiographs are helpful in the diagnosis of chronic pancreatitis.**

True. While plain abdominal radiographs cannot exclude the diagnosis, the presence of focal or diffuse pancreatic calcification (seen in approximately 30% of cases) makes the diagnosis of advanced chronic pancreatitis almost certain and obviates the need for additional testing.

○   **What osseous abnormalities are associated with chronic pancreatitis?**

Approximately 5% of patients with chronic pancreatitis demonstrate medullary infarcts or aseptic necrosis of the femoral or humeral head. The long bones of the hands and feet are affected most often. These abnormalities result from medullary fat necrosis during episodes of acute pancreatitis.

○   **When is ERCP useful in the diagnosis of chronic pancreatitis?**

Changes of early chronic pancreatitis may not be seen on ERCP. ERCP assesses ductular changes, such as irregularity, dilatation, tortuosity, stenosis, and ductal calculi, which occur in advanced chronic pancreatitis. ERCP is also useful in differentiating chronic pancreatitis from pancreatic cancer. Endoscopic ultrasound (EUS) is also capable of diagnosing chronic pancreatitis on the basis of both ductal and parenchymal changes and, thus, may be able to detect chronic pancreatitis earlier than ERCP.

○ **What are the most common complications of chronic pancreatitis?**

- Chronic abdominal pain, often leading to narcotic dependence, is the most common complication of chronic pancreatitis.
- Pancreatic exocrine insufficiency with steatorrhea.
- Pseudocysts occur in up to 25% of patients with chronic pancreatitis. In contrast with acute pseudocysts, chronic pseudocysts almost never resolve spontaneously. Hemorrhage into a pseudocyst with subsequent conversion into a pseudoaneurysm is potentially the most serious complication of chronic pancreatitis.

○ **What is pancreatic ascites?**

Pancreatic ascites occurs as a consequence of persistent leakage of pancreatic fluid from a pseudocyst or a disrupted pancreatic duct. Its incidence in chronic pancreatitis is less than 1%, but may occur in up to 15% of patients with pseudocysts. It may be distinguished from ascites secondary to cirrhosis by the finding of high ascitic fluid amylase levels greater than serum levels and high fluid protein or albumin levels.

○ **True/False: The presence of signs of fat-soluble vitamin deficiencies is highly suggestive of chronic pancreatitis.**

False. While the absorption of fat-soluble vitamins (A, D, E, and K) is diminished, marked deficiency is relatively uncommon. The clinical presence of easy bruisability, bone pain, and decreased night vision resulting from deficiencies of vitamins K, D, and A, respectively, is more suggestive of small intestinal disease with malabsorption.

○ **True/False: Patients with pancreatic exocrine insufficiency secondary to chronic pancreatitis are predisposed to nephrolithiasis.**

True. Patients with untreated steatorrhea have high concentrations of long-chain fatty acids in the colon, which bind intraluminal calcium and form insoluble calcium soaps. Consequently, less calcium is available to bind to and precipitate unabsorbed dietary oxalate as calcium oxalate and more oxalate is absorbed and excreted in the urine. Hyperoxaluria and oxalate stone formation may then develop.

○ **How should hyperoxaluria be treated in patients with chronic pancreatitis?**

Low dietary oxalate intake, low dietary long-chain triglycerides, pancreatic enzyme substitution, and increased intake of either calcium (3 g/day) or aluminum in the form of antacids (3.5 g/day).

○ **True/False: Patients with chronic pancreatitis may have vitamin B_{12} malabsorption.**

True. The probable mechanism is due to competitive binding of cobalamin by cobalamin-binding proteins (usually destroyed by pancreatic proteases). It is correctable with administration of pancreatic enzymes and occurs in 40% of patients with advanced chronic pancreatitis.

○ **True/False: Retinopathy may occur in patients with chronic pancreatitis.**

True. Nondiabetic peripheral retinopathy may occur due to a deficiency of vitamin A and/or zinc. Diabetic retinopathy and other microvascular complications of diabetes are less common. However, the prevalence of diabetic retinopathy and neuropathy in patients with chronic pancreatitis is comparable to that of patients with idiopathic diabetes mellitus if corrected for the duration of diabetes.

○ **What nonsurgical and surgical modalities of pain control are available in chronic pancreatitis?**

Cessation of alcohol intake, nonnarcotic analgesics, and celiac plexus block. Pancreatic enzyme supplementation should be utilized in all patients with chronic pancreatitis to correct exocrine insufficiency. Their utility in the management of pain in chronic pancreatitis remains controversial. The non-enteric-coated preparation is preferable for treatment of the pain associated with chronic pancreatitis. Correctable causes of pain such as the presence of a pseudocyst, duodenal or biliary narrowing, and pancreatic ductal stricture/stone should be sought. Surgery offers better longer-lasting pain control compared to endoscopic therapy. Lateral pancreaticojejunostomy (modified Puestow) is preferred in patients with ductal obstruction in the head of the pancreas with distal duct dilatation, whereas partial pancreatic resection should be considered in patients without ductal dilatation, so-called small-duct disease or localized distal (tail) disease.

○ **How much lipase is necessary in the form of pancreatic enzyme supplementation for treatment of steatorrhea?**

Malabsorption does not usually occur if more than 5% of normal maximal enzyme output is delivered to the duodenum. This requires 28,000 IU of lipase during a 4-hour postprandial period. Pancreatic enzymes are available in two forms: enteric and non-enteric-coated preparations. The advantage of enteric-coated compounds (eg, Creon, Zenpep, and Pancrease, as opposed to Viokase) is that they do not dissolve in the stomach and are less susceptible to acid-pepsin inactivation. Exogenous enzymes should be given with meals and with snacks. Their dose may need to be titrated upward.

● ● ● SUGGESTED READINGS ● ● ●

Segarra-Newnham M, Hough A. Antibiotic prophylaxis in acute necrotizing pancreatitis revisited. *Ann Pharmacother*. 2009;43(9): 1486-1495.

American Gastroenterological Association (AGA) Institute on "Management of Acute Pancreatits" Clinical Practice and Economics Committee; AGA Institute Governing Board. AGA Institute medical position statement on acute pancreatitis. *Gastroenterology*. 2007;132(5):2019-2021.

Banks PA, Freeman ML; Practice Parameters Committee of the American College of Gastroenterology. Practice guidelines in acute pancreatitis. *Am J Gastroenterol*. 2006;101(10):2379-2400.

Bornman PC, Botha JF, Ramos JM, et al. Guideline for the diagnosis and treatment of chronic pancreatitis. *S Afr Med J*. 2010;100 (12 Pt 2):845-860.

American Gastroenterological Association Medical Position Statement: treatment of pain in chronic pancreatitis. *Gastroenterology*. 1998 Sep;115(3):763-764.

Clain JE, Pearson RK. Evidence-based approach to idiopathic pancreatitis. *Curr Gastroenterol Rep*. 2002;4(2):128-134.

CHAPTER 39

Medical Aspects of Cholelithiasis

David S. Wolf, MD and
Atilla Ertan, MD, AGAF, MACG

○ **What is the prevalence of gallstones in the United States?**

Approximately 10%. Gallstones are two to three times more common in women than men. Pima Indians are at highest risk of developing gallstones in the United States followed by Hispanic women. A genetic influence is noted in gallstone formation. Pigment stones account for 10%–25% of all gallstones in the United States.

○ **What are the major roles of mucin in the formation of gallstones?**

Mucin acts as a pronucleating agent (promoting nucleation and crystallization of cholesterol from saturated bile) and acts as a scaffolding for crystal deposition during stone development.

○ **What is the pathogenesis of acute calculous cholecystitis?**

A stone is impacted in the cystic duct causing obstruction. The resultant bile stasis and increase in intragallbladder pressure damages the gallbladder mucosa, resulting in phospholipase A release and activating the inflammatory cascade.

○ **Seventy percent to 80% of gallbladder stones in the United States are composed of cholesterol. What is the composition of primary common bile duct (CBD) stones?**

Primary CBD stones are usually associated with ascending cholangitis proximal to biliary strictures and are softer brown pigment stones. They form from the enteric bacterial conversion of bilirubin and phospholipids.

○ **A 23-year-old man with sickle cell disease presents with abdominal pain located in the right upper quadrant (RUQ). An evaluation including abdominal ultrasonography reveals the presence of cholelithiasis. What is the most likely composition of the gallstones?**

Black pigment stones are most commonly associated with sickle cell disease, chronic hemolysis, and cirrhosis.

○ **True/False: Primary bile duct stones are black pigment stones and are identical to the black pigment stones, which arise in the gallbladder.**

False. Primary bile duct stones are brown and are different than the black pigment stones, which arise in the gallbladder.

○ **True/False: There has been a reported decrease in frequency of gallstones in obese patients on very low calorie diets with the use of cholestyramine.**

False. However, ursodeoxycholic acid (UDCA) 600 mg daily has been shown to decrease the frequency of gallstone development in this setting from 28% to 3%.

○ **True/False: Prophylactic use of cholecystokinin (CCK) octapeptide intravenously twice daily given to patients on long-term parenteral nutrition helps to prevent cholelithiasis and acalculous cholecystitis.**

True.

○ **True/False: The development of gallbladder sludge from the use of ceftriaxone usually disappears spontaneously after the discontinuation of the medication.**

True.

○ **True/False: Transabdominal ultrasonography is the test of first choice in the evaluation of jaundice and RUQ abdominal pain.**

True. The overall sensitivity of abdominal ultrasonography is 95% for stones that are larger than 2 mm in diameter. In contrast, the sensitivity is only approximately 50% for CBD stones.

○ **What factors may compromise the interpretation of transabdominal ultrasonograms?**

Transabdominal ultrasonographic examinations are somewhat subjective and operator dependent. They are compromised by obesity and interfering shadows caused by ribs, scars, and bowel gas.

○ **True/False: Abdominal computed tomography (CT) is not appropriate for the diagnosis of uncomplicated stone disease or evaluation of biliary colic because half of all gallstones are radiolucent on CT.**

True.

○ **When should percutaneous transhepatic cholangiography (PTC) be considered in the evaluation of patients with biliary tract obstruction?**

PTC may be favored in patients with more proximal biliary obstruction at the level of the hilum or higher. In addition, PTC may be favored in patients with distorted or altered gastroduodenal anatomy (eg, status post-Whipple, Billroth II Roux-en-Y gastrojejunostomy). PTC may also be efficacious in patients in whom endoscopic retrograde cholangiopancreatography (ERCP) was unsuccessful. PTC is generally successful in patients with dilated ducts and 75%–95% successful in patients with nondilated ducts in experienced hands.

○ **True/False: Erythromycin hepatotoxicity presents as a syndrome of pain, fever, and cholestatic hepatitis, which often mimics acute cholecystitis.**

True. It is important to elicit a history of antibiotic consumption during a review of symptoms. A compatible history and associated eosinophilia may assist in making the diagnosis.

○ **What percentage of gallstones is visible on plain abdominal x-ray?**

Fifty percent of pigment stones and 20% of cholesterol stones. However, 80% of gallstones are of the cholesterol type; therefore, only 25% of stones will be seen on plain radiographs.

○ **Distal ileal diseases, such as Crohn's disease, are recognized risk factors for the development of gallstones. What is the most common problem resulting in lithogenic bile in these diseases?**

The loss of specific bile salt transporters in the distal ileum results in excessive bile salt losses in the stool and leads to a diminished bile acid pool.

○ **Describe the pathophysiogical mechanism(s) resulting in gallstone formation in the following groups: the elderly, the obese, the pregnant, those receiving clofibrate, and those receiving parenteral nutrition.**

Elderly	– increased biliary cholesterol saturation
Obese	– increased 3-hydroxy-3-methyl glutaryl-CoA reductase activity
Pregnant	– increased biliary cholesterol saturation and impaired gallbladder motility
Clofibrate therapy	– decreased 7-alpha-hydroxylase activity with decreased bile salt production
Parenteral nutrition	– gallbladder stasis

○ **True/False: Management of an elderly frail patient with choledocholithiasis and severe gallstone pancreatitis differs from a young healthy patient.**

False. ERCP and sphincterotomy can be safely performed in the elderly. However, following sphincterotomy and successful stone extraction, some reports suggest that frail elderly patients can be successfully managed without a cholecystectomy.

○ **What is the rate of gallstone formation in obese patients who undergo bariatric surgery?**

Approximately 50%. Causes include an increased hepatic secretion of biliary cholesterol, increased mucin production in the gallbladder, and gallbladder hypomotility. UDCA can be used prophylactically in this group to prevent gallstone formation during their extreme weight loss.

○ **True/False: The most frequent site of maximal biliary pain is in the RUQ of the abdomen?**

False. Maximal biliary pain occurs in decreasing frequency in the following locations: epigastric, RUQ, left upper quadrant (LUQ), precordium, and lower abdomen. Radiation of pain occurs in half of patients to the scapula, right shoulder, or lower abdomen.

○ **What is biliary sludge (ie, microlithiasis)?**

Thickened gallbladder bile that may contain stones less than 3 mm in size. On ultrasound, it is seen as a mobile low amplitude signal with layering in the dependent portion of the gallbladder. Its presence is associated with idiopathic acute pancreatitis.

○ **What are the common conditions associated with the development of gallbladder sludge?**

Spinal cord injuries, prolonged parenteral nutrition, long-term fasting, and prolonged treatment with octreotide may cause gallbladder stasis-induced sludge. Ceftriaxone may also result in the formation of sludge. Gallbladder sludge may cause acute cholecystitis and acute pancreatitis.

○   **True/False: Mirizzi's syndrome is due to a severe drug reaction, which results in intrahepatic cholestasis.**

False. Mirizzi's syndrome is a rare complication of gallstones in which a stone becomes impacted in the neck of gallbladder or the cystic duct and extrinsically compresses the CBD resulting in jaundice. Preoperative diagnosis of this syndrome is important to avoid bile duct injury. This syndrome is rare, occurring in approximately 1% of all patients undergoing cholecystectomy.

○   **What are the two types of Mirizzi's syndrome?**

Type I: The hepatic duct is compressed by a large stone that has become impacted in the cystic duct or Hartmann's pouch. Associated inflammation may contribute to the stricture.

Type II: The stone has eroded into the hepatic duct producing a cholecystocholedochal fistula.

○   **A 37-year-old woman presents with a history of intermittent severe upper abdominal pain and a more recent problem of persistent abdominal distension with associated nausea and vomiting. What complication of gallstone disease is being demonstrated in the CT image below?**

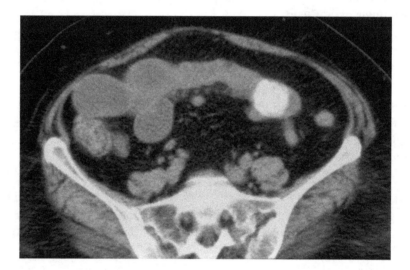

Figure 39-1

Gallstone ileus from a large gallstone obstructing the mid-ileum.

○   **What is the most common location of a bowel obstruction in patients with gallstone ileus?**

Characteristically, the obstruction occurs in the terminal ileum where the lumen is the narrowest. The majority of patients with gallstone ileus are women and older than 70 years. Recurrent gallstone ileus may occur in approximately 5% of patients and a search should be made for an additional stone(s) during surgery.

○   **What are the x-ray findings in gallstone ileus?**

An intestinal gas pattern compatible with intestinal obstruction in most patients, pneumobilia in half of all patients, and a visible aberrant gallstone in a minority.

○   **What is the size of the gallstone that causes gallstone ileus?**

Usually >2.5 cm in diameter.

○ **How does gallstone ileus present?**

Gallstone ileus should always be considered in an older patient with intestinal obstruction. It sometimes has a prior history of acute cholecystitis, but most of the stones erode slowly through the gallbladder and the symptoms may be minimal, especially in the elderly.

○ **What are the characteristics of small bowel obstruction in gallstone ileus?**

As the gallstone progresses down the length of the gut, it intermittently obstructs the lumen. Characteristically, complete obstruction occurs in the ileum, where the lumen is the narrowest.

○ **True/False: Bouveret's syndrome refers to terminal ileal obstruction due to a gallstone.**

False. Gastric outlet obstruction as a result of gallstone (Bouveret's syndrome) is a rare but serious complication of cholelithiasis.

○ **A 56-year-old man presents for evaluation of jaundice. He had been well until 3 weeks ago when he noticed the onset of mild mid-epigastric pain, which resolved spontaneously. His past medical and surgical histories were unremarkable. He reported an 8-pound weight loss, which he blamed on a lack of appetite. Examination was notable only for jaundice and icteric conjunctivae. Laboratory tests revealed a total bilirubin of 8.6 mg/dL and an alkaline phosphatase of 565 IU/L. Aminotransferases were only slightly elevated. Amylase and lipase were normal. An abdominal ultrasound demonstrated a dilated extrahepatic bile duct. What is the next most appropriate test?**

ERCP.

○ **In the previous case, an ERCP was done with the finding below. What would you do next?**

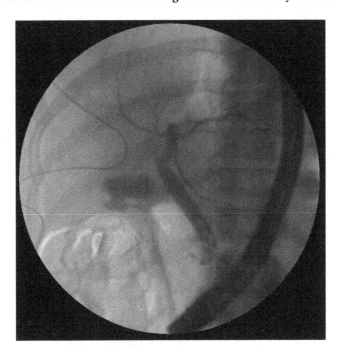

Figure 39-2

Endoscopic sphincterotomy with stone extraction.

○ A 42-year-old man with no previous health problems presented to the hospital with a 2-day history of severe intermittent epigastric pain radiating to his back with associated nausea and vomiting. He denied alcohol abuse, prior pancreatitis, or gallstones. He had lost about 35 pounds over the last 4 months and attributed the weight loss to intentional dieting and exercise. On examination, he was febrile, jaundiced, and tender to palpation over the epigastrium. Laboratory testing revealed a leukocyte count of 19,000 with a left shift, alkaline phosphatase of 650 IU/L, bilirubin of 4.8 mg/dL, and amylase of 2500 IU/L. An abdominal ultrasound showed some "sludge" in the gallbladder but was otherwise normal. What is the most appropriate therapy for this patient?

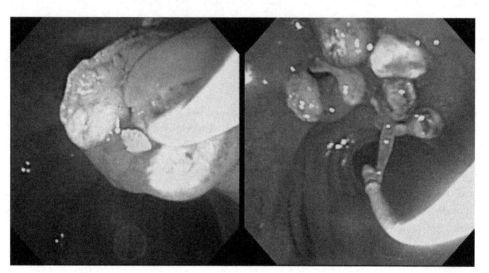

Figure 39-3 See also color plate.

Early administration of intravenous (IV) antibiotics, IV fluids, and other supportive intensive care measures are important. Endoscopic retrograde cholangiography (ERC) with sphincterotomy and stone extraction (see Figure 39-3) are also indicated in the setting of acute gallstone-related cholangitis and severe pancreatitis.

○ **What is the approach to a patient with acute bacterial cholangitis due to an obstructed bile duct?**

Initial therapy should include blood cultures with empiric use of intravenous antibiotics. About 85%–90% of patients have a response to initial antibiotic and supportive therapy before biliary interventions. Biliary drainage is mandatory. Its urgency is dictated by the response to antibiotics and supportive care. ERCP with stent, nasobiliary drain or sphincterotomy, and duct drainage is associated with significantly lower morbidity and mortality compared to surgery. If endoscopic approaches fail, then surgical or percutaneous approaches should be tried.

○ **True/False: Prophylactic cholecystectomy is recommended in the management of asymptomatic cholelithiasis.**

False. Since almost all patients with cholelithiasis develop symptoms before they develop complications, there is no evidence to support prophylactic treatment in the management of asymptomatic gallstones. Two-thirds of patients with gallstones are asymptomatic.

○ **What is the rate of development of biliary pain per year in patients with previously asymptomatic gallstones?**

Two percent per year for 5 years in one study from Michigan. A recent Italian study reported rates of 12%, 17%, and 20% at 2, 4, and 10 years, respectively. Therefore, prophylactic cholecystectomy is not indicated in an otherwise healthy person with asymptomatic gallstones. In contrast, patients with symptomatic gallstone disease have a 50% risk per year to re-experience biliary colic, and their annual rate to develop biliary complications is 1%–2%.

○ **True/False: Charcot's triad occurs in over 90% of patients with acute ascending cholangitis.**

False. The triad of fever, RUQ abdominal pain, and jaundice occurs in 50%–75% of patients with acute cholangitis. The added presence of confusion and hypotension (Reynold's pentad) is suggestive of acute suppurative cholangitis and is associated with a higher morbidity and mortality.

○ **What are the advantages and disadvantages of nasobiliary drainage?**

Advantages include the ability to repeat cholangiography and to remove it without the need of a second ERCP. The risk of infection when improperly cared for, poor patient acceptance and discomfort, and potential for electrolyte disturbances from external drainage of bile have been cited as disadvantages of this approach.

○ **What is the sump syndrome?**

The sump syndrome is a complication of choledochoduodenostomy in which food debris accumulates in the bypassed segment of the native biliary tree. Recurrent episodes of pain or cholangitis may occur. These episodes may effectively be treated by endoscopic sphincterotomy of the native ampulla with removal of the debris.

○ **Name three possible mechanisms of benign obstruction at the level of the ampulla.**

Inflammation, fibrosis, or muscular hypertonicity.

○ **True/False: Biliary obstruction due to duodenal diverticula is a common occurrence.**

False. One should be wary of attributing biliary obstruction to a duodenal diverticulum. It is much more likely that the diverticulum is an innocent bystander and that the jaundice is due to a more common cause, particularly gallstones.

○ **What is the role of percutaneous cholecystolithotomy?**

This technique is being increasingly used in elderly and high-risk patients unsuitable for laparoscopic cholecystectomy. It may be successful in achieving stone clearance but is associated with a high incidence of recurrent stone formation.

○ **Some patients undergoing laparoscopic cholecystectomy may have CBD stones that may not be suspected at the time of the procedure. What is the natural history of these unsuspected CBD stones?**

Unsuspected CBD stones are detected in 1.2%–14% of patients undergoing cholecystectomy. A number of reports have documented the spontaneous passage of CBD stones into the duodenum. Only 0.5%–0.8% of patients undergoing laparoscopic cholecystectomy will subsequently return with problems due to unsuspected CBD stones. These patients can easily be managed by ERC with sphincterotomy and stone extraction.

○ **True/False: ERC should be performed routinely prior to laparoscopic cholecystectomy.**

False. When comparing the low yield of detecting anatomic variants (3%) and clinically unsuspected stones (3.9%) versus a generally accepted 3%–7% complication rate of ERC, the routine use of ERC prior to laparoscopic cholecystectomy is unwarranted.

○ **In what situations should preoperative ERC be considered prior to cholecystectomy?**

ERC should be considered preoperatively in patients with severe gallstone pancreatitis or acute cholangitis, in those with a high probability of having CBD stones or when there is a significant possibility of other pathology.

○ **What factors predict the presence of CBD stones?**

Four independent predictors of CBD stones are: 1) Age greater than 55 years, 2) elevated bilirubin over 1.7 mg/dL, 3) dilated CBD (>6 mm) on ultrasonography, and 4) suspected or detected CBD stone on ultrasonography.

○ **What is the probability of finding CBD stones using this four-predictor model?**

When tested prospectively in patients suspected of having CBD stones, this model demonstrated that CBD stones were present in only 8% with none of the four predictors compared to 66% with two or more.

○ **As independent parameters, which of these predictors has the highest positive predictive value?**

As independent parameters, increased bile duct diameter and presence of stones on ultrasonography had the highest positive predictive value for detecting a CBD stone (64% and 78%, respectively).

○ **What is the best approach to take in patients with severe gallstone pancreatitis?**

ERCP with sphincterotomy is the therapy of choice in this situation, especially in the presence of cholangitis. Early cholecystectomy with CBD exploration is associated with high morbidity and mortality rates and is not the best initial approach in this setting.

○ **What is a characteristic radiographic finding seen with a cholecystoenteric fistula?**

Air in the biliary tree (pneumobilia), small bowel obstructive pattern (gallstone ileus), or a stone may be seen in the right lower quadrant. This fistula occurs when a large gallstone erodes through the gallbladder into the adjacent bowel.

○ **In what clinical settings should you order cholescintigraphy (hepatobiliary scintigraphy)?**

Suspected acute cholecystitis and the evaluation of suspected postcholecystectomy bile leak.

○ **What are the common clinical presentations of gallstone disease during pregnancy?**

Worsening biliary colic and acute cholecystitis are the most common clinical presentations. Jaundice and acute pancreatitis as a result of choledocholithiasis are rare.

○ **True/False: Cholelithiasis is caused in pregnant women primarily by mechanical blockage of the gallbladder.**

False. Pregnancy decreases gallbladder motility. Estrogens cause bile to supersaturate and become lithogenic due to increase in cholesterol in bile. Progesterone decreases bile acid secretion also causing supersaturated bile. More hydrophobic bile acids are produced, which reduces the capacity to solubilize cholesterol.

○ **Which imaging study demonstrated in Figure 39-4 is comparable to ERCP for detecting choledocholithiasis?**

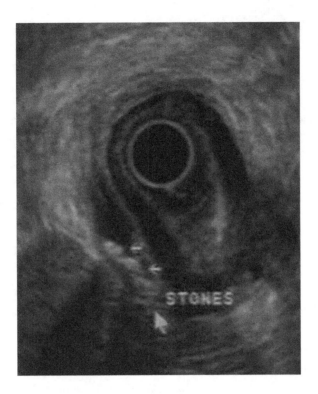

Figure 39-4

Endoscopic ultrasound (EUS) has a positive predictive value of 99%, a negative predictive value of 98%, and accuracy rate of 97% for detecting choledocholithiasis compared to ERC. Magnetic resonance cholangiopancreatography (MRCP) shown in the Figures 39-5A and B is the next best test with sensitivity and specificity of 93% and 94%, respectively.

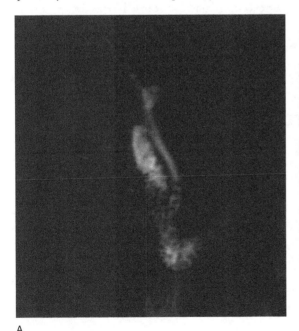

A

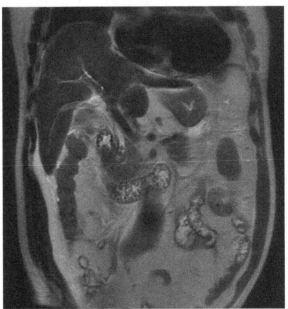

B

Figure 39-5A, B

○ **True/False: Pregnant patients with gallbladder sludge diagnosed during pregnancy have a very high risk of gallstone formation.**

False. The prevalence of sludge in pregnant women ranges from 5% to 35%. Postpartum, approximately 60% of patients will have resolution of gallbladder sludge.

○ **True/False: In the elderly, biliary symptoms usually precede the development of acute cholecystitis.**

False. However, in general, most patients with acute cholecystitis have had previous attacks of biliary colic.

○ **True/False: Gallstones are more common in diabetics.**

False. However, diabetics have a higher incidence of related complications compared to the nondiabetic population.

○ **What percentage of patients with acute calculous cholecystitis has associated choledocholithiasis?**

Choledocholithiasis is present in 5%–20% of patients with gallstone disease.

○ **What percentage of patients has concomitant gallstones in the gallbladder and the CBD?**

15%.

○ **Name two anatomic variants leading to the development of CBD stones.**

Juxtapapillary diverticulum and entry of the long cystic duct to the distal CBD.

○ **What is the recurrence rate of gallstones in patients treated with ursodeoxycholic acid?**

Recurrence is common; approximately 50% recur within a 5-year period. Patients should be monitored for gallstone recurrence by performing ultrasonography every 6 months for the first year. If all stones disappear, the treatment should be continued for 1–3 months. For recurrences, a second course may be effective.

○ **What is the most common cause of ampullary obstruction?**

Stones in the CBD.

• • • SUGGESTED READINGS • • •

van Santvoort HC, Bakker OJ, Besselink MG, et al; Dutch Pancreatitis Study Group. Prediction of common bile duct stones in the earliest stages of acute biliary pancreatitis. *Endoscopy.* 2011;43(1):8-13.

Venneman NG, van Erpecum KJ. Pathogenesis of gallstones. *Gastroenterol Clin North Am.* 2010;39(2):171-183.

Festi D, Reggiani ML, Attili AF, et al. Natural history of gallstone disease: Expectant management or active treatment? Results from a population-based cohort study. *J Gastroenterol Hepatol.* 2010;25(4):719-724.

CHAPTER 40

Surgical Aspects of Cholelithiasis

Ibraheem Mizyed, MD and
Eugene A. Trowers, MD, MPH, FACP

○ **In the era of laparoscopic cholecystectomy, what are the indications for conventional open cholecystectomy?**

Open cholecystectomy should be reserved for patients with suspected cancer of the gallbladder, cases of severe acute or chronic inflammation, liver cirrhosis with portal hypertension, severe upper abdominal adhesions following previous surgery, and in patients with biliary disease.

○ **True/False: The presence of acute cholecystitis is an absolute contraindication to laparoscopic cholecystectomy.**

False.

○ **What are absolute contraindications to laparoscopic cholecystectomy?**

Inability to tolerate general anesthesia, uncontrolled coagulopathy, suspected cancer of the gallbladder, liver cirrhosis with portal hypertension, and cholecystoenteric fistulas.

○ **What are some relative contraindications to laparoscopic cholecystectomy?**

Morbid obesity, cardiopulmonary diseases, Mirizzi's syndrome, empyema of the gallbladder, a contracted gallbladder, pregnancy, and severe acute or chronic inflammation of the gallbladder.

○ **True/False: Cholecystectomy is a reasonable consideration during weight loss operations, even without existing stones, because the subsequent development of stones can be anticipated.**

True.

○ **To which patients with asymptomatic gallstones would you recommend prophylactic cholecystectomy?**

Patients awaiting lung transplantation, patients with porcelain gallbladder, and young women of American Indian ancestry. The latter two conditions are associated with a high prevalence of gallbladder carcinoma. The risk of malignancy in calcified gallbladders exceeds 25%.

○ **True/False: Prophylactic cholecystectomy is justified in diabetics.**

False. Diabetics seem to be prone to developing both gallstones and gallstone-related complications. It has been suggested that diabetics have a high morbidity and mortality when undergoing emergency operations for gallstones. However, these perceptions have not been borne out when confounding variables such as hyperlipidemia, obesity, cardiovascular disease, and renal insufficiency are taken into account.

○ **True/False: Prophylactic cholecystectomy should be entertained for patients with asymptomatic stones prior to extended travel to remote areas.**

True. Remote areas may not have the capacity to perform a cholecystectomy if needed.

○ **True/False: Elective cholecystectomy should be considered in a patient with an 8-mm gallbladder polyp and concomitant gallstones.**

True. Polyps < 10 mm in absence of symptoms generally do not require surgery; however, a gallbladder polyp with a stone should be considered for elective cholecystectomy.

○ **True/False: Pregnancy is a contraindication to laparoscopic cholecystectomy.**

False. Improvements in anesthesia and tocolytic agents have made cholecystectomy safer during pregnancy. Complications such as spontaneous abortion and preterm labor are more common in operated women in the first and third trimesters of gestation, respectively. Laparoscopic cholecystectomy can be performed safely in a carefully controlled clinical setting.

○ **Hepatic cirrhosis is a major risk factor of morbidity and mortality in patients undergoing elective cholecystectomy. What are the major perioperative causes of death associated with this condition?**

The two major causes of death associated with this condition are intra-operative bleeding and postoperative hepatic failure.

○ **What conditions justify cholecystectomy in cirrhotics?**

Symptoms are severe and/or the cirrhosis is well compensated.

○ **What is the most common cause of death after cholecystectomy?**

Most deaths occurring after cholecystectomy are related to cardiac disease, particularly myocardial infarction.

○ **What are the complications of laparoscopic cholecystectomy performed for acute cholecystitis?**

The main intra-operative complications are perforation of the gallbladder, bleeding from the liver bed or cystic artery, bile duct leaks, and iatrogenic injuries to the bowel or vessels due to unclear anatomy. The main postoperative complications are local wound hematoma or infection and systemic hematoma.

○ **In a patient who has gallstone pancreatitis, when should cholecystectomy generally be performed?**

Cholecystectomy should generally be performed during the same hospitalization once the clinical signs of pancreatitis have resolved.

○ **What should be done if small, unsuspected stones are visualized in the common bile duct (CBD) during intra-operative cholangiography?**

Nothing. It is believed that most small stones will pass spontaneously without symptoms or complications. It is estimated that only 10% of small, unsuspected stones will become symptomatic. If they become symptomatic, endoscopic retrograde cholangiography (ERC) and endoscopic sphincterotomy with stone extraction can be performed.

○ **True/False: An endoscopic approach is most useful to treat bile leaks following cholecystectomy.**

True. A 90%–100% success rate is reported in treating biliary leaks with endoscopic management. Sphincterotomy alone, stent/nasobiliary catheter placement, or the combination of sphincterotomy and stent placement has been used successfully to reduce the intrabiliary pressure and allow fistula healing.

○ **True/False: The finding of a localized fluid collection or ascites in a patient who has recently undergone a laparoscopic cholecystectomy requires immediate surgical intervention.**

False. Postoperative ascites and edema of the gallbladder fossa on CT scan or ultrasonography is a normal postoperative change and has been reported in 19% and 22% of patients, respectively.

○ **What noninvasive test is most useful in detecting postcholecystectomy bile leaks?**

Hepatobiliary scintigraphy is highly sensitive and specific.

○ **What confirmatory test(s) should be performed if a bile leak is found on scintigraphy?**

Cholangiography, via an endoscopic or percutaneous approach, will usually confirm the presence of a leak, detect coexistent biliary strictures or retained stones, and allow for the appropriate therapeutic procedure.

○ **True/False: A CT scan can differentiate between the various types of fluid collections after cholecystectomy.**

False. CT scans have limited ability to differentiate bile from blood, ascites, pus, or lymph.

○ **What should be the first-line of investigation in a patient who presents early after laparoscopic cholecystectomy with jaundice?**

ERC.

○ **What is the best approach to take in a patient who has a postcholecystectomy bile duct injury and presents with biliary peritonitis?**

This is usually caused by infected bile. External percutaneous drainage is the best initial approach. Definitive repair of the lesion can be done after the infection has been treated.

○ **If at laparoscopy, one unexpectedly encounters an acutely inflamed pus-filled gallbladder with multiple adhesions such that the anatomy around the porta hepatis is obscured and cholecystectomy is deemed unsafe, what therapeutic laparoscopic procedure could be done?**

The fundus of the gallbladder is exposed, a trocar is inserted into the gallbladder, and the contents are aspirated. A drainage catheter can then be inserted into the gallbladder and the operation concluded.

○ **What are sites of bile duct leaks after cholecystectomy?**

Bile leaks can occur from the damaged main duct, the cystic duct remnant (most common), a gallbladder leak due to trauma to a duct during dissection of the gallbladder from the liver, clipping of the right hepatic duct proximally leaving the hepatic end free to drain, and damage to the duct of Luschka.

○ **Name three patterns of presentation in bile duct injury.**

Complete occlusion of the bile duct with rapid development of jaundice in the postoperative period; bile peritonitis; and partial duct obstruction with intermittent episodes of pain, jaundice, or cholangitis usually within 2 years of the cholecystectomy.

○ **What is the classification of bile duct injuries?**

Type A: Injuries to minor ducts without loss of continuity of biliary tree.

Type B: Injuries to aberrant right hepatic bile duct with duct occlusion.

Type C: Injuries to aberrant right hepatic bile duct with transection.

Type D: Lateral injuries that involve the main ducts and can progress to Type E injuries.

Type E: Injuries to the main duct with complete obstruction.

○ **In a patient with a bile duct injury following cholecystectomy, what is the procedure of choice if the distal CBD is found to be occluded by endoscopic retrograde cholangiopancreatography (ERCP)?**

If the distal duct is found to be occluded or transected and continuity to the proximal duct is lost, percutaneous transhepatic cholangiography (PTC) is necessary to outline the proximal ducts and to provide external biliary drainage. Surgery will eventually be necessary.

○ **What are the typical presenting symptoms in a patient with a Type A bile duct injury?**

Sixty-six percent of these patients present with a symptom complex of pain and fever. In about 33% of these cases, the presentation is that of an external bile fistula. Patients with Type A injuries are almost never jaundiced.

○ **What is the optimal approach to take in patients who present in the early postcholecystectomy period with abdominal distension suspicious of a bile leak?**

A CT scan or ultrasonography of the abdomen is used to search for intraperitoneal fluid. If a bile collection is present, it may be drained percutaneously. Biliary scintigraphy is then done to determine if a leak persists followed by therapeutic ERC if a leak is found.

○ **What is the treatment of choice for Type E injuries?**

Roux-en-Y hepaticojejunostomy.

○ **In a patient with a recent bile duct injury, what is the role of abdominal ultrasound?**

Abdominal ultrasonography may demonstrate dilated intra/extrahepatic ducts, fluid collections, or abscesses in the perihepatic region. It may also be helpful in suggesting changes of cirrhosis, splenomegaly, and portal hypertension, which are particularly important considerations in planning an intervention in any such patient.

○ **What are the situations in which the bile duct size is normal in a patient with bile duct injury?**

Presence of a biliary fistula, long-standing partial obstruction with biliary fibrosis, and cirrhosis.

○   **What is the most important cause of bile duct injury during laparoscopic cholecystectomy?**

The most important cause of bile duct injury during laparoscopic cholecystectomy is aberrant biliary anatomy found in about 3% of patients.

○   **In some patients, bile duct injury with stricture formation may appear several months after laparoscopic cholecystectomy. What is the management at this time?**

Prompt endoscopic dilatation and stenting of such strictures may lead to resolution without the need for surgical intervention.

○   **What is the significance of cholecystohepatic ducts?**

Cholecystohepatic ducts (ducts of Luschka), present in 3%–5% of cadavers, may be transected during laparoscopic cholecystectomy and are another source of biliary leakage.

○   **What factors prevent spontaneous closure of postoperative bile leaks?**

Most postoperative bile leaks heal spontaneously. The presence of distal biliary obstruction secondary to a stone or stricture contributes to the formation of leaks and bilomas and prevents spontaneous closure.

○   **Patients may have a variety of postoperative symptoms following cholecystectomy. In what group is investigation most likely to reveal a cause?**

Common postoperative symptoms include flatulence, bloating, and right upper quadrant and epigastric pain. A small percentage present with severe abdominal pain, jaundice, or emesis. Investigation in the latter group is more likely to reveal a distinct treatable cause.

○   **What happens when the gallbladder perforates into the adjacent intestine during an acute attack of cholecystitis?**

The acute attack often subsides as the inflamed organ is decompressed. If the gallstones are completely discharged and are small enough to pass rectally, an uncomplicated cholecystoenteric fistula results. However, if stones are still present in the gallbladder or CBD, chronic symptoms may arise.

○   **What are the most common sites of cholecystoenteric fistula?**

In descending order of frequency, the duodenum, hepatic flexure of the colon, stomach, and jejunum.

○   **What investigations are useful for diagnosing cholecystoenteric fistula?**

Plain abdominal x-rays may show air in the biliary tree. Barium studies often reveal the site of communication. The gallbladder does not opacify on oral cholecystography. Ultrasonography of the gallbladder can detect air in the biliary tree but not the site of the fistula. CT scans are less useful in detecting gallstones and fistulae, although they may show air in the biliary tree.

○   **What problems can be caused by a cystic duct remnant in a patient who has undergone cholecystectomy?**

In some patients, the cause of postcholecystectomy symptoms has been attributed to pathology in the cystic duct remnant. The described abnormalities include cystic duct stones, fistulae, granulomas, or neuromas. ERC is useful in delineating biliary anatomy in patients with suspected cystic duct remnant pathology. Treatment is cystic duct excision.

○   **What is the false positive rate of detecting CBD stones with intraoperative cholangiogram?**

3%–4%.

○   **What tests should be performed in a patient with postcholecystectomy symptoms?**

CBD stones are the most common cause of postcholecystectomy symptoms. Liver function tests, particularly alkaline phosphatase, may be elevated. Ultrasonography may reveal indirect signs, such as a dilated bile duct, but direct visualization of the stone is uncommon. ERC is an important diagnostic tool with which to confirm the presence of ductal stones and exclude the presence of bile duct stricture or tumor.

○   **What other biliary cause of postcholecystectomy symptoms should be considered when CBD stones and cystic duct pathology have been excluded?**

Sphincter of Oddi dysfunction, including papillary stenosis.

○   **What is the differential diagnoses of cholangitis in a patient with a history of cholecystectomy?**

Bile duct stricture and choledocholithiasis.

○   **When is surgery recommended for benign biliary strictures?**

Complete ductal transection, failed previous repair, and failure of endoscopic therapy.

○   **True/False: It is possible to differentiate between choledocholithiasis and bile duct stricture on the basis of symptoms.**

False.

○   **What radiologic evaluations should be considered in a patient with a suspected bile duct stricture?**

The evaluation should begin with ultrasonography to identify dilated ducts and/or a subhepatic fluid collection. In the early postoperative period, a ^{99m}Tc-labeled radionuclide scan may expeditiously and noninvasively demonstrate patency of the biliary tree and exclude bile leak. If these studies suggest bile duct injury, ERC is indicated to define and possibly treat the lesion.

○   **If laparoscopic bile duct injury is suspected, what is the earliest time when an ERCP can be done?**

If a biliary fistula is suspected immediately following laparoscopic cholecystectomy, diagnostic and therapeutic ERC can be performed as little as 6 hours postoperatively.

○   **How is an intrahepatic bile leak treated?**

These can be treated with biliary stents positioned below the leak.

○   **What are potential consequences of stricture development following injury to the bile duct due to laparoscopic cholecystectomy?**

Cholangitis, biliary cirrhosis, and eventual need for liver transplantation.

○   **What options are available for removal of CBD stones if preoperative ERC fails?**

If the stones are small and the laparoscopic surgeon is skilled in laparoscopic bile duct exploration, an attempt at this treatment procedure is made. If it is not successful or large stones are found, an open bile duct exploration is the treatment of choice.

○   **In cases of laparoscopic bile duct injuries, what factor is associated with the best long-term results?**

Immediate identification with immediate repair is associated with the best long-term results. Unfortunately, in one recent study, only 10% of ductal injuries were discovered and operated on in the first week. The vast majority (70%) were diagnosed within the first 6 months.

○   **What is the best initial approach to take in patients with bile duct injuries and biliary peritonitis?**

Biliary peritonitis is usually caused by infected bile. Percutaneous drainage is the best initial strategy. Definitive repair of the lesion can be done when the infection is treated.

○   **In a patient with a recurrent bile duct stricture in whom a repeat attempt at operative bypass has failed or seems unwise, what option is available?**

Consideration may be given to balloon dilation or possibly placement of metal stent across the stricture.

○   **How long should a stent remain in place in a patient with a biliary fistula and concomitant stricture?**

Biliary fistulas associated with bile duct strictures will require long-term stenting, preferably with large bore stents (10- or 11.5-French stents). These patients will need one or two 10-French stents placed with interval changes every 3 months for a mean of 10 months.

○   **If a patient has an external biliary fistula, what test should be done first?**

Fistulogram.

○   **In what situation is the best result achieved when stenting a biliary stricture?**

If the stenotic segment is short (< 1 cm) or if the stenosis is partial.

○   **What is the usual closure time of biliary leaks in the absence of stricture?**

The majority of biliary leaks (not associated with stricture) close within 7–10 days after ablation of the biliary sphincter or stent placement.

○   **True/False: Surgery is indicated for patients with chronic pancreatitis and associated biliary strictures, which produce chronic cholestasis.**

True. Surgery is indicated whenever a biliary stricture has produced chronic cholestasis or its complications. Persistent elevation of alkaline phosphastase levels, even with normal bilirubin levels, is a sufficient indication for surgery. If cholestasis is not relieved in this situation, secondary biliary cirrhosis may result.

○   **List three outcomes of gallbladder perforation.**

Localized perforation is most common and leads to a pericholecystic abscess. Next is free peritonitis followed by cholecystoduodenal or cholecystoenteric fistulae.

○   **When is cholecystectomy indicated for patients who fail gallstone dissolution with ursodeoxycholic acid?**

Cholecystectomy is recommended after the second failure.

○ **Name the four most common sites of trauma to the extrahepatic bile ducts.**

1. CBD (58.3%)

2. Common hepatic duct (23.6%)

3. Right hepatic duct (5.5%)

4. Left hepatic duct (2.8%)

○ **Name the most common presentation and treatment approach for complete blowout rupture of the fundus of the gallbladder.**

Progressive early bile ascites requires early laparotomy, whereas laparotomy can be delayed for an early seal of the perforation with delayed rupture.

○ **Name the most common presentation and treatment approach for avulsion of the gallbladder from the hepatic fossa.**

This usually results in hemoperitoneum requiring an early laparotomy.

○ **Name the most common presentation and treatment approach for contusion or incomplete blowout of the gallbladder.**

In general, minimal early symptoms occur. Late rupture of an ischemia-weakened fundus should be treated by laparotomy.

● ● ● **SUGGESTED READINGS** ● ● ●

Kianicka B, Díte P, Piskac P, Korbicka J, Vlcek P, Zák J. Endoscopic approach in diagnosis and treatment of biliary complications after laparoscopic cholecystectomy. *Hepatogastroenterology*. 2011;58(106):275-280.

Kortram K, de Vries Reilingh TS, Wiezer MJ, van Ramshorst B, Boerma D. Percutaneous drainage for acute calculous cholecystitis. *Surg Endosc*. 2011;25(11):2642-2646.

Cantù P, Tenca A, Caparello C, et al. Role of symptoms, trend of liver tests, and endotherapy in management of post-cholecystectomy biliary leak. *Dig Dis Sci*. 2011;56(5):1565-1571.

Connor S, Garden OJ. Bile duct injury in the era of laparoscopic cholecystectomy. *Br J Surg*. 2006;93(2):158-168.

Section VII   NUTRITION

CHAPTER 41 Maldigestion and Malabsorption

Parakkal Deepak, MD and
Eli D. Ehrenpreis, MD

○ **What are the common signs and symptoms of malabsorptive disorders?**

Patients usually describe diarrhea (typically large volume) and weight loss. Other symptoms may include fatigue due to anemia, gas-related symptoms like bloating and flatulence, bruising from vitamin K deficiency, skin rash from deficiencies of vitamin A, K, niacin, pyridoxine and vitamin C, muscle wasting, and paresthesias.

○ **What are the sites of carbohydrate digestion?**

Intestinal lumen (salivary and pancreatic amylase) and brush border of the enterocyte (sucrose-isomaltase, lactase, maltase (glucoamylase), trehalase, and α-limit dextrinase).

○ **What enzymes are involved in fat digestion?**

Acid lipases (lingual lipase, gastric lipase) and the pancreatic lipases. Pancreatic carboxyl ester lipase hydrolyzes triglycerides, cholesterol, vitamin esters, and other substrates. Pancreatic phospholipase A2 hydrolyzes phosphatidylcholine, phosphatidylethanolamine, phosphatidylserine, and cardiolipin.

○ **How is steatorrhea defined?**

The measurement of fat in the stools collected for 72 hours in a subject ingesting a diet adequate in fat intake (100 g/day) is required to diagnose steatorrhea. Steatorrhea is defined as a daily fecal fat output >7 g/day (7% of dietary fat intake). However, diarrhea with increased fecal output can cause secondary fat malabsorption with levels up to 14 g fecal fat/day considered as the upper limit of normal in chronic diarrhea.

○ **At what sites does protein digestion take place?**

Lumen of the stomach and small intestine (pepsin, pancreatic proteases), brush border of the enterocyte (peptidases), and cytoplasm of the enterocyte (peptidases).

○   **What tests are useful for determining enteric protein loss?**

A 24-hour stool collection for determination of chromium[51]-albumin clearance is considered the gold standard but is mainly reserved for research use. The most widely available test used clinically is measurement of the clearance of α_1-antitrypsin (AT) from the plasma during a 24-hour stool collection.

Formula: α_1-AT plasma clearance = (daily stool volume × stool α_1-AT)/serum α_1-AT. α_1-AT clearance in excess of 24 mL/day in patients without diarrhea and exceeding 56 mL/day in patients with diarrhea is considered abnormal.

○   **What clinical tests are available to test exocrine pancreatic function?**

The invasive pancreatic function tests require duodenal intubation and measurement of pancreatic enzyme secretion, volume, and bicarbonate output after pancreatic stimulation (secretin test, cholecystokinin test, and Lundh [liquid test meal]). These tests are uncomfortable, time consuming, and not widely available. "Tubeless" tests are noninvasive and include measurement of fecal chymotrypsin or elastase concentration, the fluorescein dilaurate test, the N-benzoyl-L-tyrosyl-para-aminobenzoic acid (also known as bentiromide) test, and the Stage III Schilling test. The latter three tests are either not available for use in the United States or of historical interest only.

○   **How is the stool pH a useful test in suspected malabsoprtion?**

A pH of less than 5.6 in the stool of a patient with diarrhea serves as a qualitative indicator of carbohydrate malabsorption.

○   **Name some causes of lactase deficiency.**

Acquired deficiency in adulthood, small intestinal disease or resection, and autosomal recessive congenital deficiency.

○   **What is the role of genetic testing in lactose intolerance?**

In Caucasians, a single-nucleotide polymorphism (SNP) −13910 T/C upstream of the gene coding for the enzyme lactase-phlorizin hydrolase (*LPH* gene) has been found to be involved in the regulation of LPH. The CC genotype of the SNP −13910 T/C upstream of the *LPH* gene is associated with adult-type hypolactasia. The sensitivity and specificity are 93% and 100%, respectively, which is comparable to the accuracy of both the lactose tolerance test and breath hydrogen test. However, the test is expensive and may not be useful for patients of African origin.

○   **How are breath tests for lactose intolerance performed?**

Lactose malabsorption is diagnosed if an increase in breath hydrogen concentration of greater than 20 parts per million (ppm) over baseline occurs after ingestion of 25 g of lactose. Exhaled breath measurements are performed every 30 minute after ingestion for up to 4 hours. Up to 20% of patients are hydrogen nonexcretors; a lactose tolerance test needs to be carried out in this group unless the breath is simultaneously monitored for methane.

○   **How is the lactose tolerance test performed?**

This test involves oral administration of a 50-g test dose in adults (or 2 g/kg in children), followed by blood glucose levels drawn at 0, 60, and 120 minutes. An increase in blood glucose of less than 20 mg/dL (1.1 mmol/L) and the development of symptoms such as abdominal pain, bloating, flatulence, diarrhea, and/or vomiting are diagnostic of lactose malabsorption/intolerance.

○   **What clinical features suggest a functional cause in chronic diarrhea?**

Duration of symptoms greater than 1 year, lack of significant weight loss or nutritional deficiencies, absence of nocturnal diarrhea, and normal laboratory testing.

○ **Name some diseases associated with chronic diarrhea that may be diagnosed by small intestinal biopsy and the characteristic findings on histology.**

- **Diffuse alteration of small bowel mucosa:**
  - o Abetalipoproteinemia (lipid accumulation and vacuolization of enterocytes)
  - o Collagenous sprue (collagenous band below atrophic epithelium)
  - o *Mycobacterium-avium* complex infection (acid-fast bacilli, foamy macrophages)
  - o Whipple's disease (foamy macrophages with period acid-Schiff [PAS]-positive inclusion bodies)
- **Patchy distribution in small bowel mucosa:** These diseases may therefore be missed on endoscopic small bowel biopsy.
  - o Amyloidosis (congo red–stained deposits with apple-green birefringence in polarized light)
  - o Crohn's disease (epithelioid granulomas and characteristic focal inflammation)
  - o Eosinophilic gastroenteritis (eosinophilic infiltration)
  - o Lymphangiectasia (ectatic lymph vessels)
  - o Lymphoma (clonal expansion of lymphocytes)
  - o Mastocytosis (diffuse infiltration with mast cells)
  - o Parasites (*Giardia lamblia*, *Strongyloides stercoralis*)
  - o HIV enteropathy (focal enterocyte vacuolization)
  - o Celiac disease (villous atrophy, intraepithelial lymphocytes (IELs), may be diffuse, diagnosis requires serologic confirmation)

○ **How is the fecal osmotic gap calculated and how is it used?**

Measurement of the fecal osmotic gap is performed on a randomly collected stool specimens analyzed for sodium and potassium concentrations. The following formula is used: Fecal osmotic gap = $290 - 2 ([Na^+] + [K^+])$. The normal osmolality of stool is estimated to be 290 mOsm/kg. Measured stool osmolality in collected specimens is inaccurate because bacterial fermentation of unabsorbed carbohydrates produces osmotically active organic acids that raise the measured stool osmolality. An osmotic gap > 125 mOsm/kg is suggestive of pure osmotic diarrhea, whereas an osmotic gap < 50 mOsm/kg suggests a pure secretory diarrhea.

○ **A 44-year-old man with chronic diarrhea has a fecal osmotic gap < 50 and fecal sodium > 90. What form of diarrhea is this? If the diarrhea ceases with fasting, name a possible cause.**

The fecal osmotic gap and sodium concentration are consistent with a secretory diarrhea. However, the cessation of diarrhea with fasting argues against secretory diarrhea. Ingestion of sodium sulfate or sodium phosphate (such as can occur with a factitious cause) would cause an osmotic diarrhea that mimics a secretory diarrhea because of the high sodium content.

○ **Describe a bedside test for laxative use/abuse.**

Alkalinization of 3 ml of stool supernatant or urine with one drop of concentrated (1 N) sodium hydroxide will result in a pink or red color if phenolphthalein is present and turns purple blue in the presence of bisacodyl. More sophisticated stool and urine tests are available for the detection of other laxatives. Stool sulfate, phosphate, and magnesium analysis detects factitious diarrheas caused by osmotic cathartics. Urine laxative screens detect common laxatives such as diphenolic laxatives (bisacodyl), anthraquinones (senna, cascara), magnesium, and phosphate. Stool laxative screens detect these and in addition, castor oil and mineral oil. Polyethylene glycol-containing laxatives require a separate stool or urine specimen.

○   **What is pancreatic cholera?**

Pancreatic cholera is a rare type of secretory diarrhea caused by the release of vasoactive intestinal peptide (VIP) into the circulation by a neuroendocrine tumor (ie, VIPoma). It should be suspected in diarrhea lasting longer than 4 weeks with the clinical features of secretory diarrhea, a stool volume always greater than 1 L/day, marked hypokalemia, hypochlorhydria, and severe dehydration.

○   **Describe some extra-intestinal manifestations of celiac sprue.**

In addition to the signs and symptoms common to all malabsorptive disorders, the following may also be seen:
- Cutaneous
  - Dermatitis herpetiformis (DH)
  - Ecchymoses and petechiae (vitamin K deficiency; rarely, thrombocytopenia)
  - Edema (hypoproteinemia)
  - Follicular hyperkeratosis and dermatitis (vitamin A and B complex malabsorption)
- Endocrinologic
  - Amenorrhea, infertility, and impotence (malnutrition and hypothalamic-pituitary dysfunction)
  - Secondary hyperparathyroidism (calcium/vitamin D malabsorption)
  - Thyroid disorders
- Hematologic
  - Anemia (iron, folate, vitamin B12, or pyridoxine deficiency)
  - Hemorrhage (vitamin K deficiency; rarely, thrombocytopenia due to folate deficiency)
  - Thrombocytosis, Howell–Jolly bodies (hyposplenism)
- Hepatic
  - Elevated liver biochemical test levels
- Muscular
  - Atrophy
  - Tetany
  - Weakness
- Neurologic
  - Peripheral neuropathy (deficiencies of vitamin B12 and thiamine)
  - Ataxia (cerebellar and posterior column damage)
  - Demyelinating central nervous system lesions
  - Seizures
- Skeletal
  - Osteopenia (calcium/vitamin D malabsorption)
  - Osteoarthropathy
  - Pathologic fractures

○   **What serologic tests are available for the diagnosis of celiac sprue?**

The anti-endomysial (EMA) IgA antibody, detected by indirect immunofluorescence, is the gold standard serological test for reliability with sensitivity of 90%, specificity of 99%, and reproducibility of 93%. Human antitype 2 tissue transglutaminase (tTG) ELISA is the other recommended serological test with sensitivity of 93%, specificity of 95%, and reproducibility of 83%. ELISA antigliadin IgA and IgG antibodies are inexpensive but less sensitive and specific and are no longer recommended for routine screening. Importantly, the prevalence of IgA deficiency is increased approximately 10-fold among patients with celiac sprue and testing for total IgA levels should be considered during the first step of serological testing if using an IgA-based test. Once IgA deficiency is established; testing for IgG anti-tTG antibodies or IgG anti-EMA is the next step.

○ **What is the auto-antigen recognized by the anti-endomysial antibody?**

The antigen is tTG, a calcium-dependent enzyme that catalyzes cross links between glutamine and lysine residues in substrate proteins. tTG is believed to cross-link gliadin, rendering it immunogenic.

○ **True/False: The prevalence of IgA deficiency is increased approximately 100-fold among patients with celiac sprue compared to the general population.**

False. The prevalence of IgA deficiency is increased approximately 10-fold.

○ **What is the relationship between celiac sprue and DH?**

More than 90% of patients with DH with a granular pattern of IgA deposition at the derma-epidermal junction, and at least 10% of patients with a linear pattern of IgA deposition at the derma-epidermal junction have coexisting celiac sprue. Many lack significant symptoms of the disease because the lesion is often mild and limited to the proximal intestine. Conversely, fewer than 10% of patients with celiac sprue have DH.

○ **True/False: Gluten-free diet (GFD) is a major component of the treatment of DH.**

True.

○ **Describe the classic endoscopic appearance of the small intestine in celiac sprue.**

Scalloping, multiple fissures or a mosaic-like appearance where the fissures circumscribe areas of mucosal nodularity, and/or absence of the small intestinal plicae (circular folds). However, the mucosa most commonly looks normal on endoscopy recognizing the need for biopsy and histologic examination if suspicion is high based on positive serology or clinical presentation.

○ **Name other diseases where scalloping of the mucosa is seen?**

Scalloping is not specific for celiac disease, and may be seen in:
- Eosinophilic enteritis
- Giardiasis
- Amyloidosis
- Tropical disease
- Human immunodeficiency virus enteropathy

○ **What are the classic findings suggestive of celiac disease on histological examination?**

Intraepithelial lymphocytosis, crypt hyperplasia, and villous atrophy.

○ **True/False: The mucosal lesions seen in celiac sprue are specific for that disorder.**

False. However, a completely flat mucosa is most suggestive of celiac sprue.

Intraepithelial lymphocytosis is also seen in:
- Giardiasis
- Tropical sprue
- Autoimmune diseases
- *H. pylori* gastritis
- Crohn's disease
- Bacterial overgrowth
- NSAID use

Villous atrophy is also seen in:
- Cow's milk protein intolerance (children)
- Postgastroenteritis syndrome
- Giardiasis
- Peptic duodenitis (including Zollinger–Ellison syndrome)
- Crohn's disease
- Small intestinal bacterial overgrowth (SIBO)
- Eosinophilic gastroenteritis
- Radiation or cytotoxic chemotherapy
- Tropical sprue
- Severe malnutrition
- Diffuse small intestinal lymphoma
- Graft versus host disease
- Hypogammaglobulinemia
- Alpha chain disease

○ **Name some diseases associated with celiac sprue.**
- **Clear-cut association**
  - Bird-fancier's lung
  - DH
  - Diabetes mellitus type 1
  - Down's syndrome
  - Epilepsy with cerebral calcification
  - Fibrosing alveolitis
  - Hypothyroidism or hyperthyroidism
  - Idiopathic pulmonary hemosiderosis
  - Immunoglobulin A deficiency
  - Immunoglobulin A mesangial nephropathy
  - Inflammatory bowel disease
  - Microscopic colitis
  - Recurrent pericarditis
  - Rheumatoid arthritis
  - Sarcoidosis

- **Possible association**
  - o Addison's disease
  - o Autoimmune hemolytic anemia
  - o Autoimmune liver diseases
  - o Cavitary lung disease
  - o Congenital heart disease
  - o Cystic fibrosis
  - o Immune thrombocytopenic purpura
  - o Iridocyclitis or choroiditis
  - o Macroamylasemia
  - o Myasthenia gravis
  - o Polymyositis
  - o Schizophrenia
  - o Sjögren's syndrome
  - o Systemic and cutaneous vasculitides
  - o Systemic lupus erythematosus

○ **What is the role of genetic testing in the diagnosis of celiac disease?**

Almost all patients with celiac disease are positive for human leukocyte antigen (HLA) DQ2 or DQ8. However, 35% of the persons of European ancestry in the general population are also positive for one of these. Hence, testing is useful to exclude celiac disease in the *absence of the specific loci* in the following conditions:
- Patients started on a gluten-free diet empirically without confirmation with serology or characteristic intestinal histology before starting a gluten challenge.
- Patient with celiac-like intestinal histology but negative serologies in which case a negative result indicates the need for alternative diagnosis.

○ **When is a gluten challenge reasonable to consider in clinical practice?**

Gluten challenge may be useful in two scenarios:

1. Patients started on a gluten-free diet empirically without confirmation with serology or characteristic intestinal histology, if HLA DQ2/DQ8 positive.
2. Diagnosis of celiac disease made during childhood based on positive intestinal histology with negative serology.

○ **Describe how to conduct a gluten challenge.**

Baseline serologic studies, such as IgA anti-tTG, should be performed. HLA typing for DQ2 and DQ8 may be considered, because if negative, these exclude celiac disease. A small bowel biopsy may be obtained as a baseline. Initially, a small amount of gluten (cracker or one quarter of a slice of bread) is given, which if tolerated, is doubled every 3 days until ingesting the equivalent of at least four slices of bread daily (10 g gluten). This is continued for at least 6 weeks or until more severe symptoms redevelop, at which time both serologies and/or small bowel biopsies are performed.

○ **What is nonresponsive celiac disease (NRCD)?**

Persistence of symptoms, signs, or laboratory abnormalities typical of celiac disease despite adherence to a GFD for at least 6 months. At least 10% of celiac patients are unresponsive at diagnosis or following a period of initial response to GFD.

○ **How should NRCD be evaluated?**

The commonest cause for NRCD is continued gluten ingestion, suggested by a persistent elevation of anti-tTG antibodies. The next most common cause to be ruled out is intolerance to disaccharides (eg, lactose and fructose). After these are ruled out, small bowel biopsies should be performed.

- If normalization or near normalization of small bowel histology is seen on GFD, consider:
  - o IBS
  - o Microscopic colitis
  - o SIBO
  - o Eating disorders
  - o Food intolerances
  - o Peptic ulcer disease
  - o Gastroparesis
  - o Pancreatic insufficiency
- If persistence of small bowel histological abnormalities is seen on GFD, consider:
  - o Refractory celiac disease (RCD)
  - o SIBO
  - o Peptic duodenitis
  - o Common variable immunodeficiency
  - o Crohn's disease
  - o Tropical sprue
  - o Giardiasis
  - o Post-gastroenteritis
  - o Eosinophilic gastroenteritis
  - o Autoimmune enteropathy

○ **Name some gastrointestinal complications specific to celiac sprue?**

Refractory sprue, collagenous sprue, ulcerative jejunoileitis, and development of malignancy (small bowel lymphoma [T and B cell], extra-intestinal lymphoma, small bowel adenocarcinoma, esophageal squamous cell carcinoma, oropharyngeal, and liver cancers).

○ **What is RCD and what are its types?**

Symptomatic, severe small intestinal villus atrophy that mimics celiac disease but does not respond to at least 6 months of a strict GFD and is not accounted for by other causes of villus atrophy or overt intestinal lymphoma.

- Type I RCD: Normal IELs and/or absence of T cell receptor (TCR) γ chain rearrangement.
- Type II RCD: Aberrant IELs and clonal TCRγ rearrangement.

○ **Describe the treatment of RCD.**

Glucocorticoids (budesonide) are the first line treatment for RCD, which generally improve the symptoms but may not reverse histology. Budesonide has also been used to treat RCD. Other medications include steroid-sparing agents (azathioprine and cyclosporine) and infliximab.

○ **What is the risk of enteropathy-associated T cell lymphoma (EATL) with RCD and how is it diagnosed?**

Type I RCD has an 80% 5-year survival with no risk of developing EATL, whereas Type II RCD has a 45% 5-year survival with 67% of the patients developing EATL. Poor prognostic factors include age ≥65, albumin ≤3.2, and hemoglobin ≤11.2.

EATL can be ruled out through molecular and immunohistochemical studies of small intestinal biopsies. Small intestinal radiology, enteroscopy with biopsy of the mucosa at multiple levels, capsule endoscopy, and CT or MR scanning may be helpful. As a last step, full-thickness biopsy of the small intestine can be done with lymph node biopsy at laparoscopy. Positron emission tomography (PET) scan as an addition to CT has recently been shown to increase the sensitivity of diagnosing such complications of celiac disease.

○ **What is collagenous sprue?**

Collagenous sprue is a rare disorder that presents with symptoms identical to celiac sprue. However, small intestinal biopsies show excess collagen deposition in the lamina propria beneath the epithelial layer. Patients with this condition have a poor prognosis as they do not respond to a GFD.

○ **Describe ulcerative jejunoileitis.**

Clinical features include weight loss, abdominal pain, and diarrhea unresponsive to GFD. Patients typically experience recurrent episodes of intestinal ulceration and strictures resulting in obstruction with gradual weight loss despite surgery and strict adherence to GFD. Diagnosis is made by enteroscopy, contrast studies of the small intestine, abdominal CT, capsule endoscopy, or laparotomy. Surgical excision of the worst-affected segments of small intestine is the most effective treatment; glucocorticoids and azathioprine have also been used. Increased risk of transformation to diffuse or multifocal EATL is present; 5-year survival rate is less than 50%.

○ **Which measurement used in the D-xylose test is preferable: the 1-hour serum test or the 5-hour urine test?**

The 1-hour serum D-xylose test is preferable. The 5-hour urine test can be falsely abnormal in patients with renal insufficiency, incomplete urine specimen collection, and a variety of other conditions.

○ **What is hypogammaglobulinemic sprue?**

Common variable immunodeficiency presents with chronic diarrhea, recurrent sinopulmonary infection, and meningitis. Small bowel biopsy shows decreased plasma cells in lamina propria or nodular lymphoid hyperplasia. Common intestinal infections include Giardiasis, *Isospora belli*, Cryptosporidium, and Microsporidia. Treatment is with intravenous immunoglobulin.

○ **A 25-year-old male recently migrated from the Middle East presents with a 3-month history of abdominal pain, weight loss, diarrhea, and digital clubbing on examination. What is the diagnosis?**

Immunoproliferative small intestinal disease (IPSID). This is a disease caused by a clonal proliferation of cells that produce an abnormal alpha heavy chain immunoglobulin that can be detected in the serum. Infection with *Campylobacter jejuni* has been causally associated with IPSID. Mucosal small intestinal biopsy shows dense cellular lymphoplasmacytic infiltrate in lamina propria that effaces the crypts. Premalignant forms (stage A) can be treated with long-term tetracycline, whereas the advanced stages of lymphoplasmacytic and immunoblastic lymphoma require chemotherapy or total abdominal irradiation.

○ **What is autoimmune enteropathy?**

In this condition, patients present with severe high output diarrhea and malabsorption. Diagnosis is based on ruling out other conditions such as celiac disease and histologic changes on intestinal biopsy such as partial or complete villous blunting, deep crypt lymphocytosis, increased crypt apoptotic bodies, and minimal intraepithelial lymphocytosis. Serum antibodies to enterocytes and goblet cells may be seen. Treatments include glucocorticoids and immunosuppressive drugs along with appropriate nutrition support.

○ **What is the suggested pathophysiology of "diabetic diarrhea"?**

Since most patients with diabetic diarrhea also have autonomic neuropathy, this condition was classically thought to be due to disordered motility. More recently, sympathetic denervation with decreased enterocyte α-2 adrenergic receptors has been described and this is thought to result in decreased intestinal absorptive function. Steatorrhea and bile salt malabsorption may also occur in these patients. Other causes of diarrhea in diabetic patients include bacterial overgrowth, celiac sprue, microscopic colitis, pancreatic dysfunction, and, rarely, islet cell tumors (glucagonoma, VIPoma, and somatostatinoma).

○ **Describe eosinophilic gastroenteritis.**

Eosinophilic gastroenteritis may involve any layer of the gut wall, from the mucosa to the serosa. Manifestations of eosinophilic gastroenteritis include nausea, vomiting, diarrhea, weight loss, iron deficiency, malabsorption, protein-losing enteropathy, pyloric outlet or intestinal obstruction, and eosinophilic ascites. Immunologic evidence of underlying allergy is usually lacking unless a convincing history of symptoms triggered by food and presenting with immediate reactions (IgE mediated), or is accompanied by eczema or asthma. A trial of elemental diet can be used to rule out food hypersensitivity.

○ **What conditions are associated with the occurrence of vitamin B12 malabsorption?**

Inadequate dietary intake, pernicious anemia, small bowel bacterial overgrowth, old age (incomplete release of food-bound vitamin B12 due to gastric atrophy), gastric surgery (achlorhydria, decreased intrinsic factor), therapy with proton pump inhibitors and H$_2$ receptor antagonists (incomplete release of food-bound vitamin B12), HIV infection (enteropathy, ileal disease, achlorhydria), Crohn's disease (ileal disease or resection > 60 cm), helminthic infection (*Diphyllobothrium latum*), chronic pancreatitis and Zollinger–Ellison syndrome (both due to incomplete cleavage of the R protein–vitamin B12 complex), and congenital diseases with selective ileal malabsorption of vitamin B12 despite normal ileal histology due to abnormalities of the vitamin B12 receptor (Imerslund–Gräsbeck syndrome).

○ **How is the Schilling test performed?**

Of note, this test is mainly of historical interest in the present day. An intramuscular dose of nonlabeled vitamin B12 (usually 1000 μg) is administered to saturate liver binding sites. Oral radiolabeled vitamin B12 is then administered and urine radioactivity is measured over 24 hours. Appearance of less than 10% of the radiolabeled vitamin B12 in the urine is considered diagnostic of vitamin B12 malabsorption. If vitamin B12 malabsorption is corrected by administration of intrinsic factor, it establishes intrinsic factor deficiency (Stage II Schilling test). If vitamin B12 malabsorption is corrected with pancreatic enzymes (Stage III) or with antibiotics (Stage IV), then the test establishes pancreatic insufficiency or bacterial overgrowth, respectively. If the test does not correct with any of these maneuvers, then the cause of malabsorption is ileal disease or resection.

○ **A 72-year-old woman presents with memory loss and a borderline low vitamin B12 level (< 250 pg/mL) is found. How can a definitive diagnosis of vitamin B12 deficiency be made?**

Elevated serum methylmalonic acid and/or homocysteine levels establish the presence of vitamin B12 deficiency at the tissue level. Elevated homocysteine levels may also indicate the presence of folic acid deficiency.

○ **Name the clinical conditions associated with SIBO.**

- Small intestinal stagnation due to anatomical derangements (Billroth II gastrectomy, duodenal or jejunal diverticulosis, surgical blind loop, and obstruction).
- Motor disorders (scleroderma, intestinal pseudo-obstruction, and diabetic gastroenteropathy).
- Abnormal connection from colon to proximal small bowel (intestinal fistulae or resected ileocecal valve).
- Achlorhydria (medications, atrophic gastritis, and vagotomy).
- Others (cirrhosis, celiac disease, chronic pancreatitis, chronic kidney disease, radiation enteritis, rheumatoid arthritis, and cystic fibrosis).

○ **What is the most consistent laboratory abnormality that may occur in SIBO?**

An elevated folate with or without vitamin B12 deficiency is the most common abnormality. Serum folate levels are frequently elevated because of bacterial production of folate, whereas B12 levels are reduced due to bacterial consumption.

○ **What tests are available to diagnose SIBO?**

The "gold" standard for the diagnosis of bacterial overgrowth is quantitative small bowel culture. Bacterial concentrations greater than 10^5 colony forming units/mL indicates bacterial overgrowth. Several different breath tests (C^{14}-D-xylose, glucose-H_2, and lactulose-H_2) are also available; however, there is controversy regarding the sensitivity and specificity of these tests. Because of limited availability and known problems inherent in the above-mentioned tests, a therapeutic trial of antibiotics is often used as a "diagnostic" tool in clinical practice.

○ **What are the mechanisms of malabsorption that can occur in patients with scleroderma?**

Bacterial overgrowth often occurs secondary to small intestinal stasis, loss of the migrating motor complex, and the presence of small intestinal diverticula. Villous atrophy, enterocyte dysfunction, and submucosal collagen deposition may also be present. Pancreatic insufficiency may also occur.

○ **True/False: Octreotide has a role in the management of SIBO.**

True, at least in patients with scleroderma and associated intestinal dysmotility. Octreotide at a low dose of 50 mcg every evening for 3 weeks has been shown to induce migrating motor complexes, reduce bacterial overgrowth, and relieve abdominal symptoms in SIBO associated with systemic sclerosis.

○ **How is tropical sprue treated?**

Initial treatment includes correction of fluids, electrolytes, and deficient nutrients. Tetracycline (250 mg four times a day) or doxycycline (100 mg once daily) and folic acid are given as pharmacotherapy. The beneficial effect of treatment with folic acid on both macrocytic anemia and villous atrophy suggests that folate deficiency plays a role in perpetuating the intestinal lesion of tropical sprue. It is recommended that treatment be continued for 6 months. A GFD is not needed.

○ **How does ileal resection lead to diarrhea and what is the treatment?**

Resection of less than 100 cm leads to bile salt wasting. Bile salts are deconjugated in the colon where they cause a secretory diarrhea. Bile salt wasting is compensated by increased bile salt synthesis in the liver, leading to normal fat absorption. Treatment includes bile salt binders such as cholestyramine.

Resection of greater than 100 cm of ileum leads to depletion of the bile salt pool resulting in impaired micelle formation, fat malabsorption, steatorrhea, and diarrhea. Treatment theoretically consists of exogenous conjugated bile acid supplements (eg, cholylsarcosine 2–4 g with meals or desiccated ox bile 500 mg capsule with meals); however, these are not readily available. Therefore, a fat-restricted diet with or without medium-chain triglyceride oil supplementation is the primary treatment. Bile salt binders should be avoided as they exacerbate the problem by further depletion of the bile salt pool.

○ **What mechanisms may be responsible for diarrhea in Crohn's disease?**

Small bowel inflammation, small bowel bacterial overgrowth, surgical resection, fistulae, cholerrhetic diarrhea, and steatorrhea.

○ **Explain the mechanism of calcium oxalate stone formation in Crohn's disease.**

This condition is termed enteric hyperoxaluria. Bile salt malabsorption due to ileal disease or resection may result in fat malabsorption. Intraluminal fatty acids bind calcium cations, which would otherwise bind to intestinal oxalate. Free oxalate thus enters the colon where it is absorbed and then renally excreted, causing calcium oxalate stones. Prevention of calcium oxalate stones in patients with Crohn's disease involves limitation of fat and oxalate intake, as well as calcium supplementation. A patient who has undergone a colectomy cannot develop enteric hyperoxaluria.

○ **What are some common ingredients of prescription and nonprescription medications that may cause malabsorption?**

Polyols (sorbitol, mannitol, and xylitol), gluten, and lactose.

○ **A 15-year-old boy presents with chronic diarrhea and steatorrhea. You elicit a history of recurrent upper respiratory infections. What laboratory test is recommended?**

A sweat test to rule out cystic fibrosis. If this were negative, testing for common variable immunodeficiency (quantitative immunoglobulins) should be considered.

○ **What medications may result in malabsorption of vitamins and other nutrients?**

Antacids, H2 blockers, proton pump inhibitors, mineral oil, cholestyramine, methotrexate, chemotherapeutic agents, phenytoin, orlistat, sulfasalzine, and sucralfate.

○ **Name some medications that can cause secretory diarrhea.**

Laxatives, cholinergic agents, quinidine and quinine, colchicine, metoclopramide, misoprostol, olsalazine, theophylline, lubiprostone, tegaserod, and thyroid preparations.

○ **What enteric infections may present with malabsoprtion?**

- Protozoan infections
  - o Giardiasis (*Giardia lamblia*)
  - o *Cryptosporidium parvum*
  - o *Isospora belli*
  - o *Cyclospora cayetanensis*
  - o Microsporidia (*enterocytozoon bieneusi* and *encephalitozoon intestinalis*)
  - o Visceral leishmaniasis
- Helminthic infections
  - o *Strongyloides stercoralis*
  - o *Capillaria philippinensis*

○ **What are the mechanisms causing diarrhea in Zollinger–Ellison (ZE) syndrome?**

High volume of secreted hydrochloric acid, fat maldigestion due to inactivation of pancreatic lipase, and bile acid precipitation due to the low duodenal pH. Diarrhea occurs in up to one-third of patients with the ZE syndrome, may precede the other symptoms, and may be the major clinical manifestation of the disease.

○ **What is the Cronkhite–Canada syndrome?**

The Cronkhite–Canada syndrome is a noninherited polyposis syndrome characterized by hamartomatous polyps found throughout the gastrointestinal tract and by a severe protein-losing enteropathy due to a diffuse mucosal injury of obscure etiology. Clinical features also include cutaneous hyperpigmentation, alopecia, and nail atrophy.

○   **Describe the clinical features and genetic defect of abetalipoproteinemia?**

Abetalipoproteinemia is a rare autosomal recessive disorder of lipoprotein metabolism characterized by extremely low levels of serum cholesterol and triglycerides and the absence of apoB-containing lipoproteins. Clinical manifestations include intestinal malabsorption, neurological symptoms such as spinocerebellar dysfunction, and retinopathy that causes impairment of night and color vision. Mutations of the microsomal triglyceride transfer protein have been shown to cause abetalipoproteinemia. Peripheral blood smear shows the presence of acanthocytes and low plasma chylomicrons, and small bowel biopsy shows lipid accumulation with vacuolization of enterocytes.

○   **What are the clinical features of intestinal lymphatic obstruction?**

Findings of protein-losing enteropathy including hypoalbuminemia, hypoglobulinemia, lymphopenia, peripheral edema, ascites, and possibly anasarca. The differential diagnosis of intestinal lymphatic obstruction includes congenital intestinal lymphangiectasia, cardiac disease, Whipple's disease, Crohn's disease, mesenteric tuberculosis, mesenteric sarcoidosis, lymphoma, and lymphenteric fistula.

○   **What are the causes of iron deficiency occurring after gastric surgery?**

Gastric acid dissociates iron salts from food and dissolves them. The achlorhydric stomach cannot release food-bound iron. In addition, patients who have undergone antrectomy have defective meat digestion so that heme proteins (myoglobin and hemoglobin) cannot be digested properly by pancreatic proteases to liberate the heme–iron complexes. Finally, iron deficiency may result from decreased food intake and blood loss from gastritis.

○   **Name some systemic diseases associated with malabsorption.**

Thyrotoxicosis, hypothyroidism, Addison's disease, hypoparathyroidism, diabetes mellitus, scleroderma, and HIV infection.

○   **What are clinical and diagnostic features of Whipple's disease?**

Diarrhea with steatorrhea, fever, arthritis, lymphadenopathy, pericarditis, endocarditis, myocarditis, dementia, depression, choreoathetosis, and ophthalmoplegia. This condition, which typically affects older men, is caused by a Gram-positive bacillus called *Tropheryma whippelii*. Polymerase chain reaction (PCR) analysis of small intestinal biopsies is now the preferred test. Treatment usually consists of an induction phase (first 10–14 days) using penicillin G plus streptomycin or a third-generation cephalosporin (eg, Ceftriaxone) followed by treatment with double-strength trimethoprim-sulfamethoxazole twice daily for 1 year.

○   **What are the causes of PAS-positive macrophages present in the lamina propria seen on intestinal biopsy?**

In the past, the finding of lamina propria PAS-positive macrophages was diagnostic of Whipple's disease. More recently, it has been recognized that PAS-positive macrophages are also seen with atypical mycobacterial infections. The acid-fast stain distinguishes between the two.

○   **What are the most common causes of short bowel syndrome in children?**

Congenital defects (eg, intestinal atresia) (75%) and necrotizing enterocolitis (25%).

○   **What are the most common cause of short bowel syndrome in adults?**

Crohn's disease requiring multiple bowel resections and acute mesenteric ischemia.

○   **Describe the pathophysiology and clinical features of D-lactic acidosis?**

D-lactic acidosis is a rare complication of short bowel syndrome that occurs as a result of carbohydrate overfeeding and, possibly, small bowel bacterial overgrowth. Malabsorbed carbohydrate is metabolized by colonic bacteria to short-chain fatty acids and lactate, which, in turn, lower colonic pH. A lower colonic pH favors the growth of D-lactate-producing enteric flora. D-lactate is absorbed but is poorly metabolized due to a lack, in humans, of D-lactic acid dehydrogenase.

Patients present with anion gap metabolic acidosis with a normal L-lactate level, nystagmus, ophthalmoplegia, ataxia, confusion, and inappropriate behavior. The mediator of the neurologic symptoms is unknown. Initial treatment consists of bicarbonate administration and fasting. Prevention may be attempted with a low carbohydrate diet and, possibly, antibiotics and/or probiotics.

○   **What pancreatic enzyme formulations are used for the treatment of the pain of chronic pancreatitis?**

Although controversial, non-enteric-coated formulations are potentially beneficial in the treatment of chronic pain in some patients with chronic pancreatitis. Some data suggest that the protease components of these supplements reduce the pain of chronic pancreatitis. Enteric-coated formulations are used to treat pancreatic maldigestion. To prevent steatorrhea, the recommended dose is 30,000 IU (90,000 USP units) of lipase in the prandial and postprandial portions of each meal.

○   **What are the mechanisms of diarrhea in patients with radiation enteritis?**

Altered absorption of fluids and electrolytes, bile-salt malabsorption, bacterial overgrowth due to stasis, entero-enteric fistulae, and short bowel syndrome secondary to resection.

○   **What is the rationale for using medium-chain triglycerides (MCTs) as nutritional supplements in patients with fat malabsorption syndromes?**

Normal fat digestion and absorption require a multistep process including emulsification in the stomach, release of free fatty acids by gastric acids, breakdown of triglycerides by pancreatic lipases, formation of micelles with bile salts in the duodenum, and enterocyte absorption. MCTs are rapidly hydrolyzed and absorbed directly without requiring pancreatic lipase, bile salts, or micelle formation.

● ● ● SUGGESTED READINGS ● ● ●

Hogenauer C, Hammer HF. Maldigestion and Malabsorption. In: Feldman F, Friedman LS, Brandt LJ, eds. *Sleisinger and Fordtran's gastrointestinal and liver disease: pathophysiology, diagnosis and management.* 9th ed. Philadelphia, PA: Saunders-Elsevier; 2010: 1736-1767.

Farrell RJ, Kelly CP. Celiac Disease and Refractory Celiac Disease. In: Feldman F, Friedman LS, Brandt LJ, eds. *Sleisinger and Fordtran's gastrointestinal and liver disease: pathophysiology, diagnosis and management.* 9th ed. Philadelphia, PA: Saunders-Elsevier; 2010: 1797-1819.

CHAPTER 42 Short Bowel Syndrome

Carol Rees Parrish, MS, RD and Nora Decher, MS, RD, CNSC

○ **Adults with what remaining length of small intestine are at risk of developing malabsorption consistent with short bowel syndrome?**

Approximately 200 cm (6.5 ft). This length is often used as a guideline for the definition of short bowel syndrome; however, the absolute length varies considerably among individuals.

○ **True/False: The length of small bowel differs between men and women.**

True. The length of small intestine is approximately 630 cm in men and approximately 590 cm in women. The length of colon is about 150 cm in both sexes.

○ **What are the major causes of short bowel syndrome in adults?**

Postoperative complications, mesenteric infarction, radiation enteritis, Crohn's disease, trauma, and volvulus.

○ **What is the leading cause of short bowel syndrome in children?**

Congenital abnormalities such as intestinal atresia, gastroschisis, malrotation with midgut volvulus, and aganglionosis.

○ **What is the difference in villi shape in different parts of small intestine?**

The villi are taller and crypts deeper in the jejunum than the ileum. The activity of microvillus enzymes and nutrient absorptive capacity per unit length of intestine is several-fold higher in the proximal than in distal small bowel.

○ **True/False: The majority of digestion and absorption of most nutrients occurs in the distal ileum.**

False. The digestion and absorption of most macro- and micronutrients occur in the first 100 cm of jejunum. Therefore, patients with short bowel syndrome in general can maintain nutritional balance on oral feeding if more than 100 cm of jejunum remains. Conversely, most patients with a jejunal length of less than 100 cm will require long-term parenteral nutrition (PN), depending on the presence of the colon.

○ **Where is the site of absorption of macronutrients (fat, protein, and carbohydrate) and micronutrients (calcium, magnesium, and iron)?**

The primary site for iron and folate absorption is the duodenum. Macronutrients and most other micronutrients, including calcium, are absorbed in the proximal jejunum. Bile acids and food-bound vitamin B12 are only absorbed in the ileum (synthetic B12 is absorbed throughout the small intestine). Electrolytes and water are absorbed in both the small and large intestines.

○ **What is the absorptive efficiency of fluids received by the small intestine?**

The proximal small intestine receives about 9 L/day of water and electrolytes from food and secretions. About 8 L of this is reabsorbed throughout the small intestine.

○ **What is an appropriate concentration of sodium and glucose in oral rehydration solutions to achieve net sodium and water absorption in the jejunum?**

A mixture of 13–20 g glucose and 75–90 mEq (1725–2070 mg) sodium per liter.

○ **True/False: Moderate bile acid malabsorption can occur with less than 100 cm of ileum resected.**

True. More extensive resection causes bile acid depletion resulting in fat malabsorption and steatorrhea.

○ **What length of terminal ileal resection may result in vitamin B12 deficiency?**

More than 50–60 cm.

○ **True/False: Unabsorbed hydroxylated fatty acids and bile salts following extensive ileal resection cause diarrhea by stimulating colonic secretion and motility.**

True. The stimulation of colonic electrolyte and water secretion is sometimes referred to as "cholerrheic diarrhea."

○ **What is the effect of extensive small intestinal resection on the serum gastrin level during the first 6–12 months postoperatively?**

Hypergastrinemia occurs within 24 hours of extensive small bowel resection and may last up to a year. This may lead to gastric acid and volume hypersecretion, peptic complications, inactivation of pancreatic enzymes, and destabilization of bile salts.

○ **What is the most prominent clinical symptom in patients with short bowel syndrome?**

Diarrhea, steatorrhea, or both.

○ **What type of solution should be started postoperatively in patients with high output end-jejunostomy syndrome?**

Oral rehydration solution. Hypotonic solutions may result in paradoxical jejunal sodium and water secretion.

○ **A 59-year-old man with ischemic bowel disease underwent intestinal resection 9 months ago and the total length of jejunum remaining is 120 cm with an intact colon. He has lost a substantial amount of weight despite eating his previous diet. What type of oral diet should be recommended for this patient?**

A hyperphagic diet high in complex carbohydrates and low in fat is recommended. Oxalate restriction is also recommended in this setting.

○ **What is the first-line treatment of diarrhea in a patient with limited ileal resection less than 100 cm?**

Cholestyramine to bind unabsorbed bile salts.

○ **What is the first-line treatment of diarrhea in a patient with extensive ileal resection more than 100 cm?**

Fat restriction.

○ **What is the effect of resection of the ileocecal valve on absorption of nutrients?**

Although conflicting evidence exists, loss of the ileocecal valve is thought to facilitate small bowel bacterial overgrowth, which can lead to maldigestion.

○ **True/False: A patient with a remaining jejunal length of 150 cm and an intact colon should be able to avoid the need of permanent PN support.**

True. Patients with a jejunal length of 100 cm in continuity with the colon can usually be managed by oral intake alone depending upon the health of the remaining bowel. Permanent PN support will likely be needed in those with <100 cm jejunum without any colon remaining.

○ **What medications may be useful in a patient with an end-jejunostomy whose stomal losses exceed liquid intake?**

Antisecretory agents such as H_2 receptor antagonists, proton pump inhibitors, and somatostatin analogues may be useful in this setting. High doses of nonspecific antidiarrheals may also be of benefit.

○ **What is the risk of oxalate kidney stones in patients with short bowel syndrome and colectomy?**

None. Oxalate requires an intact colon for absorption.

○ **How is hyperoxaluria in patients with short bowel syndrome and preserved colon treated?**

Restriction of oxalate-containing food products such as tea, chocolate, cola beverages, certain fruits, and vegetables. Adequate fluid intake is to ensure a urine output greater than 1200–1500 mL/day. Oral calcium citrate may also be helpful to bind oxalate and prevent its absorption.

○ **A patient with short bowel syndrome and a preserved colon presents with episodes of confusion, ataxia, and inappropriate behavior. What is the most likely diagnosis?**

D-lactic acidosis is a rare complication observed only in short bowel patients with an intact colon. The episodes of acidosis are usually precipitated by an increased oral intake of refined carbohydrate. Malabsorbed carbohydrates are metabolized by colonic bacteria to short chain fatty acids and lactate.

○ **What is the appropriate management of a patient with D-lactic acidosis?**

Correction of acidosis by sodium bicarbonate and restricting concentrated carbohydrate intake. The potential benefit of oral antibiotics is debated.

○ **What is the nutritional value of a clear liquid diet in patients with short bowel syndrome?**

None. In addition, it is hyperosmolar and may provoke osmotic diarrhea.

○ **What is the value of a full liquid diet in patients with short bowel syndrome?**

None. A full liquid diet may be poorly tolerated because it contains lactose, is highly osmotic, and in those who are fat intolerant, can aggravate fat malabsorption. It is important to note that not all patients with short gut are lactose intolerant; many can take small amounts over the day without exacerbating symptoms.

○ **Where is the border between the jejunum and the ileum?**

In general, the proximal two-fifths (about 240 cm) of the small bowel is called the jejunum and the distal three-fifths (about 360 cm) the ileum.

○ **What are the major bowel factors responsible for adaptation in short bowel syndrome?**

Amount of intestine remaining, the sections remaining, the presence of an ileocecal valve, and the condition of the residual intestine. In addition to bowel factors, a number of nutritional and hormonal factors play a role in the adaptation process.

○ **What are the major mechanisms by which enteral nutrients stimulate intestinal adaptation?**

Direct contact with epithelial cells, stimulation of trophic gastrointestinal hormone secretion, and stimulation of pancreatic and biliary secretions.

○ **What are the adaptive changes to the small intestine after an extensive small intestinal resection?**

Luminal dilation, thickening and lengthening of gastrointestinal tract, and hyperplasia of the crypt-villus axis leading to increased surface area. This occurs primarily in the ileum, less so in the jejunum.

○ **Which hormones have a trophic effect on the small intestine?**

Gastrin, secretin, cholecystokinin, epidermal growth factor, corticosteroids, enteroglucagon, prostaglandins and growth hormone releasing factor, and glucagon-like peptide 2(GLP-2). Somatostatin has a negative effect on gut adaptation.

○ **Resection of which part of small intestine has only a limited effect on the ability of the small intestine to adapt?**

Jejunum. The ileum has the greatest capacity for adaptation and is able to compensate for and take over almost all of the jejunum's absorptive function. Unfortunately, the ileum is most often resected in patients with short gut.

○ **What are the major regulatory hormones in the proximal gastrointestinal tract?**

Gastrin, cholecystokinin, secretin, motilin, and gastrin inhibitory peptide.

○ **What are the major regulatory hormones in the distal gut?**

Peptide YY, GLP-1, and GLP-2.

○ **Why do some patients with short bowel syndrome have rapid gastric emptying of liquids and rapid intestinal transit time?**

Lack of GLP-1 and peptide YY secreted by the L-cells of the resected distal ileum (ileal brake slows gastric emptying and small bowel transit) and proximal colon.

○   **True/False: A barium contrast small bowel series is the best way to estimate the length of a patient's remaining bowel.**

False. The most accurate assessment of remaining small bowel length is to measure it at the time of surgery. Unfortunately, this is often not done or only the length resected is measured. A small bowel series is useful as an alternative.

○   **What are the major electrolyte and trace element losses in a patient with a high output end-jejunostomy?**

Sodium, potassium, calcium, magnesium, iron, zinc, and copper.

○   **Why are patients with short bowel syndrome prone to develop cholesterol gallstones?**

Decreased hepatic bile secretion, supersaturation of bile with cholesterol, gallbladder hypomotility, and formation of gallbladder sludge. The use of medications such as somatostatin analogues may also contribute.

○   **What is the time period of maximal small intestinal adaptive response in humans after extensive small intestinal resection?**

One year, although adaptation may occur over a longer period of time.

○   **What segment of small intestine has the highest adaptive capability?**

Ileum.

○   **What is the most critical determinant of the need for permanent PN support after extensive small bowel resection and colectomy?**

Length of remaining ileum. Patients with ileal length of less than 100 cm cannot maintain adequate nutrient absorption. These patients will usually require long-term PN. Jejunal resection is better tolerated than ileal resection due to unique characteristics of the ileum and its potential for adaptation.

○   **What type of magnesium supplement is most likely to be tolerated best in patients with short bowel syndrome?**

Magnesium gluconate is less likely to cause an osmotic diarrhea than other magnesium-containing compounds.

○   **What are the major vitamin deficiencies in a patient with extensive jejunal resection?**

The fat-soluble vitamins A, D, E, and K.

○   **What is the ideal caloric intake in a patient with short bowel syndrome?**

Caloric needs for patients with short bowel syndrome may range from 30 to 40 kcal/kg/day, depending on the patient's absorptive capacity, and the amount necessary for maintenance of the patient's goal weight.

○   **What percentage of patients with short bowel syndrome requires total PN in the immediate postoperative period?**

100%.

○   **What are the indications for small bowel transplantation in short bowel syndrome?**

Permanent need for PN support along with one or more of the following serious complications of PN: progressive liver disease, loss of vascular access sites, and recurrent episodes of central venous catheter sepsis (single episode of fungal sepsis).

○ **What trophic factor has recently shown promising results in promoting mucosal growth in patients with short bowel syndrome and may become available for use in the relatively near future as an aid to weaning PN?**

GLP-2 analogue (teduglutide). Recombinant human growth hormone with or without glutamine is currently approved for use for the same indication.

○ **What are the major causes of morbidity and mortality following small bowel transplantation?**

Infection and graft rejection.

○ **What nontransplant surgical options exist to enhance the function of the existing bowel in selected short bowel patients?**

Intestinal lengthening (eg, Bianchi procedure and serial transverse enteroplasty [STEP]), intestinal tapering, and reversed intestinal segment. Performance of these procedures is also referred to as autologous gastrointestinal reconstruction.

○ **What is the single most effective surgical procedure to allow discontinuation of PN support in short bowel syndrome?**

Restoration of bowel continuity.

○ **True/False: Plasma citrulline level is a reliable marker for a patient's potential to be weaned from PN.**

False. Citrulline may reflect remnant intestinal mucosal mass and has been shown to correlate with the need of permanent PN support in short bowel patients; however, it does not reflect how well the patient will utilize this mass. It is unlikely that the citrulline concentration reflects the various aspects of gut absorption since the latter involves not only the small bowel mucosa but also the trophic effects of pancreatic-biliary secretions, gut motility, and colonic absorption. Finally, given the alternative, making every effort to wean a patient from PN should always be attempted as opposed to relying on a lab value or other biomarker.

● ● ● SUGGESTED READINGS ● ● ●

Langnas AN, Goulet O, Quigley EMM, Tappenden KA, eds. *Intestinal Failure: Diagnosis, Management and Transplantation*. Malden, MA: Blackwell Publishing; 2008.

Parrish CR. The Clinician's Guide to Short Bowel Syndrome. *Practical Gastroenterology*. 2005;XXIX(9):67.

Efsen E, Jeppesen PB. Modern treatment of adult short bowel syndrome patients. *Minerva Gasterol Dietol*. 2011;57(4):405-417.

Clinical Nutrition, Enteral, and Parenteral Nutrition Support

CHAPTER 43

Carol Rees Parrish, MS, RD and Joe Krenitsky, MS, RD

○ **Some individuals with achlorhydria may need supplementation of which vitamin? Why?**

Vitamin B12. Both acid and intrinsic factor are produced in the gastric parietal cell. In some conditions (eg, pernicious anemia), the parietal cell has diminished, or absent, production of both acid and intrinsic factor leading to achlorhydria and vitamin B12 deficiency.

○ **Macrocytic anemia may result from deficiencies of which two B vitamins?**

Folate and vitamin B12.

○ **What biliary factors may contribute to fat malabsorption?**

Any condition that decreases bile flow or excretion, or disrupts the enterohepatic circulation of bile salts in the ileum.

○ **True/False: An individual with a more than 100-cm terminal ileal resection is at risk of developing vitamin D deficiency.**

True. Disrupted enterohepatic cycling of bile acids in those with more than 100 cm of distal ileum removed may result in bile salt deficiency that can lead to fat malabsorption, including fat-soluble vitamins (A, D, E, and K).

○ **What individuals are at risk of developing refeeding syndrome?**

Anyone with an unintentional, chronic (>10 days) inadequate intake.

○ **What classical electrolyte disturbances occur with refeeding syndrome?**

Hypokalemia, hypophosphatemia, and hypomagnesemia.

○   **In patients at nutritional risk, especially alcohol abusers, which vitamin should be given prior to the administration of intravenous glucose? Why?**

Thiamine (vitamin B1). Thiamine is a cofactor for several enzymes essential for optimal glucose utilization and metabolism. Thiamine requirements depend on metabolic rate, with the greatest need during periods of high metabolic demand and high glucose intake. This is manifest by the precipitation of Wernicke's encephalopathy in susceptible patients by administration of intravenous glucose before thiamine supplementation.

○   **What conditions are associated with thiamine deficiency and what conditions are they at risk of developing?**

Alcoholism, anorexia nervosa, hyperemesis of pregnancy, prolonged fasting or starvation, gastrointestinal surgery (eg, gastric bypass), long-term parenteral nutrition, AIDS, transplantation, and hemodialysis. Thiamine deficiency may be complicated by the development of Wernicke's encephalopathy (triad of encephalopathy, oculomotor dysfunction, and gait ataxia) and Korsakoff's psychosis.

○   **What endogenous substance initiates the cascade of events that causes refeeding syndrome?**

Insulin.

○   **True/False: Wet beriberi and dry beriberi are both the result of niacin deficiency.**

False. Beriberi results from thiamine deficiency. Wet beriberi refers to the type with prominent cardiac manifestations, whereas dry beriberi refers to the type with prominent neurological manifestations.

○   **How much fat is required in the diet to prevent essential fatty acid (EFA) deficiency?**

3%–4% of the total calories.

○   **How much fat is required in the diet to have adequate absorption of fat-soluble vitamins?**

10%.

○   **Neutropenia may be caused by which trace element deficiency?**

Copper. Copper deficiency is an underrecognized cause of anemia, neutropenia, and bone marrow dysplasia. Neuromuscular disturbances may also occur. Zinc toxicity and prior gastric surgery (resection in particular) have been described as the causes of copper deficiency. Cytopenias typically resolve with the correction of the copper deficiency.

○   **True/False: Vitamin E is produced in the gut on a daily basis.**

False. Vitamin K is produced by intestinal microbes.

○   **What is an acceptable gastric residual volume (GRV) for a patient receiving gastric tube feeding?**

Up to 500 mL. However, if GRV is used, it should be in addition to abdominal assessment for distention, nausea, and vomiting. Despite its common use, very little data exist to support the practice of checking GRV.

○   **Why is it inappropriate to bolus tube feed into the small intestine?**

The small intestine is very sensitive to volume/distension.

○   **Medium chain triglyceride (MCT) oil is sometimes offered to patients with severe fat malabsorption as a calorie supplement. What are the potential gastrointestinal side effects of excess MCT oil in the diet?**

Excess gas, bloating, diarrhea, and anal seepage.

○   **True/False: The main advantage of MCTs over long chain triglycerides (LCTs) is their ability to be absorbed directly across the small bowel mucosa.**

True. MCT does not require micelle formation for absorption.

○   **True/False: MCT does not contain EFAs, so those receiving supplemental MCT will still require a source of EFA.**

True. Another disadvantage of MCTs over LCTs is that they provide fewer calories (8 versus 9 kcal/g).

○   **True/False: Residual volumes should be checked in a patient receiving nasoduodenal feedings.**

False. The small bowel has no reservoir and therefore checking for residuals is unnecessary.

○   **True/False: Accumulating evidence supports a preference of parenteral over enteral nutrition support in the critically ill patient with severe acute pancreatitis.**

False. Compared to parenteral nutrition support, enteral nutrition support has been shown to result in better outcomes (including a Cochrane Review), particularly when the feeding is administered distal to the ligament of Treitz.

○   **What nutritional laboratory parameters need to be monitored closely in a patient with pancreatitis who is receiving parenteral nutrition with lipids?**

Serum triglycerides and blood glucose levels. Elevated serum triglyceride level is often a function of hyperglycemia as lipoprotein lipase activity decreases along with clearance of triglycerides from the bloodstream beginning as glucose rises over 150 mg/dL.

○   **True/False: A 63-year-old man has been tolerating tube feeding for 3 weeks and suddenly develops a stool output of 950 mL/day. The enteral formula is the most likely cause of the sudden increase in stool output.**

False. In this situation, especially if tolerance had been good, an investigation for other causes of diarrhea should be initiated. Potential causes include gut infections, particularly *Clostridium difficile*, and the use of medications given through the feeding tube that contain sorbitol or other sugar alcohols.

○   **With regard to the previous question, what changes could you make to the tube feeding regimen without compromising his/her nutritional status?**

Nothing. The problem is rarely related to the tube feeding itself.

○   **True/False: Whenever possible, all medications administered through a feeding tube should be given as solutions or elixirs.**

True. Crushed medications have the potential to clog the feeding tube. However, elixirs can precipitate diarrhea due to sugar alcohol content.

○   **In a patient with severe acute pancreatitis requiring enteral nutritional support, name the jejunal access options.**

Nasojejunal, combined nasogastric-jejunal tube (for gastric venting and jejunal feeding), percutaneous endoscopic/radiologic gastrostomy-jejunostomy, direct percutaneous endoscopic/radiologic jejunostomy, and surgical jejunostomy.

○   **Skin site infections occur in approximately what percentage of patients following percutaneous endoscopic gastrostomy (PEG) placement?**

5.4%–30%.

○   **True/False: An overly tight external bolster is the biggest risk factor associated with buried bumper syndrome.**

True.

○   **A 54-year-old woman is hospitalized 1 year status post Roux-en-Y gastric bypass surgery with severe ataxia, peripheral neuropathy, and myeloneuropathy. What micronutrient deficiency is the most likely cause of these symptoms?**

Copper.

○   **True/False: The initial nutritional management for a chyle leak consists of a very low fat diet or enteral formula prior to using parenteral nutrition.**

True. Chyle, containing ingested fat and protein, electrolytes, lymphocytes, and other substances, is absorbed from the GI tract into the lymph system where it travels and ultimately is returned to the circulation via the subclavian vein over a period of several hours.

○   **True/False: If a patient with a chyle leak requires parenteral nutrition support, intravenous lipids must be withheld.**

False. Intravenous lipid emulsions are infused directly into the blood stream and do not enter the lymph system.

○   **True/False: EFA deficiency can be determined by checking a triene:tetraene ratio.**

True. A triene:tetraene ratio >0.4 is generally considered to indicate an EFA deficiency.

○   **True/False: The EFAs are linoleic acid (omega-6) and linolenic acid (omega-3).**

True. Linoleic is the primary EFA. Corn, flaxseed, soybean, and sunflower oils are all high in EFA.

○   **True/False: Serum proteins such as albumin or prealbumin are accurate indicators of nutritional status in hospitalized patients.**

False. Serum proteins are inverse acute phase reactants and do not correlate with nutrition intake, and should not be used as a marker of nutritional status.

○   **What conditions, other than malnutrition, may result in decreased serum albumin and prealbumin?**

Renal disease, liver disease, hydration, chemotherapy, blood loss, or any physiologic stress such as a surgical procedure or infection that results in an acute phase response.

○   **What clinical factors are most likely to indicate compromised nutrition status?**

Unplanned weight loss and decreased oral intake (below 50%–75% of normal) for 1 week or greater.

○   **True/False: Obese patients are rarely malnourished.**

False. Obese patients may have poor oral intake for a prolonged period with significant weight loss that is not initially apparent because they remain obese. Considering the increasing incidence of obesity in the United States, it is likely that the incidence of malnourished obese patients seen in practice will increase.

○   **True/False: All patients receiving mechanical ventilation require a specialized pulmonary enteral formula.**

False. Use of specialized pulmonary formulas has not been demonstrated to decrease time requiring mechanical ventilation or improve other outcomes in randomized, controlled studies.

○ **What are the macronutrient characteristics that make a pulmonary enteral formula unique and theoretically beneficial to the mechanically ventilated patient?**

High fat and low carbohydrate. This theoretically results in reduced carbon dioxide levels and a reduced work of breathing, thereby facilitating weaning from the ventilator. These benefits have not been borne out in clinical practice.

○ **List factors that may contribute to aspiration in a gastrostomy tube-fed patient.**

Head of bed elevation less than 30 degrees during formula infusion, delayed gastric motility, depressed cough reflex, and a rapid infusion of large bolus feeding.

○ **What are clinical implications of providing excess parenteral dextrose?**

Exacerbation of hyperglycemia, which may cause hypertriglyceridemia and increase the risk of infection, and hepatic steatosis with elevated liver tests.

○ **How many days after the initiation of parenteral nutrition support will a rise in liver tests typically occur?**

Ten to twelve days.

○ **True/False: Critically ill patients who do not tolerate full enteral nutrition support within 2–3 days should be started on parenteral nutrition to prevent malnutrition.**

False. An early start of parenteral nutrition support has recently been shown to result in increased complications without apparent benefit.

○ **List the mechanisms through which hyperglycemia can impair or negate efforts to improve nutrition status.**

Increased catabolism and muscle breakdown, decreased gastric motility with impaired food intake or impaired enteral feeding tolerance, and calories lost through glucosuria.

○ **True/False: Only long-term hyperglycemia affects gastric motility.**

False. Acute hyperglycemia decreases motility in the stomach, duodenum, and jejunum.

○ **How long does it take to develop biochemical evidence of an EFA deficiency on a fat-free diet?**

Three weeks.

○ **What two organs are storage sites for vitamin A?**

Adipose tissue and liver.

○ **Name one complication that can result from megadoses of vitamin D.**

Soft tissue calcium deposition.

○ **True/False: Patients with end-stage kidney disease receiving maintenance hemodialysis or peritoneal dialysis should receive a reduced-protein feeding formula.**

False. Patients receiving maintenance hemodialysis have increased losses of amino acids, peptides, and proteins during the dialysis process and thus have increased protein needs of 1.3–1.4 g protein/kg compared to the healthy adult protein requirements of 0.8–1.0 g protein/kg.

○ **What specific nutritional characteristics of a renal enteral formula make it clinically useful in a patient with end-stage renal disease?**

Lower amounts of potassium, magnesium, and phosphorus, and increased caloric density to provide more calories in less volume. All patients on dialysis should receive increased protein.

○ **Why is the total amount of calcium and phosphorus limited in a parenteral nutrition solution?**

An excess in the total calcium/phosphate product will cause precipitate formation in the solution.

○ **List the advantages of continuous enteral feeding into the jejunum compared to the stomach.**

Potentially lower risk of aspiration, particularly for those patients with poor gastric motility.

○ **What are feeding restrictions of jejunal feedings?**

Very rapid infusions (>150 mL/h) or very hyperosmolar (>750 mOsm/L) formulas may not be well tolerated initially. Most standard polymeric, nutrient-dense, or fiber-containing feedings are well tolerated in patients with a normal GI anatomy and function when the formulas are started at reduced rates and then increased. High fiber, nutrient-dense formulas can clog very small caliber tubes (<8 French) used for jejunal feeds.

○ **What are potential complications of a surgical jejunostomy?**

Infection, bowel obstruction, bowel torsion, dislodgement, leakage, bowel necrosis, and the general risks of surgery and anesthesia.

○ **A 45-year-old woman on long-term home parenteral nutrition for short bowel syndrome has a total bilirubin of 17.8 mg/dL and is receiving a standard multiple trace element additive (eg, MTE-5). What two trace elements should be monitored to avoid toxicity?**

Copper and manganese. Both are excreted via the biliary tract. Copper and manganese levels should be monitored and these trace elements should be removed from the parenteral nutrition formula if serum or whole blood levels are increased. Copper and manganese should not empirically be removed from the parenteral nutrition solution because severe copper deficiencies have been reported when trace elements were removed without first checking for toxicity.

○ **A 37-year-old man with newly diagnosed chronic intestinal pseudo-obstruction is sent home from the hospital on long-term parenteral nutrition. The parenteral nutrition provides a standard multivitamin additive and multiple trace element additive that provides zinc, copper, chromium, and manganese. Why is the patient at risk for cardiomyopathy?**

Patients receiving long-term parenteral nutrition are at risk for selenium deficiency if selenium is not provided. Fatal cases of cardiomyopathy related to selenium deficiency have been reported in patients that did not receive selenium in the parenteral nutrition.

○ **What trace mineral may be required in increased amounts when patients have persistent loss of small bowel fluids related to a fistula, short gut, or new ileostomy?**

Zinc. Zinc losses in small bowel fluids are approximately 12 mg/L of small bowel fluid lost and can exceed the amount of zinc provided in a normal diet, tube feeding, or parenteral nutrition in patients with large volume losses.

○   **What macromineral may need to be supplemented to standard tube feedings or parenteral nutrition if a patient has persistent large volume small bowel fluid losses related to a fistula or new ileostomy?**

Sodium. All tube feedings and most standard parenteral nutrition solutions provide a limited amount of sodium, while jejunal and ileal fluid losses contain 100–120 mEq/L of sodium. Persistent large volume small bowel fluid losses can result in greater sodium loss than is provided with standard parenteral nutrition or enteral feeding formulas.

○   **A 27-year-old woman with idiopathic gastoparesis who has been receiving jejunostomy feedings as the primary source of nutrition for 1 year begins to develop significant alopecia. What nutrient deficiencies should be suspected?**

Iron and zinc are primarily absorbed in the proximal small bowel and patients on long-term enteral nutrition who bypasses the duodenum are at increased risk of deficiencies, which can result in alopecia. Iron and zinc compete for absorption; therefore, care should be taken to prevent iatrogenic deficiencies if supplemental doses of one or the other mineral are provided.

○   **What macromineral deficiency can be anticipated in patient with a gastric outlet obstruction receiving jejunostomy feedings while continuously venting endogenous gastric secretions from a gastostomy?**

Chloride. In a complete gastric outlet obstruction, patients will lose more chloride as hydrochloric acid than is provided with tube feedings, even while receiving a proton-pump inhibitor, due to the modest chloride provision in enteral nutrition formulas. Failure to provide additional chloride (generally as sodium chloride) with the feedings in the setting of persistent high-volume gastric fluid losses will result in metabolic alkalosis.

○   **How many calories are there in a 500-mL container of 20% lipids? How much protein is in the bottle?**

1000 calories. There is no protein.

○   **True/False: A 20% lipid emulsion can be given through a peripheral intravenous line.**

True. All intravenous lipids are isotonic.

○   **What food allergies may serve as a contraindication to the use of parenteral lipid emulsions?**

Severe egg or soy allergies.

● ● ●   SUGGESTED READINGS   ● ● ●

Practical Gastroenterology Nutrition Series. Available at the University of Virginia Health System GI Nutrition Website: www. ginutrition.virginia.edu.

Gottschlich MM, ed. *The A.S.P.E.N. Nutrition Support Core Curriculum: A Case Based Approach—The Adult Patient.* Silver Spring, MD: American Society for Parenteral and Enteral Nutrition; 2007.

Buchman AL, ed. *Clinical Nutrition in Gastrointestinal Disease.* Thorofare, NJ: SLACK Incorporated; 2006.

CHAPTER 44 Obesity and Eating Disorders

David J. Frantz, MD, MS and
Tamar Ringel-Kulka, MD, MPH

○ **What are the types and subtypes of eating disorders (EDs)?**

The Diagnostic and Statistical Manual of Mental Disorders IV (DSMV-IV) defines three categories of EDs: anorexia nervosa (AN), bulimia nervosa (BN), and EDs not otherwise specified (NOS). AN is further divided into restricting and binge-eating/purging subtypes. BN subtypes are purging and non-purging. Binge eating disorder (BED) is an entity currently part of NOS and may be considered as a separate entity in the future. The International Classification of Diseases 10 (ICD-10) uses different categories including AN, BN, and atypical ED.

○ **What are the underlying mechanisms of EDs?**

AN and bulimia are multifactorial disorders that result from a combination of biologic, genetic, psychological, familial, social, and environmental influences. Psychiatric comorbidities are common among the EDs.

○ **What are the DSM-IV criteria for AN?**

- Refusal to maintain body weight at or above 85% of expected body weight for age, height, and sex.
- Fear of gaining weight and becoming fat despite being underweight.
- Distorted body weight and shape.
- Amenorrhea or absence of at least three menstrual cycles.

○ **What are the DSM-IV criteria for BN?**

- Recurrent episodes of binge eating.
- Engagement in compensatory behavior to prevent weight gain.
- Occurrence of episodes twice weekly for at least 3 months.
- Disproportionate estimation of body size.
- No AN episodes.

○ **What are some characteristics of BED?**

- BED is more common than AN and BN.
- Occurrence of episodes at least twice weekly for 6 months.
- Patients feel lack of control over eating, feel guilty, and/or disgust from their behavior.
- Patients do not engage in compensatory behavior to prevent weight gain.
- Patients are often obese [body mass index (BMI) >30].

○ **What are the major differential diagnostic considerations in EDs?**

- Inflammatory bowel disease (IBD)
- Celiac disease
- Malabsorption
- Marked increased physical activity
- Diabetes mellitus
- Hyperthyroidism
- Chronic infections
- Pituitary prolactinoma
- Pregnancy (hyperemesis gravidarum)
- Addison disease
- Substance abuse
- Depression and/or obsessive compulsive disorder (OCD)
- Malignancy including central nervous system (CNS) tumor
- Superior mesenteric artery syndrome (also a sequela)
- Gastric outlet obstruction

○ **What is the incidence and prevalence of AN in the United States? Has it changed over the years?**

Incidence rates for females 15–19 years of age range from 20 to 74 per 100,000 person years. The incidence rate is believed to have been increasing over the past 50–60 years, particularly in women aged 15–24. There is mixed data regarding the last few decades, partly due to more strict definitions of the disorder. The lifetime prevalence is approximately 0.9% among women and 0.3% among men in the United States. Most authors agree that only a fraction of patients with the disorder come to medical attention.

○ **When is the usual onset of presentation of the EDs?**

Median age of onset of all EDs is between 18 and 21 years; however, they can occur at all ages.

○ **What is the male to female ratio in AN?**

The difference in lifetime prevalence between females and males with anorexia is thought to be less than previously reported in the literature. In one recent study, the ratio in the United States was reported as 3:1.

○ **Describe the differences in attitude concerning weight in patients with other psychiatric or organic disorders compared to patients with EDs.**

Those with disorders other than EDs:
- Are concerned about their weight loss.
- Do not try to prevent weight gain by restricted diet.
- Do not engage in excessive exercise.
- Do not have distorted body image.

○ **True/False: Anorectic patients will engage in self-induced vomiting or take purgatives.**

True. In bulimic-type AN, weight loss is accomplished in these ways about half of the time rather than with restriction and exercise.

○ **True/False: Anorectic patients do not experience the sensation of hunger.**

False. Anorectic patients do feel hunger; however, in their pursuit of thinness, they struggle against hunger to achieve an unrealistic degree of weight loss.

○ **What physiologic measures are decreased in anorectic patients?**

Core temperature, blood pressure, pulse rate, bowel sounds, and gastric emptying rate.

○ **What is the most common endocrine abnormality in AN?**

Amenorrhea is the most common endocrine abnormality in anorectic patients. The origin of amenorrhea is due to hypothalamic-pituitary dysfunction. Serum levels of estradiol, follicle-stimulating hormone, and luteinizing hormone are lower than in healthy individuals.

○ **True/False: Amenorrhea may precede weight loss.**

True. In about one-third of the patients, amenorrhea precedes weight loss. Stress appears to cause psychogenic amenorrhea prior to the onset of weight loss.

○ **True/False: Amenorrhea always resolves after achieving ideal body weight.**

False.

○ **What signs of health compromise in ED patients should prompt recommendation of hospitalization?**

Urgent care is based on the existence of medical, psychiatric, and behavioral factors that do not enable treatment in outpatient facilities. Specific criteria may include the following:
- Weight Criteria:
  o <85% of healthy body weight for age, height, or sex
  o Excessive decline in weight together with food refusal regardless of current BMI
  o BMI <13 kg/m^2 or BMI <2nd percentile
- Physiologic Criteria:
  o Blood pressure <80/50 mmHg
  o Postural hypotension drop >10–20 mmHg
  o Heart rate <40 beats/min
  o Oxygen saturation <85%
  o Electrolytes below minimal normal level
  o Body temperature <34.5°C
  o Electrocardiogram abnormalities such as a prolonged corrected Q-T interval (QTc) or T wave changes
  o Subjects needing supervision due to suicidality, and/or supervision during or after meals
  o Patients who are uncooperative and/or poorly motivated

○ **What are the causes of death in EDs?**

There are limited data on the specific causes of death, but in aggregate, it is thought that about half of the patients die from complications of their EDs such as starvation, heart failure, cardiac arrhythmia, or renal failure. Less than a third commit suicide and about a fifth die from unknown causes.

○ **True/False: Electrocardiographic abnormalities are common in AN.**

False. Although various electrocardiographic abnormalities have been described in AN, most patients who are not chronically vomiting or abusing laxatives will have a normal electrocardiogram. Prolongation of the QTc interval is the main predictor of risk of sudden death especially when combined with hypokalemia.

○ **True/False: The primary goal of nutritional intervention in AN is to slowly get the patient to a body weight out of the range of medical risk.**

True. The refeeding should be slow and the patient must be carefully monitored for refeeding syndrome. Weight gain should be gradual rather than rapid. Initially, patients generally require a soft diet with both multivitamin and mineral supplementation.

○ **What are the common long-term morbidities associated with AN?**

Osteoporosis is a common morbidity due to hypoestrogenemia along with nutritional deficiencies. Other common sequelae are dental problems, growth retardation, infertility, perinatal complications, and increased psychosocial impairment.

○ **What behaviors may BN patients exhibit to prevent weight gain?**

- Regularly self-induce vomiting
- Abuse of laxatives, diuretics, diet pills, and other medication in efforts to reduce weight
- Excessive exercise
- Fasting

○ **True/False: Constipation is one of the acute gastrointestinal complications in patients with BN.**

False. Constipation is a chronic complication of AN. Mallory–Weiss tears with acute gastrointestinal bleeding and Boerhaave's syndrome are potential acute gastrointestinal complications of BN.

○ **What is a common metabolic complication seen in BN patients?**

Hypochloremic, hypokalemic metabolic alkalosis. This is due to regular/excessive vomiting.

○ **What are typical signs that can be recognized on physical examination in BN patients?**

Russell sign (excoriation on the dorsum of hands or fingers), loss of dentine on the lingual and occlusal surface of the teeth, and parotid gland hypertrophy.

○ **True/False: The incidence and prevalence of BN are lower than that of AN.**

False. The incidence and prevalence of BN are higher than that of AN. The lifetime prevalence of bulimia is 1.5% in females and 0.5% in males.

○ **True/False: Unlike anorectic patients, BN patients have normal body size.**

True. Bulimic patients usually have normal body weight, less body image distortion, greater awareness that their secret compulsive behaviors are aberrant, and greater acceptance of treatment compared to anorectic patients.

○ **True/False: Satiety interrupts binging episodes in bulimic patients.**

False. The binge-purge cycle is an eating compulsion associated with failure to achieve or respond to normal satiety. The episodes occur secretly, are planned, and are terminated by a feeling of guilt or physical discomfort.

○ **What predicts the long-term prognosis of EDs?**

For AN patients, the younger the onset and the shorter the duration, the better the outcome. In BN, the opposite is true; the longer the duration of the illness, the higher the recovery rate. One study found that about a third of BN and BED patients continue to have active ED 12 years after diagnosis. Another study showed that about a fifth of anorectic patients continued to have difficulties in everyday life 10–20 years after onset.

○ **True/False: Multidisciplinary treatment is recommended for AN.**

True. Multidisciplinary treatment is the experts' recommended treatment for AN. Family-based therapy (Maudsley) gained moderate level of evidence on its efficacy. Pharmaceutical intervention with atypical antipsychotic drugs to target dopaminergic dysregulation and comorbid features reduce distorted cognitions and anxiety symptoms, and therefore reduce the resistance to weight gain.

○ **What is the recommended treatment for BN and BED?**

There is strong evidence of efficacy for cognitive behavioral therapy (CBT) in treating BN and BED. For the acute phase of BN, selective serotonin reuptake inhibitors (SSRIs) appear efficacious; however, there is not enough data on their long-term utility. There is moderate evidence for the use of pharmacotherapy in the treatment of BED. This includes the use of antidepressants (SSRIs—slight benefit) and anticonvulsants (topiramate—moderate benefit) to reduce binge episodes. Appetite suppressants such as sibutramine show a moderate benefit on weight loss.

○ **True/False: AN has increased mortality and persistent psychiatric disorders compared to other EDs.**

True.

○ **True/False: Fifty percent of obese people who lose weight on a well-designed program of diet and exercise will maintain their achieved weight.**

False. Ninety to 95% of persons who lose weight subsequently regain it within 5 years.

○ **What measure is commonly used to define obesity?**

Body mass index (BMI).

$$BMI = \frac{weight\ in\ kilograms}{(height\ in\ meters)^2}$$

○ **What are the BMI classifications of normal weight, overweight, and obesity?**

Category	BMI (kg/m²)
Normal	18.50–24.99
Overweight/Pre-obese	25.00–29.99
Obese	≥30.00
Obese Class I	30.00–34.99
Obese Class II	35.00–39.99
Obese Class III	≥40.00

○ **What health risks are associated with obesity?**

The risk of stroke, ischemic heart disease, and diabetes mellitus in patients with a BMI > 28 is three to four times the risk of that seen in the general population. In addition, obese patients are at increased risk of obstructive sleep apnea, osteoarthritis, gout, cancer, chronic kidney disease, gallstones, nonalcoholic fatty liver disease (NAFLD), and gastroesophageal reflux disease (GERD).

○ **True/False: The distribution of fat over the body is important with respect to morbidity and mortality.**

True. A higher risk of morbidity and mortality is more strongly associated with a central distribution than with a peripheral distribution of body fat.

○ **True/False: Adipose tissue is an endocrine organ.**

True. Active research into obesity has revealed that adipose cells have a potent endocrine function producing multiple adipokines, which primarily work in conjunction with central nervous system and gut hormones to control hunger, satiety, and lipid metabolism. Adipokines exert a pleiotropic effect on the body and may play a role in inflammation, immune response, vasoregulation, insulin resistance, and the development of metabolic syndrome. Three important adipokines include leptin, adiponectin, and tumor necrosis factor (TNF)-alpha.

○ **True/False: The goal when treating obesity is to achieve normal body weight.**

False. The goal is reduction of health risks. Even modest weight loss can alleviate symptoms from obesity-related comorbidities.

○ **True/False: A calorie- and fat-reduced diet is the most successful nonsurgical treatment for obesity.**

False. Data are insufficient to recommend any specific diet. A multidisciplinary individualized approach including nutrition counseling, regular activity, and reinforcement of behavioral modification is considered the most successful nonsurgical approach.

○ **When is bariatric surgery recommended?**

The consensus guidelines from NIH published in 1991 are still generally accepted today. These include the following:
- Well-informed and motivated patient.
- Patient's BMI >40.
- Patient's BMI >35 and existence of serious comorbidities such as sleep apnea, cardiomyopathy, joint disease, or diabetes.
- Patient has acceptable risk profile for surgery.
- Patient failed previous nonsurgical methods of weight loss.

○ **What are the roles of the counter regulatory hormones ghrelin and leptin?**

Ghrelin is produced in the stomach and promotes hunger. In contrast, leptin is derived from adipocytes and helps reduce hunger. In obesity, these counter regulatory roles become perturbed. In obese individuals, ghrelin is not suppressed after eating, which results in continued hunger. In addition, leptin levels are elevated in obese individuals, but the body becomes resistant to its effects, and thus, leptin does not reduce satiety as it does in nonobese individuals.

○ **True/False: Pharmacotherapy is recommended for all patients with obesity.**

False. Drug treatment can be useful in combination with diet and exercise. It is recommended for people with BMI >30 with no comorbidities or BMI >27 with comorbidities.

○ **Which neuropeptide plays a major role in the central control of appetite?**

Neuropeptide Y—a potent-appetite stimulant.

○   **True/False: Roux-en-Y gastric bypass is the most common surgical procedure recommended in the treatment of obesity.**

True. Roux-en-Y gastric bypass surgery and the adjustable gastric band have become the most common bariatric procedures used in severely obese patients.

○   **True/False: Jejunoileal bypass for morbid obesity is rarely performed because of a high incidence of serious intestinal and liver complications.**

True. In addition, a characteristic arthropathy may complicate the postoperative course.

○   **True/False: Morbidly obese individuals are at lower risk of malnutrition than normal weight individuals.**

False. Overweight individuals are at higher risk of malnutrition. Up to 30% of obese individuals will be vitamin D deficient. In addition, obese patients may be deficient in antioxidants, calcium, and other important nutrients.

○   **List nutritional deficiencies in identified patients who have undergone Roux-en-Y gastric bypass.**

The main nutritional deficiencies include:
- Protein
- Vitamin D
- Calcium
- Iron
- Thiamine
- Vitamin B12
- Folic acid
- Copper

○   **True/False: Kidney stones are a long-term complication of gastric bypass surgery.**

True. Patients who have undergone gastric bypass surgery commonly have problems with calcium and vitamin D absorption and develop secondary hyperparathyroidism, which may result in metabolic bone disease and kidney stones.

○   **True/False: Weight loss after Roux-en-Y gastric bypass surgery generally continues for 2–3 years before the weight stabilizes.**

False: Most patients' weight stabilizes approximately 12–18 months after surgery. Continued weight loss may be a sign of a complication of the surgery.

○   **What is the generally accepted short-term mortality of bariatric surgery?**

The 30-day mortality from bariatric surgery appears to be less than or equal to 1%. One recent prospective cohort study from 10 centers in the United States captured 6118 patients who underwent primary bariatric surgery. Eighteen deaths (0.3%) occurred within 30 days of surgery.

According to the most recent Cochrane review, bariatric surgery appears beneficial, but long-term morbidity and mortality studies are ongoing and data are limited.

● ● ● SUGGESTED READINGS ● ● ●

Treasure J, Claudino AM, Zucker N. Eating disorders. *Lancet.* 2010 Feb 13;375(9714):583-593.

Flegal KM, Carroll MD, Ogden CL, Curtin LR. Prevalence and trends in obesity among US adults, 1999–2008. *JAMA.* 2010;303(3): 235-241.

NIH conference. Gastrointestinal surgery for severe obesity. Consensus Development Conference Panel. *Ann Intern Med.* 1991;115(12): 956-961.

American Gastroenterological Association medical position statement on obesity. *Gastroenterology.* 2002;123(3):879-881.

Bal B, Koch TR, Finelli FC, Sarr MG. Managing medical and surgical disorders after divided Roux-en-Y gastric bypass surgery. *Nat Rev Gastroenterol Hepatol.* 2010;7(6):320-334.

Section VIII HEPATOLOGY

CHAPTER 45 Acute Liver Failure and Liver Transplantation

Timothy M. McCashland, MD

○ **What are the hallmark diagnostic signs of acute liver failure (ALF)?**

Encephalopathy and coagulopathy. When the international normalization ratio (INR) is greater than 1.5 and encephalopathy is present within 8 weeks of the beginning of the illness, the diagnosis is secure.

○ **Criteria for poor outcome in cases of acetaminophen-induced ALF include:**

Prothrombin time > 50 s, pH < 7.3, and grade 4 encephalopathy.

○ **A 43-year-old woman with Wilson's disease presents with grade 3 encephalopathy and jaundice. Family members discover that she has not taken her penicillamine over the last few weeks. What treatment does her current clinical condition require?**

Liver transplantation. Restarting penicillamine has shown little efficacy in this setting.

○ **A 25-year-old woman in her third trimester of pregnancy presents with jaundice, confusion, and right upper quadrant (RUQ) pain. Laboratory evaluation reveals marked anemia, severe thrombocytopenia, and elevated liver tests. What would be the most appropriate management?**

Rapid delivery of the baby with appropriate clotting factor support. HELLP syndrome (hemolysis, elevated liver enzymes, and low platelets) is associated with rapid liver failure, usually in the third trimester of pregnancy, and is a medical emergency.

○ **When should a patient with ALF be transferred to a transplant center?**

Any patient with encephalopathy of grade 2 or more.

○ **What are the most common causes of ALF in the United States?**

Acetaminophen toxicity, indeterminate, other medications, and acute viral hepatitis (types A and B).

○ **What is the most common cause of death in ALF while awaiting liver transplantation?**

Cerebral edema. Cerebral edema is reported in 80% of those dying from ALF.

○   **True/False: Survival after liver transplantation for ALF is comparable to transplantation for end-stage liver disease.**

False. Survival after transplantation for ALF ranges from 46% to 89% (66% average). The lower survival is related to the presence of multiple organ failure at the time of transplantation.

○   **The neurological exam of a patient with ALF begins to deteriorate. What should you do?**

Sequential management of cerebral edema includes elevation of head of bed 10–20 degrees, hyperventilation, administration of mannitol, and induction of a pentobarbital coma. Intracranial pressure monitoring may be very helpful in this situation.

○   **True/False: Survival of patients with ALF is related to their grade of encephalopathy at the time of transplantation.**

True. Grade 1—90%, grade 2—71%, and grade 3 or 4—48%.

○   **Poor prognostic variables in non-acetaminophen-induced ALF include:**

An INR >3.5, age <10 or >40, drug-induced, indeterminate cause, duration of jaundice >7 days, and bilirubin >30 mg/dL.

○   **True/False: A 40-year-old man with ALF of unknown etiology (indeterminate) is febrile and has an elevated leukocyte count. He should immediately be listed for liver transplantation.**

False. Contraindications to liver transplantation include active infection and severe cerebral edema. Infection at the time of transplantation has contributed to death in about 11% of patients. Up to 36% of patients with ALF have been reported to develop bacteremia. Cerebral perfusion pressure of <40 mmHg for longer than 1 h makes neurological recovery unlikely.

○   **What are the most common infections that occur in ALF?**

Pneumonia (50%) followed by bacteremia (26%) and urinary tract infection (22%).

○   **A 35-year-old woman with acetaminophen-induced ALF is persistently febrile despite being on broad-spectrum antibiotics. What infectious organism should you suspect?**

Fungal infections are common in ALF (13%–32%). *Candida albicans* is the most common fungal organism identified.

○   **What is the cause of renal failure associated with ALF?**

Renal failure develops in 43%–80% of cases, depending on the etiology of liver failure. Acetaminophen may cause direct injury to the distal tubules of the kidney; however, most cases result from a decrease in renal blood flow as a consequence of vasoconstriction. This is similar to what occurs in hepatorenal syndrome.

○   **The use of what medications/substances, when taken chronically, results in a higher risk of ALF with concomitant acetaminophen use?**

Any medication that induces the cytochrome P450 system in the liver may enhance ALF with acetaminophen. The most common medications in this setting are alcohol, phenytoin, and antidepressants.

○   **A 20-year-old male bodybuilder presents with jaundice, confusion, and bruises. What is the most likely cause of ALF in this setting?**

Anabolic steroids, when used in high doses, may result in ALF.

○ **A family of campers that just recently returned from a camping trip presents to their physician with diarrhea and confusion. Liver tests and serum creatinine are elevated. What are your diagnosis, treatment, and prognosis?**

Amanita phalloides poisoning presents with diarrhea, neurological changes, and signs of hepatorenal failure. Children below the age of 10 have the highest rate of fatality with an overall death rate of 20%. Initial management with high-dose penicillin has shown some benefit.

○ **A 45-year-old woman presents to your office 4 days following laparoscopic cholecystectomy with nausea, vomiting, fever, and diffuse myalgias. Evaluation reveals the aminotransferase levels to be over four times greater than normal. What diagnosis do you suspect?**

Idiosyncratic hepatic injury due to anesthetic drugs is reported in up to 1 in 9000 cases. The usual interval from surgery to presentation is 3–5 days but can be up to 15 days. Halothane is considered the classic example of anesthetic-induced liver injury.

○ **What is the single most important factor limiting liver transplantation in the United States?**

The availability of cadaveric donors. Approximately 6000 liver transplants are performed each year; however, up to 10,000 potential candidates are identified each year. As many as 15% of patients die, waiting for a liver transplant.

○ **Liver transplant candidates are matched to the cadaveric donor by what variables?**

Weight (liver size limit) and blood type.

○ **How does a transplant center prioritize who receives a transplant?**

The United Network for Organ Sharing (UNOS) in 2002 implemented the Model for End Stage Liver Disease (MELD) score as the means to prioritize candidates on the waiting list. Highest priority is for fulminant liver failure as status 1 patients. All others are allocated by MELD scores, with patients with the highest score receiving the highest priority.

○ **What are contraindications to liver transplantation?**

Extrahepatic malignancy, sepsis, active alcoholism, psychosocial issues, and advanced cardiorespiratory disease.

○ **For patients with alcoholic liver disease, what is the usual period of abstinence before consideration of liver transplantation?**

Most programs require a period of abstinence of at least 6 months with adequate support systems and compliance with medical care.

○ **True/False: Spontaneous bacterial peritonitis is a contraindication to liver transplantation.**

False. Antibiotic treatment for 2–5 days is associated with high bacteriologic cure.

○ **True/False: Hepatorenal syndrome is a contraindication to liver transplantation.**

False. Hepatorenal syndrome may be reversed by liver transplantation.

○ **True/False: Waiting times for liver transplantation are equal throughout the United States.**

False. There is great variability in waiting times due to availability of donors in the UNOS designated geographical regions.

○ **What are the most common medications used for immunosuppression after liver transplantation?**

Cyclosporine, tacrolimus (FK 506), mycophelolate mofetil, and prednisone.

○ **What is the mechanism of action of cyclosporine and tacrolimus (FK 506)?**

Both inhibit early T-cell signal pathways and interleukin-2 production and release.

○ **True/False: A 32-year-old female presents to the emergency room with nausea, vomiting, and mildly decreased mental status. Liver tests are notable for an alanine aminotransferase (ALT) of 5120 U/L, aspartate aminotransferase (AST) of 3560 U/L, bilirubin of 6.9 mg/dL, and INR of 3.5. Acute viral serologies are negative, as are antinuclear antibody, antismooth muscle antibody, drug screen, and acetaminophen levels. N-Acetylcysteine use has been shown to improve the survival of patients in this scenario.**

True. Intravenous N-acetylcysteine (NAC) was shown to improve transplant-free survival in patients with early stage encephalopathy (grades I–II) in nonacetaminophen-related ALF patients. Survival in the NAC group was 52% versus 30%. Indeterminate etiology is the third leading cause of ALF in the United States.

○ **A 52-year-old female with a history of tuberculosis presents to the hospital with new onset rash, confusion, and severe jaundice. Liver tests reveal an ALT of 3210 U/L, AST of 2505 U/L, bilirubin of 20.5 mg/dL, and INR of 4.0. Further history reveals she started treatment for the tuberculosis 3 weeks prior. What are the most common causes of drug-induced liver injury–ALF (DILI-ALF)? What is the prognosis in patients with nonacetaminophen DILI?**

The most common causes of DILI-ALF are antimicrobials (antituberculosis > sulfa drugs > nitrofurantoin > antifungal), psychoactive drugs, nonprescription medications, dietary supplements, and weight loss treatments. Transplant-free survival is extremely poor, approximately 25%, in DILI cases.

○ **Multiple prognostic models have been proposed to predict outcome and requirement for emergency liver transplantation in ALF. The most common model applied is the Kings College Hospital criteria for acetaminophen and nonacetaminophen etiologies. What variables are used in the Kings College Hospital criteria?**

Nonacetaminophen: Prothombin time (PT) >100 s (INR >6.5) and encephalopathy or any three of the following: Patient age <10 or >40 years, bilirubin >30 mg/dL, duration of jaundice >7 days, PT >50 s (INR >3.5), nonhepatitis A/B, or drug etiology.

Acetaminophen: Arterial pH <7.3, PT >100 s (INR >6.5), serum creatinine >3.0 mg/dL, and encephalopathy grade III–IV.

○ **What diseases for which transplantation is performed may recur following liver transplantation?**

Hepatitis C is the most common recurrent disease. Hepatitis B can recur if not adequately treated posttransplant. Autoimmune diseases such as primary biliary cirrhosis, primary sclerosing cholangitis, and autoimmune hepatitis have also been reported to recur after transplant.

○ **At present, what liver disease represents the most common indication for liver transplantation?**

Chronic hepatitis C, followed by hepatocellular carcinoma (HCC), alcoholic liver disease, cholestatic liver disease, cryptogenic liver disease, and metabolic liver disease.

○ **How is recurrent hepatitis B prevented following liver transplantation?**

Excellent patient and graft survival is now possible with pre- and postliver transplant use of nucleos(t)ide medications with posttransplant use of hepatitis B immune globulin (HBIG).

○ **True/False: Survival following liver transplant for chronic hepatitis C (HCV) is inferior to non-HCV chronic liver disease causes.**

True. One- and five-year survival after transplantation for chronic hepatitis C is generally good; however, survival is slightly worse (10%–15% lower) compared to other nonmalignant chronic liver disease etiologies.

○ **True/False: A 50-year-old man with chronic hepatitis C presents with worsening ascites. Ultrasound reveals a single 3-cm lesion in the right lobe of the liver. This patient is still a liver transplant candidate.**

True. The following variables have been found to correlate with poor prognosis: single tumor size greater than 5 cm, multiple lesions (>3), vascular invasion, and noncircumscribed shape. Nevertheless, survival remains comparable to other etiologies for liver transplantation if the patient falls within Milan HCC criteria (single lesion <5 cm, 3 or fewer lesions, the largest <3 cm).

○ **A potential liver transplant recipient asks you during a clinic visit about differences in the risks and complications between living-related liver transplantation versus deceased-donor liver transplantation. What are the differences?**

Living-related liver transplantation in comparison to deceased-donor liver transplantation is associated with higher rates of biliary leak (31% versus 10%), unplanned re-exploration (26% versus 17%), hepatic artery thrombosis (6.5% versus 2.3%), and portal vein thrombosis (3% versus 0%). Despite these potential complications, the 1-year patient and graft survival of living-related transplantation and deceased-donor transplantation is similar.

○ **What are the two biliary anastomosis methods used in liver transplantation and when are they used?**

Choledochocholedochostomy (CDC) and Roux-en-Y choledochojejunostomy. Roux-en-Y choledochojejunostomy is commonly employed when the recipient has biliary tract disease (eg, primary sclerosing cholangitis) and in retransplants.

○ **A 45-year-old woman presents with fever, shortness of breath, and increased liver tests 20 days following liver transplantation. She had steroid resistant rejection 1 week prior and is being treated with antilymphocyte medication. What is the most likely diagnosis?**

Cytomegalovirus (CMV) pneumonitis and hepatitis is common after aggressive immunosuppression and usually occurs within the first month of transplantation. Those highest at risk are patients who are CMV-negative and receive a liver from a CMV-positive donor. Most centers now provide prophylaxis against infection with acyclovir.

○ **What are the most common biliary complications following liver transplantation?**

Biliary strictures and leaks are the most common biliary complications. Eighty percent develop within the first 6 months. Biliary strictures at the anastomosis may be dilated or stented and rarely require surgical revision. Biliary leaks are managed with nasobiliary tubes, stents, or sphincterotomy.

○ **What vaccines are not safe after liver transplantation?**

Live or attenuated vaccines should be avoided (measles, mumps, rubella, oral polio, BCG). Hepatitis A, B, and pneumococcal vaccines, if not given prior to transplantation, should be given.

○ **True/False: Pregnancy is possible in patients following liver transplantation and pregnant transplant recipients should continue their immunosuppression medications.**

True. However, pregnancy after liver transplantation is complicated by a higher rate of prematurity and low birth weight. Immunosuppressive agents should be continued throughout pregnancy.

O **What are the most common neoplasms that occur in recipients of liver transplants?**

The most common neoplasms after liver transplant are skin cancers (both squamous and melanoma) and solid organ tumors (lymphoma > colon > genital/urinary > lung > oropharyngeal/larynx).

O **A 56-year-old male returns to your clinic after receiving a liver transplant 6 months prior with pruritis, mild jaundice, and slightly elevated liver tests. The patient states he received a DCD liver and wonders if this has something to do with his symptoms. What is a DCD donor and what are the common complications associated with DCD donors?**

DCD refers to donation after cardiac death. The use of DCD donors is increasing and now composes more than 5% of all liver transplants in the United States. The most common complications associated with DCD donors are diffuse intrahepatic biliary strictures (similar to primary sclerosing cholangitis) due to ischemia to the bile ducts, a higher risk of primary graft nonfunction, and a higher risk of need for retransplantation.

O **A 60-year-old Asian male with a history of hepatitis B presents with a 4-cm single lesion in the liver by screening ultrasound. Alpha fetoprotein is 250 mg/mL and MRI shows a 4-cm lesion with a washout phase consistent with HCC. What are the listing criteria for HCC for liver transplantation?**

Listing for liver transplantation for patients with HCC is by UNOS policy of patients with T2-defined lesions (2–5 cm) with either a biopsy-proven diagnosis or imaging study consistent with HCC with a washout phase. A MELD score of 22 is assigned to the patient meeting criteria if the patient's calculated MELD score is less than 22. A sequential increase of 10% is applied to the MELD score every 3 months to those remaining on the waiting list.

O **What are the most likely causes of hyperlipidemia following liver transplantation?**

Long-term use of corticosteroids, frequent use of bolus steroids for episodes of rejection, pretransplant hyperlipidemia, and possibly the use of cyclosporine versus tacrolimus. Nearly 40% of patients develop hyperlipidemia posttransplant and require some form of treatment.

● ● ● **SUGGESTED READINGS** ● ● ●

Stravitz RT, Kramer AH, Davern T, et al. Intensive care of patients with acute liver failure: recommendations of the U.S. Acute Liver Failure Study Group. *Crit Care Med.* 2007;35:2498-2508.

Polson J, Lee WM. AASLD position paper: the management of acute liver failure. *Hepatology.* 2005;41:1179-1197.

Thuluvath PJ, Guidinger MK, Fung JJ, et al. Liver transplantation in the United States, 1999–2008. *Am J Transplantation.* 2010; 10(Part 2):1003-1019.

CHAPTER 46

Alcoholic Liver Disease and Nonalcoholic Steatohepatitis

Temitope Foster, MD, MSCR and
Ryan M. Ford, MD

○ **What are the different types of alcohol-induced liver disease?**

Bland reversible steatosis, transaminitis, steatohepatitis, acute alcoholic hepatitis (AAH), and alcohol-induced cirrhosis.

○ **What are the primary risk factors for alcoholic liver disease?**

The amount and duration of alcohol consumption are the most important. Neither the pattern of drinking nor the beverage type is necessarily a risk factor. Genetic factors, environmental factors, and other medical comorbidities also portend risk of chronic liver disease from alcohol.

○ **What percentage of the U.S. population suffers from either alcohol abuse or alcohol dependence?**

Approximately 7%–8%.

○ **What percentage of patients with chronic alcoholism in the United States go on to develop cirrhosis of the liver?**

Approximately 20%–25%.

○ **How is a standard drink of alcohol in the United States defined?**

0.6 fluid ounces of ethanol, which is found in a 12-fluid ounce beer, a 5-fluid ounce glass of wine, or a 1.5-fluid ounce shot of 80-proof spirit. It is important to note that a standard drink is different in different parts of the world (alcohol by volume, etc).

○ **Describe what is meant by "first-pass" metabolism of ethanol and how it may vary among individuals.**

The stomach contains alcohol dehydrogenase (ADH) and may account for up to 10% of "first-pass" metabolism, or oxidation of ethanol before systemic absorption occurs. The dose of ethanol, concomitant food ingestion, and gastric emptying time may affect first-pass gastric metabolism. Also, women, Native Americans, Asians, and the elderly have lower levels of gastric ADH and therefore may absorb more ethanol systemically.

○ **What are the two major pathways of ethanol metabolism in the liver?**

ADH and the microsomal ethanol oxidizing system (MEOS)/cytochrome P450 pathway (CYP2E1).

○ **What are the negative effects of acetaldehyde, a toxic metabolite of ethanol?**

It causes formation of reactive oxygen species and depletes glutathione stores, both of which contribute to ongoing cellular and DNA damage.

○ **What are the threshold levels of daily consumption of alcohol in males and females that may lead to significant liver disease?**

Twenty grams of ethanol per day in women and 80 g of ethanol per day in men.

○ **What countries in the world have the highest daily amount intake of ethanol per adult?**

Russia and Ukraine.

○ **What percentage of individuals with alcoholic liver disease also has antibody positivity to hepatitis C virus (HCV)?**

40%.

○ **What three factors must be present for a diagnosis of alcohol dependence ("alcoholism")?**

Physiological dependence, loss of control, and social/physical impairment.

○ **True/False: Alcohol abuse is the same as alcoholism.**

False. "Alcoholism" refers to alcohol dependence as defined by Diagnostic and Statistical Manual-Fourth Edition-Text Revision (DSM-IV-TR) criteria. Alcohol abuse refers to problematic drinking with consequences.

○ **What tools are available to help a physician screen someone for alcoholism?**

Detailed history, CAGE questions, and Michigan Alcohol Screening Test (MAST). The "CAGE" criteria consist of four questions referring to events occurring within a patient's lifetime. It is a commonly used and practical means of screening for alcoholism and consists of the following questions: have you ever had to "cut-down" on drinking?; have you ever been "annoyed" when people ask about your drinking?; have you ever felt "guilty" about your drinking?; and, have you ever had an "eye-opener" or had to drink alcohol in the morning to avoid feeling badly?

○ **What diseases are associated with nonalcoholic steatohepatitis (NASH)?**

Dyslipidemia, insulin resistance, diabetes mellitus, hypertension, obesity, and the metabolic syndrome.

○ **What commonly prescribed medication can result in the histologic picture of NASH?**

Drugs are responsible for less than 2% of all cases of steatohepatitis. Amiodarone has been shown to independently cause steatohepatitis. Tamoxifen, corticosteroids, and estrogens have also been associated with steatohepatitis, although a causal relationship has not been clearly established and the mechanism is likely through the exacerbation of NASH risk factors.

○ **True/False: Cirrhosis caused by alcoholic liver disease can occur in the absence of necroinflammation, that is, alcoholic hepatitis.**

True.

○ **What is the current hypothesis for the development of alcoholic cirrhosis in the absence of inflammation?**

Ethanol metabolites (ie, acetaldehyde) and products of lipid peroxidation are involved.

○ **What is the most important microsomal ethanol oxidizing enzyme related to the pathogenesis of both alcoholic liver disease and NASH?**

Cytochrome P450 2E1.

○ **True/False: Patients with AAH may show clinical signs of chronic liver disease, despite not having cirrhosis.**

True. Acute hepatic congestion and stellate cell activation can lead to transient portal hypertension. As a result, patients can develop hepatosplenomegaly, ascites, encephalopathy, and/or varices.

○ **True/False: Patients with alcoholic liver disease are at increased risk for acetaminophen toxicity.**

True, due to a lack of glutathione stores and an upregulated cytochrome P450 (CyP2E1) system.

○ **True/False: Ethanol causes only microsteatosis of the liver.**

False. Ethanol can cause both a macrosteatosis and a microsteatosis. Ethanol classically causes a potentially reversible macrosteatosis, but a more serious microsteatosis can develop in the setting of mitochondrial toxicity.

○ **True/False: Mallory's hyaline is pathognomonic for alcohol-induced liver disease.**

False. Mallory's hyaline can be seen with other inflammatory hepatitides, including NASH.

○ **True/False: AAH is more likely to occur in first-time drinkers.**

False. AAH is more likely to occur in habitual drinkers of alcohol.

○ **True/False: AAH is a self-limiting disease with a good prognosis.**

False. AAH is a serious medical condition that can be fatal.

○ **In addition to abstinence, what is the most important therapy for patients with AAH?**

Optimal nutritional support and supplementation.

○ **What is an important prognostic formula to calculate in patients who present with AAH?**

Maddrey discriminant function, which is calculated as follows: $4.6 \times$ (PT-control) + serum bilirubin (mg/dL). A value > 32 is associated with a worse prognosis.

○ **Other than the Maddrey discriminant function, what are some prognostic scoring systems to predict mortality with alcoholic hepatitis?**

Child-Pugh score, model for end-stage liver disease (MELD) score, Lille model, and the Glasgow score.

○ **True/False: A typical patient with AAH will have aminotransferase levels > 400 U/L.**

False. Transaminase levels are almost never elevated above 400 U/L in the setting of AAH alone. Additionally, aspartate aminotransferase (AST) levels generally exceed alanine aminotransferase (ALT) levels in AAH.

○ **True/False: Corticosteroids can improve mortality in some patients with AAH.**

True, in selected groups. A number of clinical trials and meta-analyses have shown benefit in a selected group of patients with AAH.

○ **In which patients should corticosteroids be considered in the treatment of AAH?**

Patients with a Maddrey discriminant function >32 and no evidence of active infection. Those with encephalopathy may also benefit. The presence of renal failure or GI bleeding may be a relative contraindication to steroids.

○ **What dose and what type of corticosteroid should be used?**

Prednisolone 40 mg daily for 4 weeks. Methylprednisolone may also be used at a dose of 32 mg per day. Prednisone 40 mg daily may also be acceptable. Steroids should be tapered down prior to discontinuation.

○ **What is another medication that has been shown to improve mortality and prevent renal failure in severe AAH?**

Pentoxifylline.

○ **True/False: Alcoholic cirrhosis is a risk factor for hepatocellular carcinoma (HCC).**

True. Patients with alcoholic cirrhosis should be screened for HCC every 6 months.

○ **In chronic alcoholics, which epidemiological characteristics have been identified as independent risk factors for HCC?**

Cirrhosis, age greater than 50, male sex, hepatitis B surface antigen positivity, and anti-HCV positivity.

○ **True/False: Alcoholic cirrhosis is currently the second most common indication for liver transplant in the United States.**

True. Hepatitis C is the most common and nonalcoholic fatty liver disease (NAFLD) is the third most common.

○ **How long does a patient need to be abstinent before he/she can be considered for a liver transplant?**

Although controversial, many transplant centers require 6 months of abstinence; however, this is not universal and somewhat arbitrary.

○ **What length of sobriety more accurately indicates a low risk of recidivism?**

5–7 years, although the longer the better.

○ **What are some risk predictors of alcohol relapse?**

Family history of alcoholism, concomitant substance abuse, prior history of relapse, coexisting psychiatric disease, poor social support/structure, noncompliance, and concomitant personality disorder.

○ **What three variables independently increase the risk of progression of alcohol-related hepatic steatosis to cirrhosis?**

Continued alcohol consumption, severity of initial histologic injury, and female gender.

○ **True/False: Patients who undergo liver transplant for alcohol cirrhosis have a lower overall survival than patients who are transplanted for other reasons.**

False.

○ **What is the approximate relapse rate of any alcohol use after liver transplant for patients with alcohol liver disease?**

5%–20%.

○ **True/False: Acetaminophen can be safely given to patients with alcohol cirrhosis. What about nonsteroidal anti-inflammatory drugs (NSAIDs)?**

True. In the setting of abstinence, acetaminophen remains the initial drug of choice to treat pain in patients with alcohol cirrhosis. Generally, the dose should not exceed more than 2–3 g/day. Aspirin and NSAIDs should be avoided due to increased risk of GI bleeding and acute kidney injury.

○ **What other general classes of drugs should be avoided in patients with end-stage liver disease?**

The most important group of drugs to avoid is aminoglycosides as they can precipitate renal failure.

○ **What are the clinical signs/symptoms of alcohol withdrawal or delirium tremens?**

Alcohol withdrawal syndrome is defined by autonomic hyperactivity, manifested by tachycardia, hypertension, diaphoresis, dilated pupils, and anxiety. Delirium tremens is a severe form of withdrawal that includes extreme agitation with delusions or hallucinations. Seizures may also be precipitated in alcohol withdrawal.

○ **What risk factors are associated with delirium tremens?**

Male sex, age >30, 5- to 15-year drinking history, history of withdrawal seizures, and previous history of delirium tremens.

○ **What are some other neurologic syndromes that can occur in alcoholics?**

Wernicke's encephalopathy (nystagmus, ataxia, and confusion), Korsakoff's syndrome (dementia with confabulation due to mamillary body destruction), and peripheral neuropathy. These problems relate to thiamine deficiency.

○ **What is the principal collagen-producing cell in the liver?**

Stellate cell.

○ **True/False: The prevalence of antibody to HCV increases with the severity of underlying alcoholic liver disease.**

True. While there is a 20% prevalence of antibody to HCV in patients with alcoholic hepatitis and 40% in patients with alcoholic cirrhosis, it is found in only 2% of alcoholic patients with normal liver biopsies.

○ **True/False: In aggregate, trials of parenteral and enteral nutritional support indicate that restricted intake of nutrients is associated with a poor prognosis in patients hospitalized with alcoholic liver disease.**

True. Feed the hospitalized alcoholic, especially those with AAH. Enteral nutrition is preferred over parenteral nutrition.

○ **True/False: When faced with a patient with steatosis who drinks some amount of alcohol and who has elevated liver tests, there is a score that can help differentiate between alcohol- and nonalcohol-induced steatohepatitis.**

True. The Mayo alcoholic liver disease/nonalcoholic liver disease index (ANI) score can be useful and uses the variables of age, gender, AST, ALT, mean corpuscular volume (MCV), and body mass index (BMI). The ANI score is most useful in patients with a MELD score less than 20.

○ **What is the typical profile of a NASH patient?**

Middle-aged female with obesity, non-insulin-dependent diabetes mellitus, with or without hyperlipidemia.

○ **Which cytokines have been implicated in the development of NASH?**

Pro-inflammatory cytokines, tumor necrosis factor α (TNF-α), and interleukin 6 (IL-6), have been shown to play a major role in the development of NASH. Levels of TNF-α and IL-6 are elevated in the liver and blood of patients with NASH, and inhibition of these cytokines has improved liver tests in animal models.

○ **True/False: Currently available imaging modalities are relatively insensitive and nonspecific for NASH.**

True. Although a number of noninvasive imaging techniques and scoring systems have been evaluated, liver biopsy remains the gold standard for confirming a clinical suspicion of NASH.

○ **True/False: NASH is histologically indistinguishable from alcohol-induced liver disease.**

True. NASH is, therefore, a diagnosis made after carefully excluding excessive alcohol use defined as greater than 20 g/day in females and 30 g/day in males.

○ **What treatments can be recommended to patients with NASH?**

Treatment consists of modifying the factors that are commonly associated with NASH—vigorous exercise with or without weight loss, actual weight loss, reduction in serum lipids and glucose, and cessation of responsible medications. Medical therapy with vitamin E as well as statin drugs have shown some promise.

○ **What counseling can be given to patients with NAFLD about their overall prognosis?**

The majority of patients with NAFLD have a benign fatty infiltrate that is considered to be nonprogressive. However, it is estimated that up to 10%–25% of those with NAFLD (or 2%–7% of the entire population) will have NASH, a combination of necroinflammation and fibrosis. About 10%–29% of those with NASH will go on to develop cirrhosis over 10 years.

○ **Define focal fatty liver, or fatty sparing.**

An important difference between NAFLD and the above named lesion is that NAFLD is diffuse. Focal fatty liver is incidentally found as a result of improved abdominal imaging techniques. This is not a pathologic diagnosis, needs no treatment, and often regresses.

○ **What are the histologic features of NASH?**

Steatosis in the presence of lobular inflammation and hepatocyte ballooning.

○ **What are the leading causes of increased mortality in patients with NAFLD?**

Currently, the number one cause of mortality is cardiovascular disease followed by nonliver malignancy, then liver-related deaths.

○ **True/False: Patients with NASH can develop HCC in the absence of cirrhosis.**

True. There is now increasing evidence of NASH patients with only stage 1 or 2 fibrosis developing HCC.

○ **What ethnic group in the United States has the highest prevalence of NAFLD?**

Hispanics, followed by Caucasians, then African-Americans.

○ **What gene is associated with the ethnic variation seen in the prevalence of NAFLD?**

Patatin-like phospholipase domain containing 3 gene (PNPLA3) also called adiponutrin. PNPLA3 accounts for approximately 70% of the variation in the prevalence of NAFLD among Hispanics, African-Americans, and Caucasians. The physiological role of PNPLA3 and the mechanism by which it influences fatty liver are not yet known.

○ **How much daily alcohol consumption would make a diagnosis of NAFLD less likely?**

More than 20 g/day in females and 30 g/day in males.

○ **True/False: Patients with NASH typically have elevated transaminases.**

False. Most patients with steatohepatitis have normal liver function tests.

○ **True/False: More than 70% of patients with diabetes have evidence of NAFLD.**

True.

● ● ● SUGGESTED READINGS ● ● ●

Cohen JC, Horton JD, Hobbs HH. Human fatty liver disease: old questions and new insights. *Science.* 2011;332(6037):1519-1523.

Vernon G, Baranova A, Younossi ZM. Systematic review: the epidemiology and natural history of non-alcoholic fatty liver disease and non-alcoholic steatohepatitis in adults. *Aliment Pharmacol Ther.* 2011;34(3):274-285.

Menon KV, Gores GJ, Shah VH. Pathogenesis, diagnosis, and treatment of alcoholic liver disease. *Mayo Clin Proc.* 2001 Oct;76(10): 1021-1029.

Lucey MR, Mathurin P, Morgan TR. Alcoholic hepatitis. *N Engl J Med.* 2009 Jun. 25;360(26):2758-2769.

Dunn W, Jamil LH, Brown LS, et al. MELD accurately predicts mortality in patients with alcoholic hepatitis. *Hepatology.* 2005;41(2): 353-358.

CHAPTER 47

Autoimmune, Cholestatic, and Overlap Liver Disorders

Thomas J. Byrne, MD

○ **What antibodies are associated with type 1 autoimmune hepatitis (AIH)?**

Anti-nuclear antibody (ANA) and/or smooth muscle antibody (SMA). Antibodies against soluble liver antigens (anti-SLA) or liver-pancreas antigen (anti-LP) may also be present in type 1 AIH, particularly in ANA/SMA-negative patients.

○ **What types of autoantibodies are usually present in individuals with type 2 AIH?**

Antibodies to liver/kidney microsomal antigen type 1 (anti-LKM1) and/or antibodies against liver cytosol type 1 (anti-LC1).

○ **True/False: Antinuclear antibodies are highly specific for the diagnosis of AIH.**

False.

○ **True/False: A negative ANA and SMA excludes the diagnosis of type 1 AIH.**

False. AIH is a clinical diagnosis. The International Autoimmune Hepatitis Group has developed criteria and scoring systems for the diagnosis of "definite" and "probable" AIH. Some of the criteria include gender (women scored higher), degree of liver test elevation, presence/degree of serum globulin elevation, type and titer of autoantibodies, viral hepatitis markers (positive serology reduces AIH probability score), use of known or suspected hepatotoxic agents, liver histology, and response to therapy.

○ **How is AIH treated?**

Corticosteroids remain the cornerstone of initial treatment, due to their rapid anti-inflammatory effects on liver histology. A long-term steroid sparing agent is usually begun concomitantly or a short time after initiation of steroids to allow as rapid a steroid taper as possible. Steroid-free management is the goal but is not always achievable. Azathioprine is the most widely used steroid sparing agent but has important potential short-term and long-term risks. Alternatives to azathioprine in selected situations include mycophenolate mofetil, cyclosporine, and tacrolimus. Emerging evidence suggests budesonide may be effective in AIH.

○ **What autoimmune condition is most commonly associated with type 1 AIH?**

Autoimmune thyroiditis. About 15%–20% of patients with type 1 AIH have a concomitant autoimmune disease, thyroid being the most common.

○ **True/False: Several studies have demonstrated an association between human leukocyte antigen (HLA) haplotypes and susceptibility to AIH.**

True. Several studies have shown an association of AIH with HLA. Specific HLA haplotypes include B8, B14, DR3, and DR4. HLA DR3 has been associated with more aggressive disease in some individuals, whereas HLA DR4 may predict a higher likelihood of extrahepatic manifestations.

○ **True/False: Antinuclear antibodies are almost never present in individuals with primary biliary cirrhosis (PBC).**

False.

○ **True/False: AIH, primary sclerosing cholangitis (PSC), and PBC are all more common in women than men.**

False. About 70% of cases of AIH occur in women and 90% of cases of PBC occur in women, but about 60%–70% of cases of PSC occur in men.

○ **True/False: Antimitochondrial antibodies (AMA) occur equally commonly in both PBC and PSC.**

False. AMA are highly associated with PBC, not PSC.

○ **AMA are detectable in the sera of about what percent of cases of PBC?**

Approximately 90%. AMA primarily recognize the E2 subunits of oxoacid dehydrogenase complexes, most frequently, pyruvate dehydrogenase.

○ **PSC is associated with ulcerative colitis in what percentage of affected patients?**

Ulcerative colitis is present in 45%–90% of PSC patients. Biopsy evidence suggests it may be present more often than realized since colonic mucosa may appear grossly normal but demonstrate compatible histological changes of chronic ulcerative colitis.

○ **True/False: The presence of c-antineutrophil cytoplasmic antibodies (c-ANCA) supports the diagnosis of PSC.**

False. Perinuclear antineutrophil cytoplasmic antibodies (p-ANCA), directed against myeloperoxidase, have been reported in 30%–80% of individuals with PSC. c-ANCA, directed against proteinase 3, is commonly present in individuals with Wegener's granulomatosis.

○ **True/False: There is a 25% chance that a sibling of an index patient with PSC will have the same disease.**

False. PSC is not inherited in a Mendelian fashion.

○ **What is the lifetime incidence of cholangiocarcinoma in patients with PSC?**

Patients with PSC have a 10%–15% lifetime incidence of cholangiocarcinoma, though autopsy studies suggest perhaps double this risk. The vast majority of cholangiocarcinoma diagnoses, however, are in patients without PSC.

○ **True/False: Biliary ductal cysts are associated with increased risk for cholangiocarcinoma.**

True. Recognized risks for cholangiocarcinoma include PSC, parasitic liver flukes, choledochal cysts, and hepatolithiasis. Recent evidence suggests metabolic syndrome may be an independent risk factor for cholangiocarcinoma.

○ **True/False: PSC patients who develop hilar cholangiocarcinoma are ineligible for liver transplantation.**

False. Highly selected patients with cholangiocarcinoma, whether or not in the setting of PSC, are eligible for liver transplantation for hilar cholangiocarcinoma. Patients must have limited disease burden radiographically, undergo chemoradiation, be free of extrahepatic disease including mandatory surgical exploration with lymph node sampling, and cannot have had a percutaneous or endoscopic ultrasound (EUS)-guided sampling of tumor due to risk of needle-seeding of cancer cells.

○ **What drug has been shown to prolong the time to death or liver transplantation in PBC?**

Ursodeoxycholic acid.

○ **What are the typical cholangiographic findings in PSC?**

Diffuse multifocal strictures of the biliary tract and multiple areas of ectasia, resulting in a "beading" pattern. Alternatively, some patients have a single or few "dominant" stricture(s) in the common bile duct, the common hepatic duct, or the main right or left biliary duct branches. Finally, small duct PSC is a variant of the disease affecting terminal branches of the biliary tree such that changes are not seen on magnetic resonance cholangiopancreatography (MRCP) or endoscopic retrograde cholangiopancreatography (ERCP) and can only be appreciated histologically.

○ **What are some causes of secondary forms of sclerosing cholangitis?**

The differential diagnosis of sclerosing cholangitis includes autoimmune cholangiopathy (in which serum IgG4 levels may be elevated, and may be associated with autoimmune pancreatitis), radiation-induced cholangitis, ischemic biliary disease (commonly seen after liver transplantation in patients with hepatic arterial stenosis), and AIDS cholangiopathy.

○ **What metabolic bone diseases are associated with chronic cholestatic liver diseases like PBC and PSC?**

Osteoporosis and osteomalacia.

○ **True/False: Intractable pruritis in the face of normal liver function is a valid indication for liver transplantation in cholestatic liver disease.**

True. Intractable itching that has failed to respond to maximal medical efforts is an accepted criterion for liver transplantation. Patients failing medical therapy can receive plasmapheresis with often dramatic and immediate success but the expense and invasive nature (intravenous catheter similar to dialysis) of plasmapheresis render this a nonideal long-term solution. In the setting of intractable pruritis with preserved liver function, patients may not be competitive for transplant via Model for End-Stage Liver Disease (MELD) score, in which case live donor liver transplantation (LDLT) has been used with success.

○ **True/False: Liver biopsy is usually diagnostic in PBC.**

False. The florid bile duct lesion, which is essentially diagnostic for PBC, is only seen in a minority of cases. Usually, the liver biopsy is "consistent with" a diagnosis of PBC.

○ **Ductular proliferation is seen in what histological stage of PBC?**

Stage 2. Stage 1 is the florid bile duct lesion, Stage 3 demonstrates progressive fibrosis, and Stage 4 displays cirrhosis.

○ **True/False: Ursodeoxycholic acid has been shown to improve survival and reduce need for liver transplantation in PSC.**

False. Some patients experience biochemical improvements with ursodeoxycholic acid, but no significant impact on progression of disease or need for liver transplantation has been demonstrated to date. Furthermore, recent data suggest that high-dose ursodeoxycholic acid for the treatment of PSC is associated with higher mortality.

○ **True/False: "Overlap syndrome" refers to the combination of NASH and hepatitis C.**

False. "Overlap syndrome" is a poorly defined term but usually refers to a clinical setting where features of more than one autoimmune and/or cholestatic disease are present. Most commonly, overlap syndrome refers to patients with histological features of AIH, yet are ANA-negative and antimitochondrial antibody-positive (AIH-PBC overlap). This is in distinction to "autoimmune cholangiopathy" in which the histological appearance is that of PBC but with negative antimitochondrial antibody and often positive ANA. Some patients respond biochemically to ursodeoxycholic acid monotherapy, others to ursodeoxycholic acid and typical AIH agents, and some are refractory to therapy. Finally, there is a recognized group of patients with histological (and occasionally serological) features of AIH and cholangiographic evidence of sclerosing cholangitis (AIH-PSC overlap).

○ **True/False: Recurrent bacterial cholangitis is a common complication of PBC.**

False. It is a common complication of PSC.

○ **What rheumatologic diseases are associated with PBC?**

Scleroderma/CREST and Sjögren's syndrome are the most common.

○ **In which liver disease might you order a Schirmer's test?**

PBC. A Schirmer's test is used to detect xerophthalmia, which is a component of Sjögren's syndrome.

○ **True/False: Celiac disease is associated with PBC.**

True, albeit a rare association.

○ **True/False: Elevated serum cholesterol concentrations in AIH are caused by synthesis of an abnormal lipoprotein known as lipoprotein X.**

False. Elevated serum cholesterol concentrations are not associated with AIH. Lipoprotein X is synthesized in association with increased serum cholesterol concentrations in long-standing bile duct obstruction. This is commonly seen in individuals with PBC.

○ **True/False: Epidemiological studies have shown an association between PBC and coronary artery disease.**

False. Although serum cholesterol concentrations are elevated in many individuals with PBC, an association with coronary artery disease has not been demonstrated.

○ **A 56-year-old woman presents with pruritis. Blood tests reveal an elevated serum alkaline phosphatase. AMA are present in serum at a titer of 1:640. Liver ultrasound is normal. What is the diagnosis and what is the role of liver biopsy in this setting?**

PBC. A positive antimitochondrial antibody is 90% sensitive for the diagnosis of PBC. Such a patient could be treated with ursodeoxycholic acid without further testing. A liver biopsy is indicated for staging purposes and to look for confirmatory histology. However, the lack of classic features on biopsy, not uncommon early in the course of PBC, does not exclude a PBC diagnosis, which is made on clinical grounds.

○ **A 43-year-old man with a history of ulcerative colitis presents with jaundice. Routine laboratory testing demonstrates an elevated serum bilirubin concentration and elevated serum alkaline phosphatase. His weight has been stable. He complains of itching. An ultrasound examination of the liver, gallbladder, and bile ducts is normal. What test should be ordered next?**

MRCP. This test has essentially replaced ERCP as the first-line diagnostic modality in cases of suspected PSC. ERCP should be done if MRCP reveals a suspicious stricture worrisome for malignancy or choledocholithiasis or is nondiagnostic.

○ **True/False: AIH is strongly associated with systemic lupus erythematosus (SLE).**

False. There is no strong association between AIH and SLE despite the historical term "lupoid hepatitis."

○ **True/False: Patients with cirrhosis as a result of PBC are generally poor candidates for orthotopic liver transplantation.**

False. PBC as a transplant diagnosis is associated with arguably the longest post transplant survival.

○ **How frequently, and by what modality, should patients with PSC be screened for cholangiocarcinoma?**

There are no evidence-based guidelines regarding whether to screen and, if so, how frequently and by what modality. This cancer should be considered with new onset PSC and in patients with high-grade strictures (in which case biliary brushings and fluorescent in situ hybridization [FISH] sampling at ERCP should be done). Finally, a change in the course of long-standing PSC, such as progressive episodes of cholangitis, progressive pruritis, anorexia, or weight loss, should prompt consideration of cholangiocarcinoma. MRCP may be used as an initial diagnostic test but cannot reliably distinguish benign from malignant stricture.

○ **True/False: CA 19-9 is considered a highly reliable marker for cholangiocarcinoma in the setting of PSC.**

False. CA 19-9 demonstrates both poor sensitivity and specificity for cholangiocarcinoma but may prompt suspicion when markedly elevated.

○ **What agents have been shown to be effective in the treatment of pruritis in individuals with cholestatic liver disease?**

Diphenhydramine, hydroxyzine, cholesterol binding resins such as cholestyramine, opioid antagonists such as naloxone and naltrexone, and rifampin. Recent studies have suggested a benefit from sertraline. Ursodeoxycholic acid is generally ineffective as an antipruritic.

○ **True/False: In about 60% of cases of AIH, infection with the hepatitis C virus is thought to be a triggering factor.**

False.

○ **The term "nonsuppurative cholangitis" best describes the histopathological lesion in what liver disease?**

PBC.

● ● ● **SUGGESTED READINGS** ● ● ●

Makol A, Watt KD, Chowdhary VR. Autoimmune hepatitis: a review of current diagnosis and treatment. *Hepat Res Treat.* 2011; 2011:390916. Epub 2011 May 15.

Boberg KM, Chapman RW, Hirschfield GM, Lohse AW, Manns MP, Schrumpf E; International Autoimmune Hepatitis Group. Overlap syndromes: the International Autoimmune Hepatitis Group (IAIHG) position statement on a controversial issue. *J Hepatol.* 2011;54(2):374-385.

Mendes F, Lindor KD. Primary sclerosing cholangitis: overview and update. *Nat Rev Gastroenterol Hepatol.* 2010;7(11):611-619.

Hohenester S, Oude-Elferink RP, Beuers U. Primary biliary cirrhosis. *Semin Immunopathol.* 2009;31(3):283-307.

CHAPTER 48 Cirrhosis and Its Complications

Bhupinderjit S. Anand, MD

○ **Define cirrhosis.**

Cirrhosis refers to a diffuse disease in which the normal architecture of the liver is replaced by abnormal nodules (pseudonodules that lack the lobular arrangement of a normal liver) that are separated by bands of fibrous tissue. In the United States, cirrhosis affects about 3.5 people out of 1000.

○ **True/False: Cirrhosis is an irreversible disease.**

False (sort of). Although it has long been held that cirrhosis is irreversible, reversal of cirrhosis has now been documented after treatment of the underlying cause of cirrhosis.

○ **What symptoms commonly occur in cirrhosis?**

Patients with cirrhosis frequently experience generalized weakness, fatigue, poor appetite, and weight loss.

○ **What are the most recognized causes of cirrhosis?**

There are many causes of cirrhosis. The most recognized causes of cirrhosis include chronic alcohol abuse, viral infections of the liver (especially hepatitis B and C), nonalcoholic fatty liver disease, hereditary hemochromatosis, primary biliary cirrhosis, primary sclerosing cholangitis, and autoimmune liver disease.

○ **What classical physical findings may be seen in the cirrhotic patient?**

Spider angioma: These consist of a central artery with radiating smaller vessels. Pressure on the artery causes the spider to disappear. When the pressure is released, blood flows back from the artery to the smaller vessels.

Palmar erythema: Erythema of the thenar and hypothenar areas with sparing of the central palms.

Gynecomastia: Enlargement of breasts in men.

Testicular atrophy.

Enlargement of liver and spleen.

Asterixis: Flapping motions of the outstretched hands.

○ **What are the common complications of cirrhosis?**

Fluid accumulation (edema and ascites), variceal bleeding, spontaneous bacterial peritonitis, hepatic encephalopathy, renal failure (hepatorenal syndrome [HRS]), coagulopathy, hepatocellular carcinoma, and malnutrition.

○ **True/False: Malnutrition is the most prevalent complication of cirrhosis.**

True. The prevalence correlates with the severity of the liver disease and the method of nutritional assessment.

○ **What are the causes of malnutrition in chronic liver disease?**

Reduced food intake, prescribed diets limited in fat and protein ("liver diets"), maldigestion, malabsorption, and hypermetabolism.

○ **True/False: The evidence supporting branched chain amino acid supplementation in cirrhosis is limited and generally nonsupportive.**

True.

○ **What is portal hypertension?**

An increase in the pressure in the portal circulation is called portal hypertension. The normal portal pressure is less than 5 mmHg. A portal pressure >12 mmHg is generally considered to constitute clinically significant portal hypertension. Since it is difficult to directly measure the portal pressure, an indirect method is used. This involves measuring the hepatic vein pressure gradient (HVPG), which is the difference between wedged hepatic vein pressure and free hepatic vein pressure. HVPG closely reflects the portal pressure.

○ **At what pressure do esophageal varices form and when do they bleed?**

An HVPG >12 mmHg is required for the formation of esophageal varices. Similarly, variceal bleeding occurs only when HVPG is >12 mmHg. The higher the HVPG, the greater is the risk of bleeding. However, there is no absolute level of HVPG that correlates with the risk of bleeding.

○ **True/False: Esophageal varices develop in 25% of patients with alcoholic cirrhosis within 10 years of diagnosis.**

False. Nearly 80% patients with alcoholic cirrhosis develop esophageal varices within 10 years of diagnosis. The risk is somewhat less in cirrhosis due to hepatitis C virus infection.

○ **What is the magnitude of the risk of bleeding in a patient with esophageal varices?**

Nearly 30% patients with cirrhosis who have large varices experience variceal bleeding, usually within the first year of diagnosis.

○ **How common are recurrent episodes of variceal bleeding?**

If left untreated, patients who have experienced an episode of bleeding have a 70% chance of recurrent bleeding within 6 months.

○ **What is the mortality rate of acute variceal bleeding?**

Variceal hemorrhage is a serious medical emergency. Each episode of bleeding is associated with about a 30% risk of death.

○ **What are the predictors of increased risk of variceal bleeding?**

Factors associated with increased risk of bleeding include large varices, presence of endoscopic stigmata on the varices such as cherry red spots and red wale sign, and advanced liver disease.

○   **What is the treatment of choice for acute variceal bleeding?**

First-line treatment consists of combination of endoscopic treatment such as endoscopic variceal ligation (EVL) or sclerotherapy, and vasoactive drugs that reduce the portal pressure. The drug used most commonly is somatostatin or its synthetic analogue, octreotide.

○   **Is there a difference in the results obtained between endoscopic sclerotherapy (EST) and EVL.**

EST (injection of a sclerosing agent into varices) and EVL (placing a rubber band on the varices) are designed to obliterate varices. EVL has become the preferred option as it is associated with fewer complications and lower rates of rebleeding, and requires fewer sessions to achieve variceal obliteration.

○   **What drugs are effective in reducing portal pressure?**

Portal pressure-reducing drugs are divided into two categories: 1) vasoconstrictors (vasopressin, somatostatin, and beta-blockers) cause splanchnic vasoconstriction and reduce portal blood flow; and 2) vasodilators (nitrates and prazosin) decrease the vascular resistance of the intrahepatic portal vessels.

○   **What is the treatment for patients with acute variceal bleeding who fail first-line (endoscopic/medical) therapy?**

About 15% patients continue to bleed despite endoscopic and medical measures. The next line of treatment is the use of the transjugular intrahepatic portosystemic shunt (TIPS) or a surgical shunt. A device to tamponade the varices (eg, Sengstaken–Blakemore and Minnesota tubes) and slow the bleeding may need to be inserted while awaiting these shunt procedures.

○   **What are the two main complications of the TIPS procedure?**

The two most important complications are development of hepatic encephalopathy and shunt closure, which may result in variceal rebleeding. With the recent introduction of covered stents, the incidence of shunt closure has decreased substantially.

○   **True/False: Patients with Child's class C cirrhosis are optimal candidates for shunt surgery.**

False. Patients with well-compensated cirrhosis (Child's class A) are the best candidates for shunt surgery, when appropriate. The distal splenorenal shunt (splenic vein to renal vein) has gained favor since it is associated with a lower risk of hepatic encephalopathy compared to a portocaval shunt.

○   **What is portal hypertensive gastropathy?**

This term refers to the development of vascular congestion of the gastric mucosa in patients with portal hypertension. Less frequently, other parts of the gastrointestinal tract may be involved (eg, portal hypertensive colopathy, when the colonic mucosa becomes congested). Portal hypertensive gastropathy may result in chronic blood loss and anemia.

○   **What is the treatment of portal hypertensive gastropathy?**

The treatment is to lower the portal pressure with the use of vasoactive agents such as nonselective beta-blockers. If this fails, the TIPS procedure has been shown to be useful and may be considered.

○   **True/False: Varices may form in areas of the gastrointestinal tract other than the esophagus.**

True. Varices can develop anywhere in the gastrointestinal tract. After the esophagus, the next most common site is the stomach. Bleeding from extra-esophageal varices is difficult to control by endoscopic means. Initial treatment is with beta-blockers. If unsuccessful, the patients are considered for TIPS, surgical shunt, or liver transplantation.

○ **How can the first episode of variceal hemorrhage be prevented?**

Individuals at high risk of bleeding (presence of large varices and advanced liver disease) should be treated with nonselective beta-blockers (eg, propranolol, nadolol, and carvedilol). Those who are unable to tolerate these drugs can be treated with EVL, which is equally effective in the primary prevention of variceal bleeding.

○ **What are the treatment options for patients with recurrent episodes of variceal bleeding?**

The best approach is combined treatment with EVL (continued until the varices are completely obliterated) and nonselective beta-blockers. If bleeding recurs despite these measures, TIPS, surgical shunt, or liver transplantation should be considered.

○ **What are the characteristics of ascites in a cirrhotic patient?**

The ascitic fluid in cirrhosis has low albumin content and the serum to ascitic fluid albumin gradient (SAAG) is ≥1.1. SAAG value of ≥1.1 is characteristic of portal hypertension but may also be seen in congestive heart failure and myxedema. By contrast, SAAG <1.1 is seen in tuberculous peritonitis, carcinomatosis, pancreatic ascites, and nephrotic syndrome.

○ **Describe the treatment of cirrhotic ascites.**

The most important step is to obtain a negative sodium balance. This is achieved by reducing the sodium intake to <88 mmol [2 g]/day. In addition, a combination of the diuretics, spironolactone and furosemide (in a ratio of 100 mg:40 mg, respectively) is given. The maximum doses are 400 mg and 160 mg, respectively.

○ **True/False: Diuretic-refractory ascites and diuretic-resistant ascites refer to the same process.**

False. Diuretic-refractory ascites refers to persistent ascites despite sodium restriction and maximal diuretic therapy. Diuretic-resistant ascites refers to the development of diuretic-induced complications, which prevent the use of effective diuretic therapy. The most common complications are renal failure and electrolyte abnormalities.

○ **What are the treatment options for diuretic-refractory and diuretic-resistant ascites?**

Treatment options include periodic large-volume paracentesis and TIPS. A less safe and efficacious technique is the placement of a peritoneo-venous shunt (PVS) (eg, Denver shunt), which drains ascitic fluid into the superior vena cava. The PVS is associated with complications such as infection, disseminated intravascular coagulation, congestive heart failure, and shunt thrombosis. All patients with diuretic-refractory and diuretic-resistant ascites should be considered for liver transplantation if otherwise appropriate.

○ **What is spontaneous bacterial peritonitis (SBP)?**

Patients with cirrhosis and ascites are prone to develop peritonitis without a precipitating cause such as bowel perforation or inflammation, hence the term "spontaneous." The diagnosis is made by the presence of an elevated ascitic fluid neutrophil count of ≥250/mm^3. A positive ascitic fluid culture is obtained in 90% patients and shows a single bacteria (most commonly *Escherichia coli*), unlike surgical peritonitis which is polymicrobial.

○ **What is the usual first-line treatment of spontaneous bacterial peritonitis?**

The antibiotic of choice is a third-generation cephalosporin (eg, cefotaxime 2 g intravenously every 8 hours) for 5 days.

○ **True/False: Recurrence of SBP is rare.**

False. Patients who have experienced an episode of SBP have a 70% probability of a second episode within 1 year. The development of SBP would be another indication for transplant referral in an otherwise acceptable candidate.

○ **True/False: Recurrent episodes of SBP can be prevented.**

True. Long-term administration of the antibiotic norfloxacin (400 mg daily), a poorly absorbed antibiotic reduces the risk of recurrent SBP to 20% from 70% in untreated patients. Trimethoprim-sulfamethoxazole has also been shown to be effective. Those with very low ascites albumin levels seem to benefit the most. However, there are concerns regarding the emergence of drug-resistant organisms with such long-term therapy.

○ **Define HRS.**

HRS is the development of renal failure in patients with advanced liver disease and portal hypertension in the absence of a specific cause for renal failure. Typically, patients have oliguria (urine volume <500 mL/24 h) and low urinary sodium (<10 mEq/L).

○ **Describe the pathogenesis of HRS.**

The pathogenetic mechanism is reduction in renal blood flow. Structurally, the kidneys are normal and can recover completely if the liver disease is reversed or after liver transplantation.

○ **What are the different types of HRS.**

There are two types of HRS. Type I is an acute process with a twofold increase in creatinine to >2.5mg% over 2 weeks. Type II is associated with a more gradual renal failure over several weeks to months.

○ **True/False: The prognosis of individuals with HRS is poor.**

True. The median survival for type I is less than 2 weeks. Survival is longer for patients with type II, but the overall prognosis remains poor.

○ **True/False: Other than liver transplantation, there is no treatment for HRS.**

False. Treatment with a combination of midodrine (alpha-1 adrenergic agonist), a systemic vasoconstrictor (7.5–12.5 mg TID), and octreotide (100–200 µg SQ TID) is associated with significant reduction in mortality compared to no treatment.

○ **What is hepatic encephalopathy?**

The appearance of neuropsychiatric symptoms (mental confusion, personality change, sleep disturbance, unconscious state, or coma) or signs (asterixis, hyperreflexia, muscular rigidity, and decerebrate posturing) in patients with liver dysfunction in the absence of a specific etiology.

○ **What is subclinical (minimal) hepatic encephalopathy?**

Subnormal performance in psychometric tests in the presence of a normal neurological examination. The most commonly performed test is the Reitan trail test in which the time taken by a patient to connect numbers (1 to 25) is determined. Subclinical hepatic encephalopathy is seen in nearly 70% patients with cirrhosis and may be of clinical importance.

○ **True/False: Blood ammonia levels are specific for hepatic encephalopathy.**

False. Hepatic encephalopathy is a clinical diagnosis and is not based on any laboratory test. Blood ammonia levels are not diagnostic of hepatic encephalopathy.

○　**What is the treatment of hepatic encephalopathy?**

The first step is to treat any precipitating factor (infection, fluid/electrolyte disturbance, drug overdose, renal failure, constipation, or high-protein diet). Classically, treatment has consisted of a low-protein diet and the laxative lactulose, in a dose which results in 2 to 3 bowel movements per day. Recently, rifaximin, a nonabsorbable antibiotic, has been approved for the treatment of hepatic encephalopathy.

● ● ● SUGGESTED READINGS ● ● ●

Ginès P, Schrier RW. Renal failure in cirrhosis. *N Engl J Med.* 2009;361:1279-1290.

Runyon BA; AASLD Practice Guidelines Committee. Management of adult patients with ascites due to cirrhosis: an update. *Hepatology.* 2009;49:2087-2107.

Garcia-Tsao G, Sanyal AJ, Grace ND, et al. Prevention and management of gastroesophageal varices and variceal hemorrhage in cirrhosis. *Hepatology.* 2007;46:922-938.

European Association for the Study of the Liver. EASL clinical practice guidelines on the management of ascites, spontaneous bacterial peritonitis, and hepatorenal syndrome in cirrhosis. *J Hepatol.* 2010;53:397-417.

Toris GT, Bikis CN, Tsurouflis GS, Theocharis SE. Hepatic encephalopathy: an updated approach from pathogenesis to treatment. *Med Sci Monit.* 2011;17:RA53-RA63.

Verslype C, Cassiman D. Cirrhosis and malnutrition: assessment and management. *Acta Gastroenterol Belg.* 2010;73:510-513.

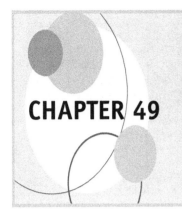

Congenital and Structural Abnormalities and Pediatric Diseases of the Liver

CHAPTER 49

Doron D. Kahana, MD, FAAP, CPNS, Chirag S. Desai, MD, and Khalid M. Khan, MBChB, MRCP

○ **What percentage of the total blood flow is received by the liver?**

About 28%. Seventy-five percent of this comes through the portal vein.

○ **What is the significance of hepatic artery blood supply to the liver?**

The hepatic artery is the sole supply to the bile duct. Thrombosis of hepatic artery can lead to complete bile duct necrosis and can lead to biloma formation and, ultimately, infection and graft loss after liver transplant.

○ **What are the major cell types in the liver?**

Hepatocytes comprise about 60% of the total cell population. Thirty-five percent is of mesenchymal origin (Kupffer, stellate, and sinusoidal endothelial cells). The remaining 5% are bile ductular epithelial cells.

○ **What is the physiological significance of the zonal division of the hepatic acinus?**

Cells are grouped into three zones based on their distance from the portal triad. Cells of zone 1 (periportal area) are closest to nutrient-rich blood and least vulnerable to hypoxia. Zone 3 is the microcirculatory periphery, first to be damaged and last to regenerate after hypoxia. In zones 1 and 2, oxidative processes predominate. In zone 3 (perivenular area), glycolysis is more active. Different pathologies of the liver affect different zones, and the pattern of damage based on zones is useful in the diagnosis.

○ **Which part of the small bowel absorbs most of the bile acids? What is the importance of this absorption in relation to the liver?**

The enterohepatic circulation of bile acids involves the distal ileum. Small amounts are also absorbed from the proximal small bowel and colon. Many drugs (eg, FK506) and nutrients (eg, long-chain fatty acids, fat-soluble vitamins) have bile acid-based absorption. Deficiency of bile acid absorption results in decreased absorption of such drugs and nutrients.

○   **Which of the commonly measured aminotransferases is more liver specific?**

Alanine aminotransferase (ALT) is found predominantly in the cytosol of hepatocytes. Aspartate aminotransferase (AST) is found in the cytosol and mitochondria of hepatocytes and in many extrahepatic tissues, such as red blood cells and muscle. Usually, both are elevated with liver cell damage; however, ALT is considered more specific to liver disease, while an increase in AST out of proportion to ALT suggests an extrahepatic cause (eg, hemolysis, muscle damage, or cardiac event).

○   **What enzymes are used to evaluate cholestasis?**

Alkaline phosphatase, gamma-glutamyl transpeptidase (GGT), and 5'-nucleotidase levels are elevated during cholestasis. The latter is the most specific but least available. Alkaline phosphatase levels may be high in pediatric patients due to active bone growth, rickets, or following a viral infection. The major clinical value of serum GGT is in conferring organ specificity to an elevated value for alkaline phosphatase since GGT activity is not increased in patients with bone disease.

○   **What coagulation factors are synthesized in the liver and what test is used to indirectly assess them?**

Factors I, II, V, VII, IX, and X are synthesized in the liver. The prothrombin time (PT), a test that evaluates the extrinsic pathway, is prolonged when any of these factors are deficient, either alone or in combination. In liver failure, these coagulation factors are significant prognosticators for recovery. Serum levels of factors V and II are extremely useful in deciding indication for transplant in fulminant hepatic failure and in many European countries they are primary indicators for listing for transplant. Typically, factors V and VIII are used in clinical practice. The latter is an endothelial factor and, therefore, should be normal in liver disease. If both are abnormal, sampling issues should be excluded.

○   **In addition to liver synthetic failure, what are the other causes of a prolonged PT?**

Congenital coagulation factor deficiency, consumptive coagulopathy, disseminated intravascular coagulation, treatment with coumadin, and vitamin K deficiency.

○   **What are the vitamin K-dependent coagulation factors?**

Factors II, VII, IX, and X. In theory, comparison of factors V and VII levels should differentiate liver disease from vitamin K deficiency. Clinically, a factor V level after administration of intravenous vitamin K is the most practical way to assess the nature of a prolonged PT.

○   **True/False: The liver edge is normally palpable in children.**

True. The right lobe may be up to 3.5 cm below the costal margin during the first 6 months, 3 cm below before 4 years, and 2 cm below before 12 years. The upper border is usually in the fifth intercostal space. The latter is important to be aware, particularly in patients with asthma or obstructive airway disease. Percussion of the upper border can help to differentiate true hepatomegaly from downward displacement of the liver with hyperinflation of the lungs.

○   **What is the major source of bilirubin?**

Hemoglobin metabolism accounts for about 80% of produced bilirubin in mammals. Other heme-containing proteins that are degraded to bilirubin include the cytochromes, catalases, and muscle myoglobin. Daily production of bilirubin in a healthy, full-term infant is about 6–8 mg/kg/day and in a healthy adult, it is about 3–4 mg/kg/day.

○ **What is the first enzyme in the pathway converting hemoglobin to bilirubin?**

Microsomal heme oxygenase. This enzymatic reaction results in reduction of the porphyrin iron (Fe^{3+} to Fe^{2+}) and hydroxylation of the alpha methane (=C-) carbon.

○ **True/False: Albumin serves the purpose of bilirubin transport from sites of production to the liver and has a very high affinity for bilirubin?**

True. Bilirubin is taken up into the hepatocyte from the hepatic sinusoids where it is bound by another protein carrier, glutathione S-transferase.

○ **Bilirubin is conjugated within the endoplasmic reticulum with glucuronic acid, the donor of which is?**

Uridine diphosphate (UDP). The enzyme responsible for this conjugation is bilirubin glucuronosyltransferase (BGT).

○ **How do metalloporphyrins prevent neonatal jaundice?**

They block heme oxygenase and prevent bilirubin formation.

○ **What are the two main bile acids in humans?**

Cholic acid and chenodeoxycholic acid are found at a ratio of approximately 1:1 and make up about 75%–80% of the bile acid pool.

○ **Approximately what percentage of the bile acid pool is newly synthesized in adults?**

2%–5%. This percentage can be increased in patients with impaired bile acid reabsorption. About 30 g of bile acids is reabsorbed by the intestines every day (enterohepatic circulation) with about 0.2–0.6 g eliminated in the stool.

○ **True/False: Bile acids make up the majority of the solute load of bile.**

True. Other bile components that exert a solute load and passively draw water into the canaliculi include phospholipids, organic and inorganic anions (eg, chloride), and cholesterol.

○ **What is the rate-limiting enzyme for bile acid synthesis?**

Cholesterol 7α-hydroxylase.

○ **The final step of primary bile acid synthesis is their conjugation with which amino acids?**

Taurine and glycine are added to bile acid intermediates to form conjugated primary bile acids.

○ **What prevents adults from reabsorbing bilirubin via the enterohepatic circulation?**

Bacterial conversion of bilirubin conjugates to urobilinoids. Neonates are at risk for increased intestinal absorption of bilirubin for several reasons including increased amount of beta-glucuronidase in the lumen, which hydrolyzes bilirubin conjugates to bilirubin, absence of intestinal flora to convert bilirubin conjugates to urobilinoids, and a significant amount of bilirubin in meconium.

○ **What constitutes physiological jaundice in the newborn?**

Increased bilirubin levels to 6–8 mg/dL on days 3 to 4. This is likely due to greater mass of erythrocytes, which carry a shorter life span. Most normal neonates experience unconjugated bilirubin levels greater than 1.4 mg/dL in the first few days. Moderate jaundice (>12 mg/dL) occurs in about 12% of breast-fed infants and 4% of formula-fed infants. Severe jaundice (>15 mg/dL) occurs in 2% of breast-fed infants and 0.3% of formula-fed infants.

○   **Which characteristics of neonatal jaundice should lead to further evaluation?**

- Infant appears ill.
- Jaundice <36 h of age.
- Jaundice >10 days of age.
- Bilirubin >12 mg/dL at any time.
- Direct bilirubin >2 mg/dL at any time.

○   **What is breast-feeding jaundice and breast milk jaundice?**

Early onset jaundice (days 2 to 4) is considered breast-feeding jaundice and is likely a consequence of suboptimal fluid and calorie intake in the first days of life coupled with meconium excretion. Breast milk jaundice develops after the first week of life and is thought to be caused by inhibition of bilirubin excretion by factors in breast milk. In some cases, evaluation of hemoglobin, reticulocyte count, peripheral blood smear, liver tests, and coagulation studies may be necessary as blood group incompatibility, hemolysis, and hypothyroidism need to be excluded.

○   **What hereditary hyperbilirubinemias are caused by defects of bilirubin conjugation?**

The autosomal recessive Crigler–Najjar's syndrome type 1 in which bilirubin glucuronyl transferase is completely absent has the worst prognosis. In the autosomal dominant Crigler–Najjar's syndrome type 2 (Arias' syndrome), residual glucuronidase activity provides for a much better prognosis. Gilbert's syndrome is autosomal dominant and benign with hepatic bilirubin clearance reduced by approximately 50% due to impaired glucuronidation.

○   **At what age are familial unconjugated hyperbilirubinemias typically recognized?**

Crigler–Najjar's syndrome types 1 and 2 are recognized in the newborn period while Gilbert's syndrome is usually not discovered until after puberty.

○   **How can Crigler–Najjar's syndrome types 1 and 2 be differentiated from each other?**

By the clinical response to phenobarbital, which induces residual enzyme activity in type 2 and causes a significant drop in total serum bilirubin level.

○   **What is the main risk of Crigler–Najjar's syndrome type 1?**

Kernicterus. Serum bilirubin levels typically range from approximately 15 to 45 mg/dL, and there is risk of both neonatal and later kernicterus.

○   **What is the mainstay of daily treatment while awaiting transplantation for individuals with Crigler–Najjar's syndrome type 1?**

Phototherapy.

○   **True/False: Liver biopsy is indicated for the diagnosis of Gilbert's syndrome.**

False. Unless other biochemical abnormalities are present, a modestly elevated serum unconjugated bilirubin without hemolysis or other laboratory indication of liver disease does not require any further evaluation.

○   **How does bile composition differ in Gilbert's syndrome from normal?**

In Gilbert's syndrome, there are more bilirubin monoglucuronides and less diglucuronides than in normal bile.

○ **What is the genetic marker for Gilbert's syndrome in Caucasians?**

Homozygous state for an extra TA in the TATA promoter region of the BGT gene.

○ **What liver serologies are abnormal in Gilbert's syndrome?**

Total and indirect bilirubin levels.

○ **What is the cause of Dubin–Johnson's syndrome?**

A genetic mutation causing deficient canalicular multispecific organic anion transport (cMOAT) protein in the apical canalicular membrane (cMOAT is also known as MRP2 [multidrug resistance protein]).

○ **How does hepatic pigmentation differentiate Dubin–Johnson's syndrome from Rotor's syndrome?**

Dubin–Johnson's syndrome has black pigment in hepatocytes while Rotor's syndrome does not.

○ **What is the inheritance pattern, treatment, and prognosis of Dubin–Johnson's and Rotor's syndromes?**

Both are autosomal recessive, have good prognoses, and do not require treatment.

○ **Measurement of what urinary component enables differentiation of Rotor's syndrome and Dubin–Johnson's syndrome?**

Urinary coproporphyrins. Total coproporphyrin (I and III) is normal in Dubin–Johnson's syndrome but over 80% is type I. Total coproporphyrin (I and III) is elevated two- to fivefold in Rotor's syndrome and less than 80% is type I.

○ **What is the single test that helps differentiate cholestasis from other forms of jaundice?**

Direct bilirubin: a direct fraction >2 mg/dL or >20% of total bilirubin indicates cholestasis.

○ **What are the three most common causes of cholestasis in infants?**

Extrahepatic biliary atresia (EHBA) and idiopathic neonatal hepatitis are each responsible for about one-third of the cases. Alpha-1 antitrypsin deficiency is found in about 17% of the cases.

○ **What is the best nonsurgical method to differentiate EHBA from idiopathic neonatal hepatitis?**

Liver biopsy. Histological features of EHBA include bile duct proliferation and bile duct plugs, portal fibrosis and edema, and preservation of normal lobular architecture. In neonatal hepatitis, typically there is inflammatory infiltration of the lobule, hepatocellular necrosis, lobular disarray, and mild portal tract disarray. Multinucleated giant cells and pseudoglandular transformation (cells arranged around a dilated canaliculus) can be present in both.

○ **True/False: There is good concordance for EHBA between siblings.**

False. The occurrence of EHBA in siblings is extremely rare.

○ **True/False: Visualization of the gallbladder rules out EHBA.**

False. There still may be distal atresia.

○ **True/False: Pigmented stools exclude EHBA.**

False. Usually pigment in the stool is proof of biliary patency; however, in some cases of severe hyperbilirubinemia, bilirubin can be excreted through the bowel wall and stools can be mildly pigmented even in the presence of EHBA.

○ **True/False: Newborns with EHBA are ill-appearing at birth.**

False. Most are full-term and in good condition. Stools may be pale from the outset but may be initially pigmented in 15%–20%.

○ **What is the Kasai procedure? What is the most effective time for Kasai's procedure to get optimum results and avoid the need for liver transplantation?**

Surgical excision of the whole extrahepatic biliary system and Roux-en-Y anastomosis of an intestinal conduit to the denuded porta hepatis (portoenterostomy). This procedure is best done before 8–10 weeks of age to have a good outcome.

○ **What are the major late complications of the Kasai procedure?**

Cholangitis develops in 40%–60% of the patients during the first year. Portal hypertension leads to esophageal varices in 39% of patients.

○ **True/False: Biliary atresia is the most common indication for liver transplant in pediatrics.**

True, followed by Alagille's syndrome and fulminant hepatic failure.

○ **What is the classical triad of symptoms characteristic of choledochal cysts?**

Abdominal pain, mass, and jaundice. However, this occurs in only 38% of pediatric patients. Frequently, it presents as cholestasis indistinguishable from EHBA, recurrent abdominal pain, recurrent pancreatitis, or acute abdomen resulting from cholangitis or perforation.

○ **What is the most common type of choledochal cyst?**

Type 1, which is saccular or fusiform dilatation of extrahepatic bile duct (EHBD), accounts for 80%–90%.

○ **What is the preferred surgical treatment of choledochal cysts?**

Radical cyst excision, if possible. If there is complicating hepatic disease, portal hypertension, and cholangitis, an initial drainage procedure may be needed with later revision.

○ **What is the histological criterion for the diagnosis of intrahepatic biliary atresia (paucity of interlobular bile ducts [PIBD])?**

The normal ratio of interlobular bile ducts to portal tracts is 0.9–1.8; a ratio less than 0.6 suggests PIBD.

○ **What is Alagille's syndrome?**

Alagille's syndrome is also referred to as arteriohepatic dysplasia or syndromic PIBD. In these patients, intrahepatic biliary atresia is associated with cardiac, facial, ocular, and/or vertebral abnormalities.

○ **What studies are important in the diagnosis of Alagille's syndrome?**

Echocardiography, renal ultrasound, vertebral imaging, and ophthalmologic exam. A liver biopsy, after the first 3 months of life, should be notable for dysplastic or hypoplastic bile ducts.

○ **Alagille syndrome is caused by mutations in which gene?**

Jagged 1 on chromosome 20p12 codes for a ligand in the Notch signaling pathway and is believed to be responsible for the majority of cases. The inheritance is autosomal dominant with variable expression. The estimated incidence is 1:100,000 live births.

○ **What is the typical cardiac defect in Alagille's syndrome?**

Peripheral pulmonary artery stenosis is most common. A cardiac murmur is present in almost all patients.

○ **What eye abnormality is associated with Alagille's syndrome?**

Posterior embryotoxon.

○ **What are some treatment options for pruritus associated with cholestasis?**

Cholestyramine, colestipol, rifampin, phenobarbital, antihistamines, and ursodeoxycholic acid. A diet rich in polyunsaturated fatty acids may promote fecal excretion of bile acids. Ultraviolet light is also believed to be helpful. Opiate antagonists may provide some relief but have not been studied in children. Refractory cases may benefit from partial external diversion of bile flow.

○ **What problems are associated with the administration of cholestyramine?**

Poor palatability, interference with absorption of fat-soluble vitamins, and constipation.

○ **What are the criteria for diagnosing idiopathic neonatal hepatitis?**

Proof of biliary patency and exclusion of all other causes of neonatal cholestasis.

○ **True/False: Giant cell transformation is pathognomonic of idiopathic neonatal hepatitis.**

False. Although more frequently observed in infancy, it can accompany various liver diseases in different ages. The histogenesis of the hepatic giant cell is not clear.

○ **What does the acronym TORCH stand for?**

It was introduced as a reminder of the serologic testing for infectious agents that might cause neonatal hepatitis. T (Toxoplasma), O (Other, eg, syphilis, HIV), R (rubella), C (CMV, coxsackie), H (Herpetoviridae: CMV, EBV, HSV). In practice, the most important infectious agents to rule out are CMV, EBV, and HSV.

○ **What eye abnormality is commonly associated with infectious neonatal hepatitis?**

Chorioretinitis.

○ **Biliary atresia and intracranial calcifications suggest what diagnosis?**

Cytomegalovirus or Toxoplasmosis.

○ **What is the most frequent metabolic cause of cholestasis in infancy?**

Alpha-1 antitrypsin deficiency accounts for 17% of neonatal cholestasis cases.

○ **True/False: The quantitation of serum alpha-1 antitrypsin level is sufficient to make the diagnosis of alpha-1 antitrypsin deficiency.**

False. One of the pitfalls of diagnosis is that alpha-1 antitrypsin is an acute phase reactant and, thus, may rise to normal in cases of hepatitis. The diagnosis of alpha-1 antitrypsin deficiency is made by testing for the molecular phenotype of the protein (protease inhibitor [Pi] type).

○ **Which electrophoretic alpha-1 antitrypsin phenotype is associated with the highest probability of liver disease?**

The ZZ phenotype.

○ **The hallmark of the liver biopsy in patients with alpha-1 antitrypsin deficiency is the deposition of the diastase resistant, mutant alpha-1 antitrypsin glycoprotein that stains positive by what stain?**

Periodic acid Schiff.

○ **Deficiency of which enzyme is responsible for tyrosinemia type I?**

Fumaryl acetoacetate hydrolase—the last enzyme of tyrosine degradation.

○ **True/False: Dietary correction of tyrosinemia alters the course of the liver disease.**

False. Tyrosine probably does not play a major role in the pathogenesis.

○ **What biochemical abnormality is diagnostic of tyrosinemia type I?**

Urinary succinyl acetone. This compound can also be measured in amniotic fluid by 15 weeks of gestation.

○ **What role does succinyl acetone play in the development of symptoms in tyrosinemia type I?**

This compound is hepatotoxic and an inhibitor of delta aminolevulinic acid dehydrogenase. The latter effect is responsible for the appearance of delta aminolevulinic acid in the urine and porphyria-like symptoms.

○ **True/False: Galactosuria is diagnostic of galactosemia.**

False. Galactosuria may be seen in many severe liver diseases.

○ **What eye abnormality is associated with galactosemia?**

Cataracts.

○ **What monosaccharides make up lactose?**

Glucose and galactose.

○ **What assay is used for the diagnosis of galactosemia?**

Measurement of erythrocyte galactose-1-uridyl-transferase. This assay must be done in any jaundiced, septic, or bleeding neonate if there is history of siblings with cataracts or unexplained death.

○ **What is the significance of lactosuria in neonates?**

None. Lactosuria may normally occur in healthy newborns.

○   **What is the treatment of galactosemia?**
Galactose-free diet for life.

○   **What enzyme deficiency causes benign fructosemia?**
Absence of fructokinase. This is asymptomatic.

○   **Deficiency of which enzyme of fructose metabolism causes severe symptoms?**
Absence of fructose-1-phosphate-aldolase and fructose-1,6-diphosphatase, both cause severe symptoms.

○   **Deficiency of which enzyme of fructose metabolism causes hereditary fructose intolerance?**
Absence of fructose-1-phosphate-aldolase.

○   **What are typical fructose-containing foods?**
Fruit and honey.

○   **True/False: Patients with hereditary fructose intolerance are asymptomatic if they avoid fructose.**
True. In fact, older children develop an aversion to foods containing fructose.

○   **What are the typical presenting symptoms of hereditary fructose intolerance in infancy?**
Vomiting, pallor, lethargy, sweating, and/or convulsions following ingestion of fructose.

○   **What is the most common physical finding in hereditary fructose intolerance?**
Hepatomegaly.

○   **True/False: Patients with fructose-1,6-diphosphatase deficiency are asymptomatic if they avoid fructose?**
False. Fructose ingestion is not required in fructose-1,6-diphosphatase deficiency for symptoms to develop.

○   **What is the toxic substance that accumulates in hereditary fructose intolerance?**
Fructose-1-phosphate.

○   **How does fructose-1-phosphate cause symptoms?**
It results in hypoglycemia by inhibiting glycogenolysis and gluconeogenesis. In addition, it is cytotoxic to the liver, kidneys, and gut.

○   **What renal manifestations may develop as a result of fructose-1-phosphate nephrotoxicity?**
Renal tubular acidosis, aminoaciduria, hyperuricemia, hypophosphatemia, or hypocalcemia.

○   **What methods are used in the diagnosis of hereditary fructose intolerance?**
Enzyme assays from intestinal or liver specimens.

○   **Which glycogen storage disease is associated with the most severe liver manifestations?**
Glycogenosis type IV (branching enzyme defect) regularly progresses to cirrhosis.

○ **Which lysosomal storage disease is associated with parenchymal liver disease in children?**

Nieman–Pick type C.

○ **What metabolites accumulate in the cells of Nieman–Pick disease patients?**

Sphingomyelin and cholesterol.

○ **What is the most common cause of neonatal ascites?**

Obstructive uropathy.

○ **What are the most common causes of noncirrhotic, extrahepatic portal hypertension in children?**

Congenital hepatic fibrosis and extrahepatic portal vein thrombosis.

○ **What medical conditions are associated with congenital hepatic fibrosis and extrahepatic portal vein thrombosis?**

Congenital hepatic fibrosis is associated with autosomal recessive polycystic kidney disease. Portal vein thrombosis in children is associated with umbilical vein catheterization (ie, neonatal).

○ **What is a surgical porto-systemic shunt and what are the different types?**

To decompress esophageal varices for the control of bleeding, when all endoscopic treatment and medical management fail, a surgical shunt may be created between the portal and systemic venous system. A shunt can be selective or nonselective.

Selective shunts decompress the esophageal varices trans-splenically without decompressing the main portal axis. This shunt has a much lower incidence of hepatic encephalopathy. The distal splenorenal shunt is an example of this type of shunt. This shunt leads to augmentation of ascites and, hence, severe ascites is a contraindication for this shunt.

Nonselective shunts directly reduce portal hypertension. Portocaval shunts (end to side [end of portal vein to vena cava] or side to side), mesocaval shunts, and proximal splenorenal shunts are examples of this type of shunt. These shunts carry a higher risk of postsurgical encephalopathy in cirrhotic patients; however, they are very good shunts for noncirrhotic patients and for extrahepatic portal vein obstruction (EHPVO).

● ● ● SUGGESTED READINGS ● ● ●

McLin VA, Balistreri, WF. Approach to neonatal cholestasis. In: Walker WA, Goulet O, Kleinman RE, et al., eds. *Pediatric Gastrointestinal Disease*. Hamilton, ON, Canada: BC Decker Inc;2004;1079-1093.

Piccoli DA, Russo P. Disorders of the biliary tract. In: Walker WA, Goulet O, Kleinman RE, et al., eds. *Pediatric Gastrointestinal Disease*. BC Decker Inc;2004;1094-1145.

Yonem O, Bayraktar Y. Is portal vein cavernous transformation a component of congenital hepatic fibrosis? *World J Gastroenterol*. 2007;13(3):1928-1929.

CHAPTER 50

Drug-Induced, Granulomatous, and Other Inflammatory Hepatic Diseases

Juan F. Gallegos-Orozco, MD and Hugo E. Vargas, MD

○ **What is the prevalence of drug-induced liver injury (DILI) or hepatotoxicity as a cause of acute liver failure?**

DILI accounts for more than 50% of cases of acute liver failure. Acetaminophen is the most common cause in the United States.

○ **What is the clinical importance of jaundice in patients with DILI and elevated aminotransferases?**

It is a marker of poor prognosis, with an estimated mortality of 10%.

○ **What is the clinical importance of eosinophilia in patients with DILI?**

It is a marker of improved short-term prognosis.

○ **What are the common steps of hepatic metabolism of orally administered drugs?**

- Phase I: Allows drugs to become hydrophilic and is accomplished by oxidation, reduction or hydrolysis; catalyzed primarily by cytochrome P450 enzyme superfamily.
- Phase II: A polar group is added to allow excretion of the metabolites from phase I. This is accomplished through conjugation with glutathione, glucuronic acid, or sulfate to produce a more water-soluble product and facilitate urinary or biliary excretion.
- Phase III: Transport of drugs and drug-products into the bile. This is mediated by adenosine triphosphate (ATP)-dependent transporters located in the bile canaliculi.

○ **What two types of drug reactions have been described in DILI?**

1. Direct reactions: Dose-dependent, reproducible, and predictable course.
2. Idiosyncratic reactions: Generally manifest after a latency period of 5–90 days and are characteristically unpredictable and not dose-related and can be divided in two main categories:
   a. Metabolic.
   b. Immunologic (hypersensitivity reaction to a specific drug).

○ **What are the biochemical patterns of liver chemistries in DILI?**

- Hepatocellular: alanine transaminase (ALT) >5 times upper limit of normal (ULN), alkaline phosphatase (AP) <2 ULN; R >5 (R, ratio of serum ALT/ULN for ALT to serum AP/ULN for AP).
- Cholestatic: ALT <5 x ULN, AP >2 x ULN; R <2.
- Mixed: ALT >3 x ULN, AP >2 x ULN; R 2-5.

○ **What are some of the important enzyme systems that detoxify reactive drug metabolites produced by cytochrome P450?**

The most important protective system is glutathione and glutathione-S-transferase, which is very abundant in hepatocytes. Another important enzyme is epoxide hydrolase, which breaks down reactive epoxides produced from drugs such as phenytoin.

○ **What drugs are commonly mentioned in association with fulminant liver failure?**

Acetaminophen, amoxicillin/clavulanic acid, phenytoin, isoniazid (INH), niacin, and valproic acid are a few examples.

○ **Provide examples of medications in which concomitant chronic alcohol consumption may increase the risk of DILI.**

Chronic alcohol intake increases the risk of liver fibrosis during therapy with methotrexate and enhances acetaminophen hepatotoxicity and susceptibility to liver damage from INH, halothane, and cocaine.

○ **What other risk factors have been implicated in the development of liver fibrosis during methotrexate treatment?**

Obesity, type 2 diabetes mellitus, insulin resistance, and psoriasis.

○ **True/False: All patients with DILI require a liver biopsy.**

False. Liver biopsy is not necessary in the management of patients with DILI, although it can be useful under certain circumstances:

- Patient has chronic liver disease and clinical presentation is difficult to ascribe to DILI versus underlying liver disease.
- To characterize the histological pattern of injury of drugs not previously known to be hepatotoxic.
- To identify more severe or residual lesions, such as advanced fibrosis, which could have prognostic significance.

○ **How common is hepatotoxicity due to highly active antiretroviral therapy (HAART) in patients with HIV/AIDS?**

Up to 30% of patients on HAART experience significant aminotransferase elevations.

○ **What are the common risk factors for HAART hepatotoxicity in patients with HIV/AIDS?**

Coinfection with hepatitis C or hepatitis B virus, advanced liver disease of any cause, and elevated aminotransferase levels before initiating HAART.

○ **What are the most common HAART drugs implicated in hepatotoxicity?**

- Didanosine and stavudine (nucleoside reverse transcriptase inhibitors) have been reported to cause a rare, but potentially fatal, hepatic steatosis and lactic acidosis.
- Nevirapine (nonnucleoside reverse transcriptase inhibitor) has a black-box warning as a cause of fatal and non-fatal hepatotoxicity. It has been associated with a hypersensitivity syndrome (rash, fever, and eosinophilia).
- Ritonavir and tipranavir (protease inhibitors) can both cause hepatotoxicity and acute liver failure.

○ **What is antiretroviral-associated portal hypertension?**

It is a novel clinical condition in which patients on antiretroviral therapy present with variceal hemorrhage, ascites, and other signs of portal hypertension. Didanosine has been implicated in its pathogenesis and removal of the drug results in clinical improvement.

○ **What is the importance of antibiotics in DILI?**

As a group, antibiotics have been implicated in up to 45% of cases of DILI in the United States. The most common antibiotic associated with DILI is amoxicillin with clavulanic acid, and is second only to acetaminophen as a cause of DILI in the United States.

○ **What are the main characteristics of DILI from amoxicillin/clavulanic acid?**

Cholestasis, which may be severe, is the most common pattern of injury. Other clinical features include skin rash, eosinophilia, and fever. Hepatotoxicity associated with amoxicillin/clavulanic acid is usually mild and subsides within 12 weeks of discontinuation of the drug. Rarely can it cause chronic liver disease with cholestasis and ductopenia with prolonged use.

○ **What are the common features of INH hepatotoxicity?**

It is the most frequent antimicrobial agent implicated in cases of DILI worldwide and commonly causes hepatocellular necrosis that can lead to liver failure and death.

○ **What are risk factors for overt liver injury from INH?**

Increasing age, female gender, and heavy alcohol use. Concomitant use of rifampin results in a fourfold increase in the risk of clinical hepatitis.

○ **What are the common features of rifampin hepatotoxicity?**

Hepatotoxicity from rifampin is less common than with INH. As a competitive inhibitor of bile salt uptake and export, it causes a mild cholestatic pattern of injury.

○ **Describe the mechanism of acetaminophen hepatotoxicity.**

Acetaminophen is a direct hepatotoxin when given in excessive doses or in therapeutic doses when the protective detoxifying pathway (P450 2E1) of the liver is overwhelmed. Accumulation of the toxic metabolite *N*-acetyl-*p*-benzoquinone-imine (NAPQI) is the cause of hepatocyte necrosis.

○ **Describe the histology of the liver after an acute overdose of acetaminophen. What explains this pattern of liver injury?**

The liver shows a nearly pure necrosis, most marked in zone 3 (around the central vein). This probably results from the metabolism of acetaminophen by cytochrome P450, which is more abundant in zone 3.

○ **What is a toxic dose of acetaminophen?**

In nonalcoholic individuals, acetaminophen is toxic in doses >7.5 g/24 hours. Chronic alcoholics or malnourished individuals are more susceptible to acetaminophen toxicity even when taken in therapeutic doses. It is generally recommended that patients with chronic liver disease limit the daily dose of acetaminophen to no more than 2 g/day.

○   **List risk factors for acetaminophen hepatotoxicity.**

Regular heavy use of alcohol. Phenobarbital, INH, and other drugs that induce cytochrome P450. Obesity may also increase the risk of toxicity because it is associated with increased cytochrome P450 2E1. Fasting reduces glutathione levels.

○   **Why does alcohol increase the risk of acetaminophen hepatotoxicity?**

Alcohol induces cytochrome P450 2E1, which metabolizes acetaminophen to a toxic, reactive quinoneimine compound. Alcohol also causes depletion of glutathione, which functions to detoxify such reactive substances in the liver.

○   **What drugs or chemicals are inducers or substrates of P450 2E1?**

INH has the greatest effect on cytochrome P450 2E1 induction. Ethanol, acetaminophen, carbon tetrachloride, chloroform, halothane, cocaine, benzene, and nitrosamines are other substrates or inducers of P450 2E1. This explains some of the interactions among alcohol and a number of other toxins and carcinogens. Alcohol metabolism by P450 2E1 produces reactive oxygen species, which are thought to contribute to the toxicity of alcohol.

○   **How is prognosis estimated in patients with acute liver failure caused by acetaminophen?**

The O'Grady or King's College criteria are commonly used to predict a fatal outcome and the need for liver transplantation in patients with fulminant liver failure. For acute acetaminophen toxicity, these criteria include: pH <7.3 (irrespective of encephalopathy grade) or international normalization ratio (INR) >6.5 (prothrombin time >100 seconds), serum creatinine >3.4 mg/dL, and grade III or IV hepatic encephalopathy.

○   **What is the difference between macrovesicular and microvesicular fatty liver, in terms of lipid composition and pathophysiology?**

Macrovesicular fat is mostly triglyceride accumulated due to increased influx and decreased efflux of lipid. Microvesicular fat is mostly unesterified fatty acid, which accumulates in conditions in which mitochondrial oxidation of fatty acids is impaired.

○   **What drugs or toxins often cause macrovesicular steatosis of the liver?**

Ethanol, glucocorticoids, methotrexate, and chlorinated hydrocarbons (such as carbon tetrachloride) are good examples.

○   **What drugs or toxins result in severe microvesicular steatosis of the liver?**

Aspirin in an overdose or in Reye's syndrome, tetracycline, and valproic acid. Some nucleoside analogs used in treating HIV disease, such as zidovudine and lamivudine, can cause mitochondrial dysfunction with microvesicular steatosis. The nucleoside analog fialuridine, used in clinical trials for treatment of hepatitis B, caused severe mitochondrial dysfunction with microvesicular steatosis, lactic acidosis, and liver failure.

○   **What drugs or toxins mimic the histological features of alcoholic hepatitis?**

The best example is amiodarone. Nifedipine, diethylstilbesterol (DES), and tamoxifen can also cause Mallory's hyaline and steatosis.

○   **A liver biopsy shows extensive homogenous intracellular material in hepatocytes. Electron microscopy shows whorls of concentric intracellular membranes. What is this and what drugs or toxins can cause it?**

This is phospholipidosis, caused by amiodarone, perhexiline maleate, chlorpheniramine, and a few other drugs. A number of the drugs that cause this are lipophilic cations.

○ **What is peliosis hepatis?**

Peliosis hepatis is a condition characterized by vascular pools in the liver, from a few millimeters to a centimeter in size, perhaps related to obstruction of the sinusoidal-central vein junction. Peliosis has been associated with hepatomegaly. Such livers are prone to bleeding after biopsy. Peliosis hepatis is associated with the use of anabolic steroids, estrogens, and thiopurines.

○ **What is nodular regenerative hyperplasia (NRH) and what medications can cause this condition?**

NRH is characterized by a diffusely nodular liver without fibrosis. NRH is thought to result from diffuse obstruction of microscopic arterioles with regeneration of better perfused areas. It is associated with the use of oral contraceptives, anabolic steroids, azathioprine, busulfan, and 6-thioguanine.

○ **List some medications that may cause indirect hyperbilirubinemia.**

Rifampin interferes with the uptake of unconjugated bilirubin by hepatocytes. Nicotinic acid can increase unconjugated bilirubin in patients with Gilbert's syndrome. Elevation of unconjugated bilirubin can also be a sign of hemolysis, which could be drug induced, such as seen with ribavirin during treatment for chronic hepatitis C.

○ **What drugs may cause inflammation involving microscopic bile ducts?**

Sulfa drugs often result in some combination of cholestasis and hepatocellular injury. Sulfonylurea use may lead to a syndrome histologically resembling primary biliary cirrhosis (PBC) but with negative antimitochondrial antibody (AMA). Diclofenac has caused a number of cases resembling PBC, sometimes with positive AMA. A large number of drugs cause chronic cholestasis. Carbamazepine may result in hepatic inflammation centered on bile ductules.

○ **Explain what is meant by "vanishing bile ducts" and list some drugs that may cause this.**

This refers to the disappearance of microscopic bile ductules, which normally number one to two per portal triad on a liver biopsy. The syndrome of vanishing bile ducts occurs in advanced PBC or in chronic liver allograft rejection. Some drugs associated with this syndrome include carbamazepine, phenothiazines, and thiabendazole.

○ **What drugs cause damage or inflammation to large bile ducts?**

The best example is FUDR (5-fluoro-deoxyuridine) given by intra-arterial infusion. This results in a syndrome resembling sclerosing cholangitis and is probably due to vascular injury.

○ **What drugs can lead to a chronic hepatitis mimicking autoimmune hepatitis?**

Sulfonamides, propylthiouracil, alpha-methyldopa, nitrofurantoin, minocycline, and ecstasy (a drug of abuse, methylene-3,4-dioxy-methamphetamine [MDMA]) are examples. Some of these drugs induce antinuclear antibodies and other autoantibodies. Halothane toxicity may be accompanied by features of autoimmune hepatitis, including antimitochondrial antibodies.

○ **List drugs that may cause cirrhosis with chronic use.**
- INH
- Methotrexate
- Methyldopa
- Nitrofurantoin
- Oxyphenisatin
- Perhexeline maleate
- Trazodone

○ **What dose of vitamin A is needed to cause hepatotoxicity?**

Large doses, in the range of a million IU/day, cause acute toxicity. Chronic use of more than 40,000 IU/day for months may cause chronic hepatotoxicity. Lower doses may be toxic in heavy alcohol users and persons with hyperlipidemia and elevated chylomicrons.

○ **What is the appearance of vitamin A toxicity on liver biopsy?**

The liver biopsy shows vitamin A droplets in sinusoidal fat-storing cells (Ito cells or hepatic stellate cells), Kupffer cell activation, inflammation, and fibrosis. This fibrosis can lead to portal hypertension without accompanying cirrhosis.

○ **What liver neoplasms may be drug-induced and name the drugs implicated?**

- Hepatocellular carcinoma: anabolic steroids, oral contraceptives, Thorotrast (thorium dioxide), vinyl chloride, aflatoxin.
- Angiosarcoma: Thorotrast (thorium dioxide), vinyl chloride, arsenic, anabolic steroids.
- Adenoma: oral contraceptives, anabolic steroids.

○ **What hepatic vascular abnormalities are associated with drug toxicity?**

- Veno-occlusive disease (VOD): Bush tea from *Senecio, Crotalaria, Heliotropiu* and some comfrey tea containing pyrrolizidine alkaloids, alkylating agents (common in hematopoietic stem cell transplantation).
- Peliosis hepatis: anabolic steroids, estrogens, azathioprine, 6-thioguanine, and Thorotrast (thorium dioxide).
- Hepatic vein thrombosis (Budd-Chiari syndrome): oral contraceptives.

○ **How common is the use of herbal and dietary supplements in the general population?**

Approximately 20% of American adults self-reported using herbal or dietary supplements in 2004. Importantly, only a third of consumers reported the use of these products to a healthcare provider.

○ **How frequently are herbal and dietary supplements implicated in DILI?**

Herbal and dietary supplements are implicated in approximately 10% of all cases of DILI in the United States.

○ **What herbal medicines have been associated with hepatotoxicity?**

Creosote bush (chaparral tea), germander, kava, black cohosh, mistletoe, usnic acid, green tea extract, pyrrolizidine alkaloids (found in comfrey tea), and constituents of Chinese herbal medicines are some examples.

○ **Describe features of hepatotoxicity from nicotinic acid?**

High-dose nicotinic acid used to treat hypercholesterolemia may cause jaundice and severe hepatocyte necrosis, occasionally resulting in fulminant liver failure. Hepatotoxicity seems to be more common with sustained-release formulations.

○ **Which nonsteroidal anti-inflammatory drugs (NSAIDs) are most prone to cause hepatotoxicity?**

Sulindac and diclofenac.

○ **What are the main features of sulindac hepatotoxicity?**

Mild hepatitis with cholestasis.

○ **What are the main features of diclofenac hepatotoxicity?**

This NSAID has caused rare cases of acute hepatitis with liver cell necrosis, often with associated antinuclear antibodies. Fulminant liver failure has occurred. Some patients have developed antimitochondrial antibodies with a histologic picture similar to PBC.

○ **What determines the relative hepatotoxicity of inhalational anesthetics?**

For the halogenated alkanes, this generally is proportional to their rate of metabolism by cytochrome P450 (halothane > enflurane > isoflurane).

○ **What types of hepatotoxicity do 6-mercaptopurine and azathioprine cause?**

An acute allergic-type reaction can occur with hepatocyte necrosis and very elevated aminotransferase levels and cholestasis. Chronic use may cause NRH and peliosis hepatis, and possibly contribute to veno-occlusive disease.

○ **What are the main features of tetracycline hepatotoxicity?**

Hepatotoxicity has occurred with high-dose intravenous use of tetracycline but can also occur with oral use. On liver biopsy, there is accumulation of microvesicular fat in hepatocytes. It appears to be due to a toxic effect on mitochondria.

○ **In what setting does cocaine hepatotoxicity occur?**

Hepatocyte necrosis usually occurs in the setting of an overdose, especially in a heavy alcohol drinker. Induction of cytochrome P450 2E1 by alcohol probably causes increased metabolism of cocaine to toxic products.

○ **What toxins are found in toxic mushrooms?**

These are mainly the amatoxins and phallotoxins. The amatoxins include a variety of cyclic peptides, which inhibit RNA polymerase type II and, thus, inhibit the synthesis of messenger RNA. The phallotoxins promote the polymerization of cellular actin.

○ **What solvent used in manufacturing rubber products may cause hepatotoxicity?**

Methyl formamide, used in manufacturing rubberized cloth, has caused a type of acute hepatitis when used without proper ventilation.

○ **What type of food poisoning is associated with acute liver failure?**

Bacillus cereus is a sporulating bacterium that can cause diarrhea and vomiting when it grows in rice and other grain products that have been improperly cooked or reheated. *B. cereus* produces an emetic toxin that has led to cases of acute liver failure by interfering with mitochondrial function.

○ **What type of hepatotoxicity is associated with cyanobacteria?**

Some strains of cyanobacteria ("blue-green algae") produce microcystins. These interfere with the hepatocyte cytoskeleton and cause liver hemorrhage and necrosis. Such liver toxicity is best known to occur in cattle but multiple cases have also occurred in humans in a hemodialysis center due to contaminated water.

○ **How common are liver granulomas?**

Granulomas of the liver are found in 5%–10% of patients in liver biopsy series.

○ **What drugs may cause granulomatous hepatitis?**

Sulfa drugs, quinidine, allopurinol, nitrofurantoin, phenotiazines, carbamazepine, and phenytoin among many others.

○ **What are the main types of granulomas?**

- Lipogranulomas, which form around fat droplets associated with ingestion of mineral oil, waxes, or other lipid material.
- Epithelioid granulomas, which are usually formed in response to a hypersensitivity reaction. A special form of epithelioid granuloma is the fibrin-ring granuloma commonly described in Q-fever and allopurinol toxicity.

○ **What are the two most common causes of hepatic epithelioid granulomas in the United States?**

Sarcoidosis and tuberculosis.

○ **What is the most common symptom in patients with hepatic granulomas?**

Fever of unknown origin is the most common symptom; however, symptoms correlate with the underlying illness. Fever is present in most cases of sarcoidosis and tuberculosis.

○ **What are the most common physical findings in patients with conditions that cause hepatic granulomas?**

Splenomegaly, hepatomegaly, and moderate lymphadenopathy.

○ **What is the most common pattern seen in biochemical tests that would suggest a granulomatous liver disease?**

A moderate to marked increase in serum alkaline phosphatase (3 to 10 times normal) and a slight increase in serum aminotransferases (2 to 6 times normal).

○ **True/False: Granulomatous diseases of the liver usually result in a clinically significant alteration of hepatic function.**

False. Most diseases that cause granulomas of the liver do not cause significant alteration of hepatic function. Sarcoidosis and PBC are exceptions.

○ **Sarcoidosis is a disease characterized by epithelioid cell granulomas. What organs are affected by these granulomas?**

Granulomas occur in many organs in sarcoidosis, but mainly affect the lungs, lymph nodes, and liver.

○ **What percentage of individuals with sarcoidosis have granulomas in the liver?**

Approximately two-thirds. The majority of granulomas are located in the portal area, although they may appear anywhere within the hepatic nodule.

○ **What is the most consistently abnormal lab value in sarcoidosis?**

Elevated serum alkaline phosphatase. Other commonly abnormal lab values include elevated serum angiotensin-converting enzyme (50%–80% of cases), elevated serum calcium, and a moderate normocytic anemia.

○ **What are the names of the two inclusion bodies found in approximately half of granulomas associated with sarcoidosis?**

Schaumann bodies and asteroid bodies. Schaumann bodies are basophilic structures with concentric proteinaceous calcified laminations. Asteroid bodies are star-like radiating structures found within a clear space.

○ **What percent of patients with Hodgkin's disease have hepatic granulomas?**

Up to 12%. Up to 2% of patients with non-Hodgkin's lymphoma have hepatic involvement.

○ **What histologic characteristics are typical of Hodgkin's disease granulomas?**

These granulomas, which are seen in both portal tracts and parenchyma, are typically epithelioid without caseation and occasionally contain Langerhan's giant cells.

○ **What percentage of cases of PBC is associated with liver granulomas and/or granulomatous necrosis?**

Approximately 25%. The presence of granulomas in PBC is associated with a better prognosis.

○ **Name six drugs that have been associated with hepatic granuloma formation.**

1. Allopurinol
2. Sulfonamides
3. Quinidine
4. Chlorpropamide
5. Beryllium
6. Phenylbutazone

○ **Name findings that might suggest that liver granulomas are from a drug reaction.**

Portal location of granulomas, peripheral eosinophilia, and tissue eosinophilia. There is no pathognomonic characteristic of drug-related hepatic granulomas.

○ **What is the typical sequela after the removal of the offending drug in cases of liver granulomas?**

None. The granulomas quickly resolve without fibrosis or calcification.

○ **What systemic vasculitis that usually manifests itself in the respiratory tract is also associated with granulomatous hepatitis, elevated alkaline phosphatase, and/or aminotransferases and ascites in 15%–30% of cases?**

Wegener's granulomatosis.

○ **What percentage of patients with polymyalgia rheumatica, giant cell arteritis, and temporal arteritis has liver test abnormalities?**

Approximately one-third.

○ **True/False: Hypogammaglobinemia is associated with liver test abnormalities.**

True.

○ **True/False: Celiac disease is associated with liver test abnormalities.**

True. The abnormalities generally normalize following initiation of a gluten-free diet.

● ● ● **SUGGESTED READINGS** ● ● ●

Chang CY, Schiano TD. Review article: drug hepatotoxicity. *Aliment Pharmacol Ther.* 2007;25:1135-1151.

Lewis JH. Granulomas of the liver. In: Schiff ER, Sorrell MF, Maddrey WC, eds. *Schiff's Diseases of the Liver.* 10th ed. Philadelphia: Lipincott Williams & Wilkins; 2007:1425-1448.

Pugh AJ, Barve AJ, Kalkner K, Patel M, McClain CJ. Drug-induced hepatotoxicity or drug-induced liver injury. *Clin Liver Dis.* 2009;13:277-294.

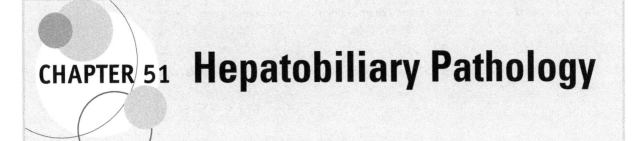

CHAPTER 51 Hepatobiliary Pathology

Cory A. Roberts, MD

○ **What liver condition is being demonstrated in the figure below? In this condition, what type of collagen is deposited to an excessive degree and what cell is its source?**

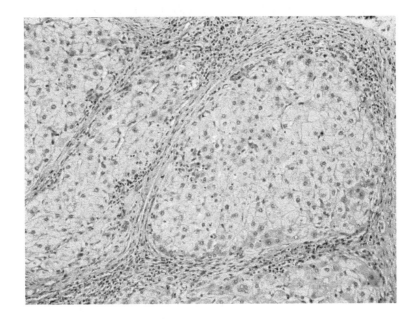

Figure 51-1

Cirrhosis. Collagen of types I and III produced by the Ito cell. The Ito cell functions as a storage vehicle, metabolizes vitamin A, and aids in the production of collagen.

○ **In ischemic liver injury, what general pattern of necrosis would be expected?**

Centrilobular necrosis. The pericentral region of the lobule (zone 3 of the acinus) is farthest from the blood supply and most susceptible to ischemic injury.

○   **What zone of the liver acinus is characteristically involved in acetaminophen toxicity?**

Zone 3.

○   **How does the pattern of necrosis in acute viral hepatitis B compare to that seen in acute viral hepatitis A infection?**

The necrosis in acute hepatitis B infection typically is centered in zone 3, whereas necrosis in acute hepatitis A characteristically involves zone 1.

○   **What specific mushroom is classically associated with liver toxicity and fulminant hepatic failure?**

Amanita phalloides.

○   **In mushroom poisoning, what zone of the acinus would you expect to see necrosis?**

Zone 1.

○   **The presence of noncaseating granulomas that are characterized by a "fibrin ring" pattern in the center should raise the diagnostic possibility of what rare type of hepatitis?**

Q-fever hepatitis caused by *Coxiella burnetii*. This histologic lesion is sometimes referred to as a "doughnut" granuloma.

○   **A 46-year-old man who admits to drinking "3 or 4 beers a day" presents with jaundice, right upper quadrant abdominal pain, and fever. A liver biopsy was eventually performed and is shown below. What is the most likely diagnosis?**

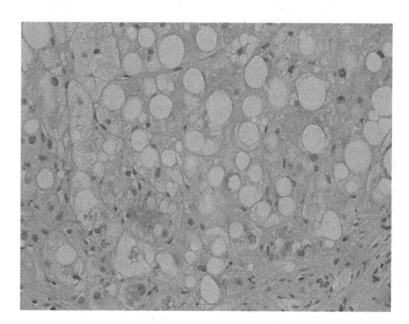

Figure 51-2

Alcoholic hepatitis. Typical features of alcoholic hepatitis include Mallory's hyaline, which is an eosinophilic inclusion within hepatocytes that stains with ubiquitin, neutrophils surrounding individual degenerating hepatocytes, sclerosing hyaline necrosis, and steatosis, predominantly macrovesicular.

○   **True/False: Mallory bodies or Mallory's hyaline are pathognomonic for alcoholic hepatitis.**

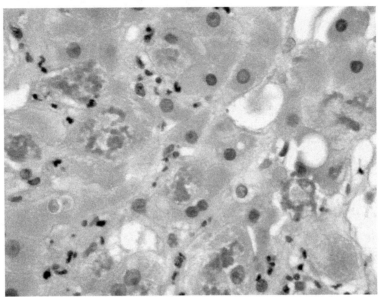

Figure 51-3

False. Few things in pathology are pathognomonic. Mallory bodies can be seen in many diseases including nonalcoholic steatohepatitis (NASH), Wilson's disease, primary biliary cirrhosis (PBC), and amiodarone toxicity.

○   **The liver biopsy specimen shown in the figure below is described in the pathology report as having nodular lymphocytic portal infiltrates, some with germinal centers. This is most suggestive of what type of viral hepatitis?**

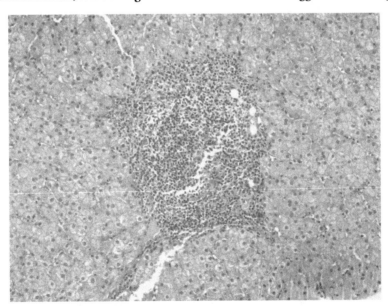

Figure 51-4

Hepatitis C. The presence of a portal area with a lymphoid aggregate or a follicle with a germinal center in a liver specimen with other features of chronic hepatitis is most suggestive of chronic hepatitis C. It should be noted that hepatitis C is notable for sometimes having some degree of bile duct involvement/injury. This can make the distinction between recurrent hepatitis C and allograft rejection difficult in some liver transplant biopsies.

○   **What two items must be described in a liver biopsy pathology report when making the diagnosis of chronic hepatitis?**

Grade and stage. The degree of inflammatory activity is referred to as the grade and the amount of fibrosis as the stage. Of course, the etiology is also included if known.

○   **What subtype of cirrhosis (micronodular or macronodular) is classically associated with alcoholic liver disease?**

Micronodular.

○   **In general, what is included in the differential diagnosis of micronodular cirrhosis?**

Alcoholic liver disease (Laennec's cirrhosis), PBC, hemochromatosis, NASH, Indian childhood cirrhosis, galactosemia, and glycogenosis type IV.

○   **What are some conditions associated with macronodular cirrhosis?**

Viral hepatitis, alpha-1 antitrypsin deficiency (A1AD), hereditary tyrosinemia, Wilson's disease, and some drug injury.

○   **What are the causes of peliosis hepatis?**

Peliosis hepatis refers to the presence of multiple large blood-filled spaces within the liver that lack an endothelial lining. Causes of peliosis hepatis include treatment with anabolic or androgenic steroids and tamoxifen, history of Thorotrast use, elevated levels of vitamin A, and infection with *Bartonella henselae*.

○   **A 36-year-old woman presents with chronic hepatitis and is found to have an HLA B8 haplotype, liver/kidney microsomal antibodies, and elevated levels of serum IgG. Her liver biopsy is shown below. What is the most likely diagnosis?**

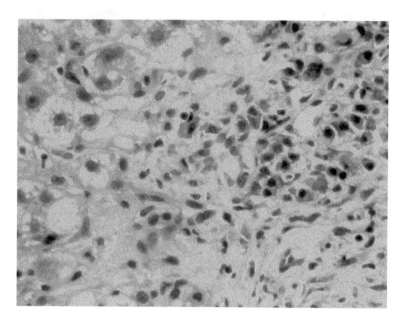

Figure 51-5

Autoimmune hepatitis (type 2).

○ **What is the most characteristic inflammatory cell seen in the infiltrate of a chronic autoimmune hepatitis?**

Plasma cell.

○ **A 45-year-old woman presents with fatigue and pruritus. Laboratory testing is notable only for an elevated alkaline phosphatase. A liver biopsy is performed. What is the diagnosis?**

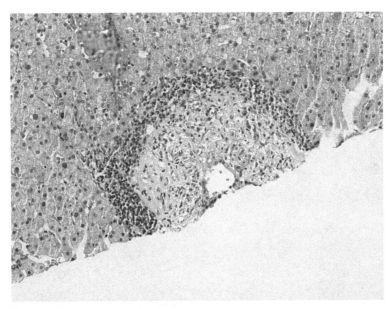

Figure 51-6 See also color plate.

PBC. The biopsy demonstrates a portal granuloma destroying a bile duct in the center of the granuloma at the edge of the tissue ("florid duct lesion"). This woman's antimitochondrial antibodies were markedly elevated.

○ **Describe the typical histologic features of PBC?**

Destruction of small original bile ducts with a portal lymphoplasmacytic infiltrate including lymphoid follicles and even granulomas. There may also be a loss of 50% or more of the original interlobular bile ducts. The fibrosis pattern is often irregular.

○ **What conditions are associated exclusively with microvesicular steatosis?**

Reye's syndrome, acute fatty liver of pregnancy, some drug reactions (eg, valproic acid), toxic shock syndrome, some familial diseases, heatstroke, and overexposure to some toxic chemicals.

○ **What HLA associations are known in primary sclerosing cholangitis (PSC)?**

HLA B8, DR3, DR2, and DRw52a. No such HLA associations are described in PBC.

○ **The finding of periductal fibrosis or sclerosis resulting in an "onion skin" pattern in the portal areas is indicative of what disorder?**

PSC.

○ **What specific antibody titer may be elevated in patients with PSC?**

Perinuclear antineutrophil cytoplasmic antibody (p-ANCA).

○ **A newborn in the neonatal intensive care unit has severe jaundice with an unconjugated bilirubin of 38 mg/dL and otherwise relatively unremarkable liver tests. The diagnosis is made and the geneticist reminds you that it is an autosomal recessive disease. What is the diagnosis?**

Crigler–Najjar type 1. These patients cannot conjugate bilirubin due to a deficiency of the enzyme uridine diphosphate-glucuronyltransferase.

○ **How can you differentiate between Dubin–Johnson's and Rotor's syndromes histologically and grossly?**

Dubin–Johnson's syndrome is characterized by a black discoloration of the parenchyma seen both grossly and histologically. Histologically, the pigment is contained within the hepatocytes in zones 2 and 3. In contrast, Rotor's syndrome is devoid of pigment and, histologically, the liver may be normal.

○ **Dubin-Johnson's syndrome and Rotor's syndrome share a common inheritance pattern. What is it?**

Autosomal recessive.

○ **Glucuronyl transferase is deficient or abnormal in what rather innocuous condition?**

Gilbert's syndrome. It is inherited in an autosomal recessive fashion.

○ **Which chemotherapeutic drug and which anti-HIV drug can reach toxic levels in patients with Gilbert's syndrome?**

Irinotecan and idinavir, respectively.

○ **On what chromosome does the defect responsible for Wilson's disease lie?**

Chromosome 13.

○ **What is the hepatic iron index and what value would you expect in a patient with hereditary hemochromatosis?**

The hepatic iron index is calculated by taking the hepatic iron concentration in mg/g dry weight, dividing it by 56 (the molecular weight of iron) and dividing that total by the patient's age. In hemochromatosis, a value greater than 1.9 is characteristic.

○ **True/False: A solitary, unilocular simple cyst of the liver is typically found in the right lobe.**

True. They are twice as common in the right lobe.

○ **Describe the two general histologic findings in the liver in a case of carbon tetrachloride toxicity.**

Steatosis and centrilobular necrosis.

○ **What is the earliest and most common histologic finding in liver biopsies of alcoholic hepatitis?**

Steatosis, predominantly macrovesicular. In addition, pericellular centrilobular fibrosis ("arachnoid" fibrosis), ballooning change of hepatocytes, sclerosing hyaline necrosis, and Mallory hyaline may be present.

○ **In a patient with ethanol-induced steatohepatitis, which histologic feature will likely disappear first if you were to rebiopsy?**

The steatosis is typically the first to develop and also the first to resolve.

○ **What is the inheritance pattern of genetic hemochromatosis?**

Autosomal recessive. The gene is on the short arm of chromosome 6.

○ **True/False: The risk of development of hepatocellular carcinoma (HCC) in patients with hemochromatosis and cirrhosis is increased.**

True. Up to 20% of patients will develop HCC.

○ **True/False: There is an association between hereditary tyrosinemia and HCC.**

True. Over one-third of patients who live beyond the age of two will develop HCC, sometimes multifocally.

○ **Foreign, polarizable material is seen in association with a foreign body giant cell reaction within expanded, fibrotic portal areas on a liver biopsy specimen taken from a patient on chronic renal dialysis. What is the foreign material?**

Silicon rubber from silastic tubing that is found in hemodialysis equipment. A similar reaction can also be seen from damaged prosthetic devices.

○ **What are some causes of hepatic granulomas or granulomatous hepatitis?**

Sarcoidosis, PBC, and drug injury are the most common causes. Other causes include polymyalgia rheumatica, unusual infections including berylliosis and Brucellosis, foreign body reaction, PSC (rarely), systemic infection, and extrahepatic malignancies. Some are also incidental findings not ever explained. Most of the latter are small microgranulomas.

○ **What is the most common parasitic disease involving the liver that can produce a granulomatous response?**

Schistosomiasis. This infection can result in the so-called "pipestem fibrosis" of portal areas and/or a granulomatous reaction in the liver.

○ **In amyloidosis involving the liver, where is the amyloid deposited?**

It can be found either within the vessel walls or the parenchyma, specifically in the space of Disse with compression of the underlying hepatocytes.

○ **What effect does Budd–Chiari's syndrome have on the caudate lobe?**

The caudate lobe is not usually involved, owing to its unique, separate venous drainage and, in fact, may exhibit compensatory hypertrophy in an attempt to "make up" for the involved liver.

○ **What are some etiologic agents of hepatic VOD?**

Ingestion of pyrrolizidine alkaloids, radiation, various cancer chemotherapies, urethane, azathioprine, dacarbazine, and hypervitaminosis A.

○ **What is Banti's syndrome?**

Also referred to as idiopathic portal hypertension, it is characterized by splenomegaly, hypersplenism, and portal hypertension.

○ **What is Zieve's syndrome?**

This refers to the triad of hemolytic anemia occurring in a patient with alcoholic hepatitis who also has hypercholesterolemia.

○   **What typical histopathologic features seen in Budd–Chiari's syndrome and veno-occlusive disease (VOD) are demonstrated in Figures 51-7A VOD and 15-7B Budd–Chiari's syndrome?**

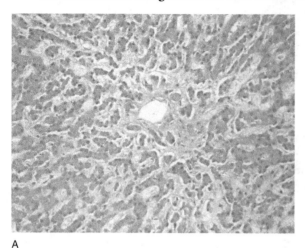   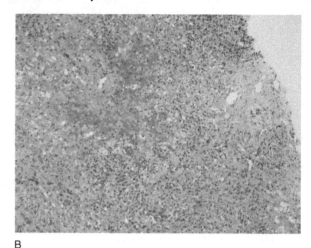

A   B

Figure 51-7

Budd–Chiari's syndrome is characterized by centrilobular congestion with associated hepatocellular dropout or necrosis. In contrast, VOD is characterized by subendothelial sclerosis of the terminal hepatic venules and intercalated veins with associated "atrophy" of the hepatocytes in the lobules.

○   **True/False: The finding of hemolysis in a young patient with liver failure is strongly suggestive of Wilson's disease.**
True.

○   **What are some causes of NASH?**

Type 2 diabetes mellitus, lipodystrophy, obesity, and some drugs such as amiodarone, tamoxifen, and highly active anti-retroviral therapy. Clinical correlation is always necessary.

○   **Differentiate between Caroli's disease and Caroli's syndrome.**

Caroli's disease is a developmental condition of intrahepatic cystic dilatation of bile ducts. The lumen of the cystic dilatations can be filled with mucin, bile, or pus if infected. Caroli's syndrome, which is more common, is Caroli's disease in association with congenital hepatic fibrosis.

○   **In what fashion is Caroli's disease inherited?**

Autosomal recessive. This is associated with autosomal recessive polycystic kidney disease. The gene is on the short arm of chromosome 6 called polycystic kidney and hepatic disease 1 (PKHD1).

○   **What are some of the main clinical manifestations of congenital hepatic fibrosis?**

In general, patients present with hepatosplenomegaly or bleeding from esophageal varices due to portal hypertension. Cholangitis is a less common presenting condition.

○   **What is Meckel's syndrome?**

It is characterized by features that are similar to congenital hepatic fibrosis with the addition of an association with encephalocele, polydactyly, and cystic kidneys.

○ **Name the two most common hepatic complications associated with autosomal dominant polycystic kidney disease.**

Infection of the liver cysts is the most frequent complication followed by cholangiocarcinoma.

○ **What are the two genes most commonly mutated in autosomal dominant polycystic kidney disease?**

PKD1 (90% of cases) on the short arm of chromosome 16 (16p 13.3) and PKD2 on the long arm of chromosome 4 (4q 21–23).

○ **What is the main gross and histologic difference in the liver in autosomal recessive versus autosomal dominant polycystic kidney disease?**

The presence of cysts. In autosomal dominant polycystic kidney disease (AKPKD), the liver is grossly and microscopically cystic and the cysts are fluid filled. The liver in autosomal recessive polycystic kidney disease (ARPKD) is usually grossly normal apart from perhaps some firmness. There are usually no cysts at all. Microscopically there are increased abnormal biliary channels but again no large cysts.

○ **What is a von Meyenburg complex?**

This is a localized collection of abnormally dilated bile ducts in a fibrous stroma background. They are generally small (a few millimeters) and are felt to be a part of the spectrum of adult polycystic liver and kidney disease.

○ **Do most people with von Meyenburg complexes have polycystic liver disease?**

No. These lesions are common (some 5% of autopsies) but they are usually incidental findings. However, it does appear that they are the progenitor of the larger, dilated cysts that people with polycystic liver and kidney disease develop.

○ **True/False: Most hydatid cysts are located in the left hepatic lobe.**

False. In general, most things are more common in the larger right lobe of the liver.

○ **Discuss the clinical and pathologic findings in mesenchymal hamartoma of the liver.**

It is a tumor that can be quite large, develops in children (average age <2, usually male), and is characterized by a loose, connective tissue (myxoid) stroma, hepatic parenchyma with admixed bile ducts and vascular structures. Large cysts can develop. A chromosomal translocation involving the long arm of chromosome 19 (19q 18.4) has been described.

○ **Which of these two benign lesions carries a greater risk of hemorrhage or rupture—focal nodular hyperplasia or hepatocellular adenoma?**

Hepatocellular adenoma.

○ **What are some of the associations with nodular regenerative hyperplasia of the liver?**

Nodular regenerative hyperplasia is associated with numerous conditions including rheumatoid arthritis; calcinosis, Raynaud's, esophageal dysmotility, sclerodactyly, and telangiectasia (CREST) syndrome; and other autoimmune diseases. It typically occurs in adults and is sometimes confused with cirrhosis.

○ **Describe the typical patient and clinical presentation of someone with a bile duct cystadenoma (hepatobiliary cystadenoma).**

They almost exclusively occur in women, typically in the fourth and fifth decades of life, are usually found in the right lobe of the liver, and often cause abdominal pain owing to their large size. Serum levels of CA19-9 are often elevated.

○ **What special stain can be used to help differentiate histologically between hepatocellular adenoma and HCC?**

A reticulin stain. Adenomas are characterized by preservation of the reticulin framework, which defines the one to two cell thick plates, whereas HCC has no such reticulin framework or it is markedly diminished and, therefore, the hepatic plates are much thicker.

○ **Typically an incidental finding and the most common benign tumor of the liver, what lesion is being shown in the figure below?**

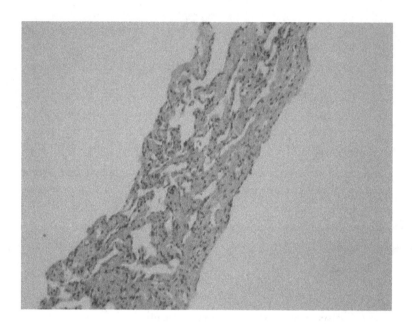

Figure 51-8

Hemangioma.

○ **What is the most common location of cholangiocarcinoma in the liver?**

The right lobe of the liver, although 30% are multifocal.

○ **What is the relationship of serum alpha-fetoprotein (AFP) to cholangiocarcinoma?**

None. The vast majority of cholangiocarcinomas have normal serum AFP.

○ **Which histologic type of HCC is characterized histologically by period acid-Schiff (PAS)-positive cytoplasmic inclusions within the tumor cells and dense fibrous strips of stroma investing sheets of tumor cells?**

The fibrolamellar variant.

○ **What are some of the unusual patient characteristics in fibrolamellar variant of HCC compared to typical HCC?**

The patients are younger (>40 years of age is rare), it is fairly evenly distributed between men and women (typical HCC is two to five times more common in men), and has a far better prognosis.

○ **In general, which is more suggestive of HCC, detection of serum AFP or immunoperoxidase stain reactivity for AFP in tissue sections?**

A markedly elevated serum AFP is much more suggestive. The reported sensitivity of AFP positivity in tissue sections varies widely but is low and can be detected in adenocarcinomas of other origins.

○ **A biopsy of a liver mass from a 14-month-old boy shows a tumor with bone formation, cartilage, and a fetal epithelial component that resembles fetal hepatocytes. What is your diagnosis?**

Hepatoblastoma (mixed type).

○ **Which histologic type of HCC occurs in young adults or adolescents, is not associated with cirrhosis, has a better prognosis, and is not associated with an elevated serum AFP?**

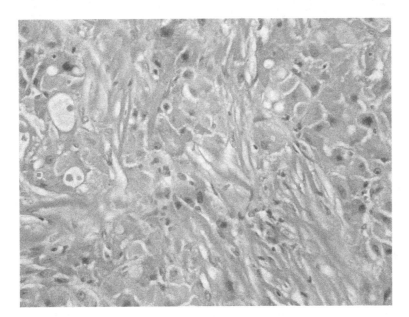

Figure 51-9

Fibrolamellar HCC. Interestingly, in contrast to many of the other lesions we have discussed, it is more common in the left lobe of the liver. Unlike typical or traditional HCC, fibrolamellar HCC is also not associated with hepatitis B or alcohol abuse. Note the histology shown above demonstrating the thick fibrous bands within the tumor.

○ **What is the gross appearance of an epithelioid hemangioendothelioma of the liver?**

They are typically multicentric, involve both lobes of the liver, and are firm and white-tan in color. Although both epithelioid hemangioendothelioma and angiosarcoma can be multifocal, the firm, white-tan appearance of the former is quite different than the hemorrhagic appearance of the latter.

○ **What are the typical demographics and presentation of a patient with epithelioid hemangioendothelioma?**

It is more common in females in the sixth decade of life. The presenting symptoms are nonspecific but include pain and jaundice. Although the tumor grows slowly, it has a 5-year survival of about 50%. Liver transplantation has been used to prolong survival.

○ **A 3-year-old boy presents with abdominal "swelling." Subsequently, a 15-cm liver mass is identified and the serum AFP is elevated. Liver biopsy is shown below. What is the most likely diagnosis?**

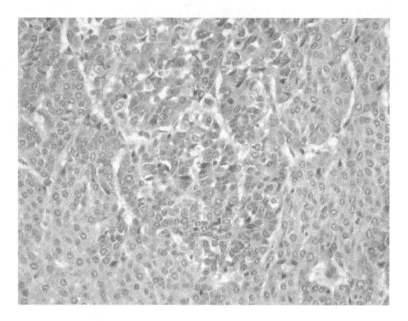

Figure 51-10

Hepatoblastoma, the most common malignancy in children. Seventy-five percent of patients are male and 90% occur before the fifth year of life.

○ **What rare liver tumor has been associated with exposure to Thorotrast, vinyl chloride monomer, arsenic, and anabolic steroids, and represents the most common primary sarcoma of the liver?**

Angiosarcoma.

○ **What are the histologic features of acute graft-versus-host disease involving the liver?**

The most noteworthy finding is that of damage to the bile ducts. In addition, individual hepatocyte necrosis may occur and endotheliitis may be present. It is very similar to acute allograft rejection.

○ **True/False: Chronic graft-versus-host disease can occur in the absence of previous acute graft-versus-host disease.**

True. This occurs in about a quarter of the cases.

○ **In bone marrow transplant patients who develop chronic graft-versus-host disease, and how frequently is the liver involved?**

Up to 60% of the time.

○ **A patient is status post bone marrow transplant and undergoes liver biopsy. The biopsy demonstrates increased stainable iron both in hepatocytes and in Kupffer cells with the latter predominating. What is the most likely etiology?**

This is a frequent finding in anyone that has received numerous blood transfusions, such as a bone marrow transplant patient. It is referred to as siderosis.

○ **Two liver biopsies are taken, each from a different patient, but they are not labeled. One patient has hemochromatosis and the other has aplastic anemia. One biopsy shows markedly increased iron predominantly in Kupffer cells and the other shows increased iron primarily in hepatocytes. Which is the biopsy from the hemochromatosis patient?**

Iron primarily in hepatocytes is typical of hemochromatosis, whereas iron found primarily in Kupffer cells is typical of transfusion-related iron overload.

○ **What is the inheritance pattern and most common mutation of classic hereditary hemochromatosis?**

It has an autosomal recessive inheritance. The mutation in 80% of the cases is C282Y. H63D is the next most common mutation and as a heterozygote with C282Y can also manifest disease effects.

○ **What substance usually binds to and detoxifies acetaminophen within the liver and becomes overwhelmed in cases of acetaminophen toxicity?**

Glutathione.

○ **True/False: B-lymphocytes are responsible for attacking the bile duct shown in this case of acute (cellular) rejection of a liver allograft.**

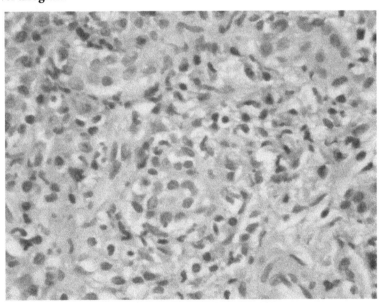

Figure 51-11

False. T-lymphocytes are responsible.

○ **What percentage of patients with A1AD characterized by a PiZZ (homozygote) phenotype have demonstrable liver disease?**

Less than 20%; however, 100% will have PAS-positive, diastase-resistant globules within the cytoplasm of hepatocytes.

○ **How is it possible for a patient with A1AD to show a normal serum A1A?**

A1A is an acute phase reactant. Therefore, inflammation of the liver or elsewhere can increase the serum levels. In a heterozygote with A1A, the serum level may actually be raised to normal or low-normal levels during the acute phase of inflammation.

○   **What are the typical histologic features of acute allograft rejection in the liver?**

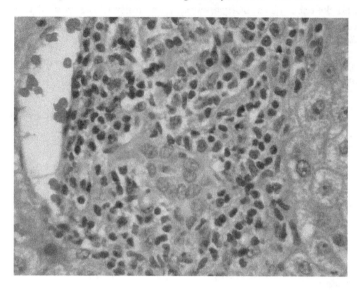

Figure 51-12

Acute rejection is characterized by a portal infiltrate composed of T-lymphocytes and eosinophils, which are generally centered around the bile ducts and portal vein. The ducts show damage (nuclear loss or vacuolated cytoplasm) and often focal infiltration by the lymphocytes. Endotheliitis is usually present involving the portal vein and characterized by subendothelial inflammatory cells causing prominence of the endothelial cells.

○   **What etiologic agent is most likely responsible for the hepatitis demonstrated in this biopsy from a 32-year-old liver transplant recipient, which shows cells with intranuclear and intracytoplasmic inclusions?**

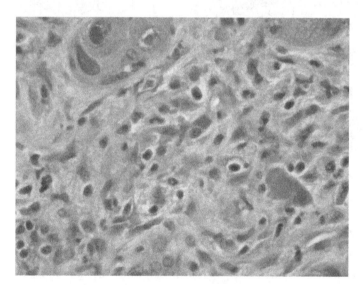

Figure 51-13

Cytomegalovirus. CMV hepatitis is characterized by hepatocytes, which contain both intranuclear and intracytoplasmic viral inclusions.

○   A 13-year-old boy presents with jaundice and evidence of liver failure and hemolysis. Liver biopsy is shown below. What is the diagnosis? What stain is shown?

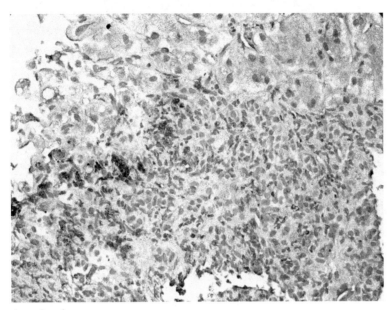

Figure 51-14 See also color plate.

Wilson's disease. Copper stain.

○   What is the liver disorder demonstrated in the following figure? What stain is shown?

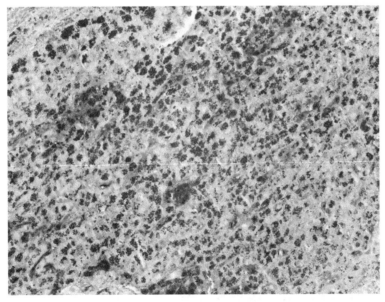

Figure 51-15 See also color plate.

Hemochromatosis. Prussian blue (iron stain). Note the panlobular staining in the hepatocytes.

○   **In the figure below, what diagnosis is most likely and what stain(s) would you use to confirm or disprove it?**

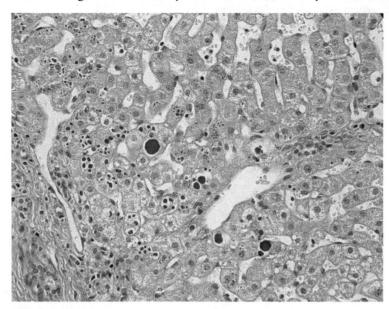

Figure 51-16 See also color plate.

A1AD. This biopsy shows eosinophilic globules within periportal hepatocytes. If it is A1AD, the globules will be PAS-positive and resist diastase digestion. Hence, a PAS and a PAS with diastase should be ordered. There is also an immunohistochemical stain for A1D that would also be expected to be positive in the case of A1AD.

○   **The liver biopsy below is taken from a 45-year-old man and your pathologist calls you excitedly to say that the biopsy shows a "classic onion skin lesion." What is the diagnosis?**

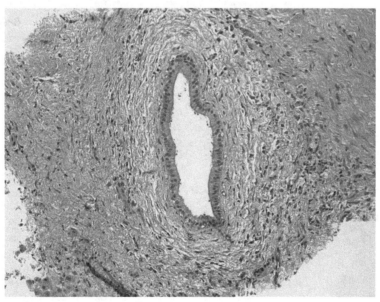

Figure 51-17 See also color plate.

PSC. The affected ducts are typically larger, medium-sized ducts, which is why this can be very difficult to diagnose on a needle biopsy simply due to sampling.

○ **True/False: It is uncommon for patients with PSC to have concomitant ulcerative colitis (UC).**

False. These two conditions coexist 70% of the time; however, patients with UC have concomitant PSC in less than 5% of cases.

○ **What gallbladder lesion is characterized by histologically normal epithelial crypts, which exist amidst a hyperplastic muscularis?**

Adenomyosis. When localized to the fundus, it is called an adenomyoma although that term is somewhat misleading as it is not a true neoplasm.

○ **A 43-year-old man presents with a liver mass that shows an abnormal vasculature (prominent arteries) and a central scar in an otherwise normal appearing liver. What is the most likely diagnosis?**

Focal nodular hyperplasia.

• • • SUGGESTED READINGS • • •

Scheuer PJ, Lefkowitch JH, eds. *Liver Biopsy Interpretation.* 7th ed. Philadelphia: Elsevier Saunders; 2006.

Burt AD, Portmann BC, Ferrell LD, eds. *MacSween's Pathology of the Liver.* 5th ed. Philadelphia: Churchill Livingstone Elsevier; 2007.

CHAPTER 52

Hepatic Infectious Disorders

Neeraj K. Sardana, MD and Nicholas Ferrentino, MD

○ **What are the clinical manifestations of amebic liver abscess?**

Patients often present with fever and right upper quadrant (RUQ) pain. Serological evaluation may reveal leukocytosis without eosinophilia, elevation in alkaline phosphatase, and elevated transaminases.

○ **How is an amebic liver abscess diagnosed?**

A patient with the appropriate clinical picture who resides in, or has traveled to, an endemic area should have imaging of the liver. Ultrasound or computed tomography (CT) imaging will reveal a single subcapsular abscess in the right lobe 70%–80% of the time. Multiple abscesses are also possible. This is usually enough to treat a patient presumptively.

Serologic testing can also be performed; indirect hemagglutination (IHA) is most sensitive. Abscess aspiration is sometimes necessary if the cyst is at risk of rupture, there has been no response to antibiotic therapy, or the diagnosis remains unclear.

○ **What percentage of patients with an amebic liver abscess have a history of dysentery or diarrhea?**

Less than 33%. Although some patients may describe a history of diarrhea in the weeks to months preceding presentation with an amebic liver abscess, less than one-third have concurrent dysentery at the time of diagnosis.

○ **True/False: All amoebae are pathogenic.**

False. *Entamoeba histolytica* is pathogenic in about 10% of infected individuals, whereas *E. dispar* and *E. moshkovskii* do not cause clinical disease.

○ **What are risk factors for developing amebic liver abscess?**
- Living in, or traveling to, an endemic area.
- Adult males; possibly due to alcoholic liver damage increasing susceptibility.
- Any condition that compromises cell-mediated immunity, including advanced age, pregnancy, corticosteroid use (or other immunosupression), malignancy, or malnutrition.

○ **What is the drug of choice for treatment of an amebic liver abscess?**

Nitroimidazoles (eg, metronidazole). Alternative therapies include dehydroemetine and choloroquine. Luminal amebicides (diloxanide furoate, diiodohydroxyquin, or paramomycin) must always be used following one of the above regimens.

○ **Which lobe of the liver is more commonly affected by liver abscesses?**

The right lobe, probably due to its larger size and blood flow. Abscesses of biliary origin are more commonly bilateral.

○ **What is the leading cause of pyogenic liver abscess?**

Biliary tract disease such as gallstones or malignant obstruction accounts for 40%–60% of cases. Other important sources include portal vein pyemia (from bowel leakage or peritonitis), trauma, or direct spread from biliary infection.

○ **What are the most common organisms isolated from pyogenic liver abscesses?**

Most pyogenic liver abscesses are polymicrobial. Gram negatives such as *Escherichia coli* and *Klebsiella pneumoniae* are most common; however, isolation of Gram-positive organisms such as *Enterococcus*, *Staphylococcus*, and *Streptococcus* has increased in frequency.

○ **What is the most common presenting symptom of a pyogenic liver abscess?**

Fever, which is present in about 90% of patients. The next most common symptom is RUQ abdominal pain. Nausea, vomiting, anorexia, weight loss, and malaise may also be present.

○ **What factors are associated with increased mortality in pyogenic liver abscesses?**

Multiple abscesses, associated malignancy, septic shock, fungal infection, presence of jaundice, hypoalbuminemia, leukocytosis, and presence of bacteremia. Advanced age, biliary etiology, and elevated aspartate aminotransferase are no longer considered to be risk factors.

○ **How are pyogenic liver abscesses treated?**

Drainage and antibiotics are the mainstays of treatment. Needle aspiration is appropriate for solitary collections <5 cm in diameter. For larger or multiple lesions, percutaneous catheter drainage is preferred. Empiric antibiotics can be used, but the regimen should ultimately be tailored to the eventual culture and sensitivity results.

○ **What is the most common infectious cause of hepatic cysts?**

Echinococcus granulosus, a species of tapeworm.

○ **What organs other than the liver are involved in echinococcal infections?**

Kidney, spleen, brain, heart, lungs, and bones.

○ **True/False: Most hydatid cysts are asymptomatic.**

True. Symptoms are unusual until a cyst reaches about 10 cm. The latency period between infection and symptoms can be up to 50 years. Many patients never become symptomatic.

○ **How are hydatid cysts diagnosed?**

A combination of imaging and serological tests can be used. Findings on CT, MRI, and ultrasound may be highly suggestive in a patient from an endemic area. Serology can be used to screen for or confirm infection. Enzyme-linked immunosorbent assay (ELISA) and immune hemagglutinin assay (IHA) are used frequently as serologic screening tests.

○ **What stages of the malarial (*Plasmodium* spp.) life cycle involve the liver?**

Pre-erythrocytic phase and exo-erythrocytic phase.

○ **What hepatic consequences can occur as a result of malaria infection?**

Mild jaundice due to hemolysis is common with infection by any *Plasmodium* spp. Hepatocyte injury, cholestasis, and severe jaundice may occur with *P. falciparum* infection but not others.

○ **Name the causative organisms of visceral leishmaniasis (VL) or "kala-azar".**

Leishmania donovani and *L. infantum.*

○ **What characteristic findings on liver biopsy are seen in cases of VL?**

A "peculiar cirrhosis" or so-called Roger's cirrhosis. This is characterized by severe intralobular fibrosis with normal architecture and no regenerative nodules. This intralobular fibrosis is completely reversible after treatment.

○ **True/False: VL in an HIV-infected person is an acquired immunodeficiency syndrome (AIDS)-defining illness.**

True. All patients found to have VL should be tested for HIV coinfection.

○ **What is the diagnostic procedure of choice in case of VL?**

Examination and culture of splenic needle aspiration has a reported sensitivity of 96%. Bone marrow or lymph nodes can also be aspirated but are less sensitive.

○ **What is the drug of choice in the treatment of leishmaniasis?**

Liposomal amphotericin B has the highest therapeutic efficacy and the best side effect profile. Second-line agents include pentavalent antimonial compounds (sodium stibogluconate) and conventional amphotericin B deoxycholate, which require increased monitoring of patients for toxicity.

○ **Name the schistosomes that affect the liver.**

Schistosoma mansoni, *S. japonicum*, *S. mekongi*, and *S. intercalatum.*

○ **What are "swimmer's itch" and "katayama fever"?**

Swimmer's itch is a localized dermatitis, usually on the lower legs or feet, at the site of schistosomal larval entry.

Katayama fever is a hypersensitivity reaction to the heavy burden of schistosomal antigens that coincide with the first 2 weeks of egg production (2–8 weeks after infection). It mimics serum sickness and can be associated with fever, chills, diarrhea, headache, arthralgias, and myalgias.

○   **What are typical clinical findings of chronic hepatic schistosomiasis?**

Normal liver architecture and cellular function in the presence of portal fibrosis and portal hypertension. Morbidity and mortality are usually related to consequences of ascites or bleeding from esophageal varices.

○   **What malignancy is associated with hepatic schistosomiasis?**

Follicular lymphoma of the spleen.

○   **What is the most useful diagnostic method in the case of active infection with schistosomiasis?**

Stool examination for eggs. This becomes negative after successful treatment.

○   **What is the drug of choice for schistosomiasis?**

Praziquantel.

○   **What is the drug of choice to treat the liver flukes, *Fasciola hepatica* and *Fasciola gigantica*?**

Triclabendazole.

○   **Name the malignancy commonly associated with the liver flukes, *Clonorchis sinensis* and *Opisthorchis* species?**

Cholangiocarcinoma.

○   **What characteristic abnormality in liver tests is seen in bacterial sepsis?**

Bacterial sepsis and the resulting systemic inflammatory response syndrome (SIRS) can trigger a "parainfectious hepatitis." Usually there is a cholestatic picture with elevation in bilirubin out of proportion to alkaline phosphatase and aminotransferases. This is commonly caused by *E. coli* but can be associated with any organism. The source of infection can be intra- or extraabdominal. It is thought that bacterial cell wall endotoxin triggers release of cytokines by bile duct epithelial cells, which in turn affects hepatocyte function.

○   **How does *Salmonella* hepatitis differ from viral hepatitis?**

Salmonella hepatitis can be indistinguishable from acute viral hepatitis; however, *Salmonella* hepatitis is associated with lower peak alanine aminotransferase (ALT) levels and higher peak alkaline phosphatase levels. High fever, relative bradycardia, and a left shift of the leukocyte count favor *Salmonella* hepatitis.

○   **What is Fitz–Hugh–Curtis syndrome?**

Perihepatitis occurring as a complication of pelvic gonorrhea or chlamydia infection. It is marked by fever, severe RUQ pleuritic pain, lower abdominal tenderness, and a hepatic friction rub.

○   **What is the most common cause of liver-associated enzyme elevation in patients with tuberculosis?**

Antituberculous therapy-related hepatotoxicity.

○   **What are the manifestations of primary hepatobiliary tuberculosis?**

Tuberculomas, ascites, porta-hepatis adenopathy, hepatic abscess, and cholangitis.

○ **What group of patients is at high risk of developing a complicated *Yersinia* infection?**

Yersinia is an iron-dependent bacterium that requires exogenous iron for growth. Therefore, patients with hemochromatosis or secondary hemosiderosis are prone to develop hepatic abscesses from *Yersinia* infection.

○ **What stages of syphilis can involve the liver?**

Syphilis can involve the liver at any stage. In early syphilis, hepatitis is characterized by elevated alkaline phosphatase with relatively mild elevations in aminotransferases. Late syphilis is uncommon in the current era but is characterized by "gummas," indolent, and granulomatous-like lesions that can affect any organ. Gummatous hepatitis may be associated with fever, epigastric pain, and tenderness over the liver, and may lead to cirrhosis. Vasculitis or endarteritis related to syphilis infection may also cause liver disease.

○ **What is Weil's disease?**

It is a severe icteric form of leptospirosis and is characterized by marked jaundice, azotemia, hemorrhagic phenomena, and hypotension. Minimal elevation of aminotransferases differentiates leptospirosis from acute viral hepatitis.

○ **What form of granuloma is seen in Q fever?**

Q fever is an infection caused by *Coxiella burnetii*. When involving the liver, it causes a "doughnut-like" lipogranuloma in which a ring of fibrinoid necrosis and lymphocytes surround a centrally-located fat vacuole. While this lesion is highly suggestive of Q fever, it is not pathognomonic. Similar lesions can be seen in VL, lymphoma, and allupurinol hypersensitivity.

○ **What are the most common infections of the liver in AIDS?**

Mycobacterium avium complex (MAC) followed by *Cryptococcus* and cytomegalovirus (CMV).

○ **What is the name of the organism known to cause bacillary peliosis hepatitis?**

The Gram-negative bacillus, *Bartonella henselae*. Peliosis hepatis refers to blood-filled cystic changes in hepatic parenchyma that may or may not have an endothelial lining.

● ● ● **SUGGESTED READINGS** ● ● ●

Reid-Lombardo KM, Khan S, Sclabas G. Hepatic cysts and liver abscess. *Surg Clin North Am.* 2010;90(4):679-697.

Kurland JE, Brann OS. Pyogenic and amebic liver abscesses. *Curr Gastroenterol Rep.* 2004;6(4):273-279.

Benedetti NJ, Desser TS, Jeffrey RB. Imaging of hepatic infections. *Ultrasound Q.* 2008;24(4):267-278.

CHAPTER 53 Metabolic Liver Disorders

Samir Parekh, MD

○ **What gene is most commonly associated with hereditary hemochromatosis (HHC) and how is it inherited?**

Approximately 90% of patients with HHC have mutations in the HFE gene located on the short arm of chromosome 6. The disease has an autosomal recessive inheritance pattern, and the most common point mutation is homozygosity for C282Y. To a much lesser degree, iron overload can occur in compound heterozygotes who have one copy of C282Y and one copy of H63D or S65C.

○ **What is the pathophysiology of HHC?**

Mutations in the HFE gene lead to decreased production of hepcidin, a peptide synthesized in the liver that plays a central role in iron regulation. Low concentrations of hepcidin result in increased intestinal absorption of iron without feedback inhibition, and subsequently iron accumulation in the liver and other organs.

○ **What values of transferrin saturation and ferritin should prompt further investigation for hemochromatosis?**

Transferrin saturation ≥45% and elevated ferritin (typically >200 µg/L for females and >300 µg/L for males).

○ **How is the transferrin saturation calculated?**

Serum iron/total iron binding capacity × 100%. An increase in transferrin saturation is the earliest laboratory finding in HHC.

○ **When is the serum iron level falsely elevated?**

After meals and at night. A fasting serum iron level collected in the morning is most useful.

○ **True/False: The serum ferritin level is both more sensitive and specific than transferrin saturation values.**

False. Ferritin is also an acute phase reactant.

○ **What hepatic conditions may also cause an elevated ferritin level?**

Chronic viral hepatitis (including Hepatitis C), alcoholic liver disease, and non-alcoholic steatohepatitis.

○ **True/False: In patients with elevated transferrin saturation and ferritin, the next step in the evaluation for HHC is liver biopsy.**

False. The next step in testing for HHC should be HFE gene testing.

○ **True/False: A negative HFE gene test rules out a diagnosis of HHC.**

False. Approximately 10% of HHC patients may be HFE negative. Recently, several other genes and proteins of iron metabolism have been identified as the causes of HHC, although much rarer than HFE-related hemochromatosis. These include mutations in ferroportin (ferroportin disease), transferrin receptor 2 (TfR2 hemochromatosis), and hemojuvelin (HJV hemochromatosis).

○ **In what scenarios should a liver biopsy be considered in HHC?**

In patients with elevated transaminases or ferritin levels > 1000 μg/L and age > 40, a liver biopsy might be helpful to rule out advanced fibrosis or cirrhosis. In addition, a liver biopsy is useful when the diagnosis is in doubt or non-HFE hemochromatosis is suspected.

○ **What stain is used to examine liver tissue for iron?**

Perl's Prussian blue stain.

○ **True/False: In patients with genetic hemochromatosis, excess iron deposition is found predominantly in parenchymal cells (hepatocytes) with very little iron in cells of the reticuloendothelial (RE) system.**

True. This differs from other, secondary, causes of iron overload.

○ **How do you calculate the hepatic iron index (HII)?**

The HII is calculated by taking the hepatic iron concentration and dividing by the patient's age in years. Keep in mind that the hepatic iron concentration must be in μ mol iron/g of dry weight of liver. Remember that the molecular weight of iron is 56.0 because the hepatic iron concentration may be reported in μg iron/g of dry weight of liver. A value > 1.9 is consistent with homozygous HHC. A value < 1.5 is not due to homozygous HHC.

○ **What is the typical HII of a patient with alcoholic liver disease? What is a normal index value?**

1.1 to 1.6; < 0.7 to 1.1.

○ **Patients with ineffective erythropoiesis who require transfusions will have iron deposition in which liver cell populations?**

In both RE cells and parenchymal cells. Secondary iron overload predominantly affects storage of iron in the RE cells.

○ **Which of the organ(s) involved in genetic hemochromatosis will not improve with phlebotomy?**

Patients with advanced cirrhosis, arthropathy, and hypogonadism do not improve with therapy.

○ **Which members of a family should be screened for genetic hemochromatosis when it has been diagnosed in one member?**

The siblings of the proband and all first-degree relatives.

○ **What is the best screening test to identify relatives of individuals with genetic hemochromatosis?**

For siblings, HFE gene testing. For children, one option is to perform the HFE gene test on the other parent and screen the children only if the C282Y or H63D gene is present.

○ **Recall all the possible rheumatoid conditions associated with HHC.**

Arthropathies involving the second and third metacarpophalangeal joints, joint space narrowing, chondrocalcinosis, subchondral cyst formation, osteopenia, and joint swelling.

○ **What infections are more common in iron-loaded patients?**

- *Vibrio vulnificus*
- *Listeria monocytogenes*, and
- *Pasteurella pseudotuberculosis.*

○ **How much iron is typically needed to be removed by phlebotomy in a patient with HHC?**

10 to 20 g.

○ **How many phlebotomies will this require?**

Each unit of whole blood removed = 250 mg of iron; therefore, at least 40 to 80 units will need to be removed.

○ **How many units of blood should be removed per week to treat patients with HHC?**

Usually 1 or 2 units/week. After achieving adequate iron depletion, most patients require approximately four maintenance phlebotomies per year.

○ **What are the goal values for transferrin saturation, serum iron, and ferritin during maintenance phlebotomy in patients with HHC?**

Transferrin saturation <50%, low serum iron level, and ferritin <50 µg/L.

○ **The presence of which two hemochromatosis-related conditions decreases life expectancy compared to the general public?**

Diabetes and/or cirrhosis.

○ **True/False: Due to the low risk of hepatocelluar carcinoma (HCC) in patients with HHC and cirrhosis, HCC screening is not recommended for this patient population.**

False. 30% of patients with HHC and cirrhosis develop HCC representing a 200-fold increased risk. Therefore, these patients should be aggressively screened for HCC.

○ **True/False: The survival rate in patients with genetic hemochromatosis following orthotopic liver transplantation (OLT) is comparable to that of patients who undergo OLT for other indications.**

True. In the past, patients with HHC had a significantly decreased survival after transplant compared to other patients because of cardiac arrhythmias related to iron overload in the myocardium and infectious complications. Currently, survival rates are comparable due to earlier diagnosis of HHC and iron depletion through phlebotomies prior to transplant.

○ **What is the least likely liver disease to also cause hepatocellular carcinoma?**

Wilson's disease.

○ **True/False: Children less than age 3 should be screened for Wilson's disease.**

False. Clinical manifestations are rarely, if ever, seen before age 5.

○ **In addition to the liver, brain, and joints, what other vital organ can be affected by Wilson's disease?**

Although the heart, pancreas, and eyes have been reported to be involved, the most important other vital organ involved is the kidney. Wilson's disease can cause Fanconi's syndrome resulting in low serum phosphorus and uric acid, and failure to excrete acid in the urine.

○ **True/False: A gene for Wilson's disease has been determined.**

True. ATP7B localized to human chromosome 13. Over 300 different mutations of the ATP7B gene have been identified.

○ **True/False: The Wilson's disease gene is expressed in the liver and kidney.**

True. It is also expressed in the brain, lungs, and placenta.

○ **What causes Wilson's disease?**

There is a gene mutation in the major copper transport protein, ATP7B found in hepatocytes that results in decreased biliary excretion of copper and toxic accumulation in the liver, brain, cornea, and other organs.

○ **What other gastrointestinal disease is associated with copper storage overload and what molecular mechanism is defective?**

Menke's disease affects the copper transporter in the proximal small intestine and results in hyperabsorption of copper.

○ **True/False: Wilson's disease is inherited in a Mendelian fashion as an autosomal dominant allele.**

False. Although Wilson's disease is inherited in a Mendelian fashion, it is inherited as an autosomal recessive allele.

○ **Name two extrahepatic manifestations that often accompany acute liver failure due to Wilson's disease.**

Renal failure and hemolytic anemia.

○ **How is the diagnosis of Wilson's disease made?**

The diagnosis requires a constellation of findings including at least two of the following: 1) Low ceruloplasmin level, 2) presence of Kayser–Fleischer rings, 3) typical neurologic symptoms, and 4) liver biopsy with a hepatic copper content of 250 μg per gram of dry weight.

○ **True/False: The serum ceruloplasmin is always decreased (ie, < 20 g/L) in patients with Wilson's disease.**

False. Remember that up to 5% of Wilson's patients will have low-normal range of serum ceruloplasmin levels. In addition, a ceruloplasmin level > 30 essentially excludes the disease.

○   **True/False: Only half of patients with Wilson's disease and liver involvement have the clinical finding shown in the accompanying figure.**

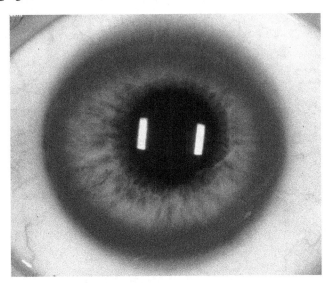

Figure 53-1 See also color plate.

True. This compares to approximately 95% of patients who have neurologic involvement. The figure shows a slit-lamp examination demonstrating the classical Kayser–Fleischer ring which are brownish or gray-green rings that represent fine pigmented granular deposits of copper in Descemet's membrane in the cornea close to the endothelial surface.

○   **What foods are to be avoided in patients with Wilson's disease?**

Organ meats, shellfish, nuts, chocolate, and mushrooms, all of which are high in copper.

○   **Up to 30% of patients with Wilson's disease develop a side effect of D-penicillamine that necessitates a change of treatment. What are the most common side effects that would necessitate stopping treatment?**

Dermatologic-rashes, pemphigus, nephrotic syndrome, Goodpasture syndrome, myasthenia syndrome, aplastic anemia (rare), leukopenia, thrombocytopenia, and systemic lupus erythematosus-like syndrome. Gastrointestinal side effects are most common but usually mild.

○   **What are alternative treatments to D-penicillamine for Wilson's disease?**

Trientine, zinc, and ammonium tetrathiomolybdate.

○   **What other drug must be administered with D-penicillamine?**

Pyridoxine (vitamin B_6, 25 mg/day).

○   **True/False: D-penicillamine should be stopped during pregnancy.**

False. Therapy must be continued but at a lower dose. Stopping therapy can result in significant exacerbations.

○   **True/False: D-penicillamine therapy should be continued for life.**

True. After initial high doses, lower maintenance doses (0.75 to 1 g/day) are instituted.

○   **How is screening performed in the siblings of Wilson's disease patients?**

Serum copper and ceruloplasmin measurements, 24-hour urinary copper measurement and a slit-lamp examination. Children younger than 5 or 6 are usually not affected and should be rechecked at intervals over the next 5 to 10 years. If the mutations of the index case are known, genetic testing should be performed. Siblings have a 25% chance of having the disease.

○   **True/False: Severe neurologic manifestations of Wilson's disease are an accepted indication for liver transplantation.**

False. Given the uncertain improvement and outcome in neurologic symptoms posttransplant, this is not an indication. Indications for liver transplant include acute liver failure and end-stage liver disease unresponsive to medical therapy. Liver transplantation is curative as it corrects the underlying metabolic defect of the disease.

○   **What is the normal phenotype for the alleles expressing the α_1-antitrypsin protease inhibitor (Pi)?**

PiMM is normal and PiZZ results in the lowest levels of α_1-antitrypsin.

○   **How common is α_1-antitrypsin deficiency?**

α_1-antitrypsin deficiency occurs in approximately 1 in 2000 individuals.

○   **Where is the abnormal gene located in α_1-antitrypsin?**

The gene, located on chromosome 14, results in the single amino acid substitution of glutamate by lysine at position 342 leading to a deficiency in sialic acid.

○   **What is the pathophysiology of α_1-antitrypsin that leads to liver disease?**

The gene mutation results in an abnormal folding of the α_1-antitrypsin protein and failure of secretion from the hepatocyte endoplasmic reticulum. The defective protein accumulates in the hepatocyte and forms polymers, leading to cellular stress and liver damage.

○   **True/False: Cirrhosis occurs in less than 20% of patients with the PiZZ phenotype.**

True. The PiZZ phenotype, in several studies, caused cirrhosis in only 12% of patients. In contrast, chronic obstructive pulmonary disease occurs in roughly 75% of these patients.

○   **Do other α_1-antitrypsin phenotypes, that is, heterozygotes, result in chronic liver disease?**

It must be remembered that certain heterozygous states can result in chronic liver disease. For instance, patients with PiSZ and PiZZ can develop cirrhosis. MZ heterozygotes usually do not develop disease unless there is some other superimposed liver condition, such as alcoholic liver disease or chronic viral hepatitis. Liver disease due to other causes may progress more rapidly in individuals who have an MZ phenotype.

○   **What is an effective treatment for patients with α_1-antitrypsin deficiency?**

The only treatment for α_1-antitrypsin-related liver disease is symptomatic management of complications and liver transplantation. With liver transplantation, the phenotype becomes that of the transplanted liver. Recall that the liver is the site of production of this protease inhibitor, and therefore, liver transplantation is curative. α_1-antitrypsin replacement therapy has no effect on liver disease since liver injury is related to accumulation of the mutant protein within the hepatocyte and not a lack of circulating antiproteases.

○ **True/False: The α_1-antitrypsin level is the best test to detect deficiency states associated with cirrhosis.**

False. The best diagnostic test is obtaining the phenotype. The level may be low-normal even in states of homozygous deficiency. Also, α_1-antitrypsin is an acute phase reactant and levels may rise in the setting of illness or other types of inflammatory stress.

○ **What is the characteristic finding of α_1-antitrypsin deficiency on liver biopsy?**

Presence of eosinophilic, periodic acid-Schiff-positive, and diastase-resistant globules in the endoplasmic reticulum of periportal hepatocytes.

○ **What is the frequency of genetic hemochromatosis, of Wilson's disease, and of α_1-antitrypsin deficiency?**

Genetic hemochromatosis (1 in 250 individuals); Wilson's disease (1 in 30,000 individuals); α_1-antitrypsin deficiency (1 in 2000 individuals).

○ **What is the most common of the acute porphyrias?**

Acute intermittent porphyria (AIP) occurs in 5 to 10 per 100,000 people. Its inheritance pattern is autosomal dominant with incomplete penetrance.

○ **What is the enzyme deficiency in AIP?**

There is a 50% reduction in porphobilinogen (PBG) deaminase activity.

○ **What are the major manifestations of AIP?**

Derangements in the autonomic nervous system.

○ **What are the predominant heme by-products in the urine of a patient with an acute attack of AIP?**

PBG and 5-aminolevulinic acid (ALA). PBG quantities are higher than ALA. These levels may be normal between attacks.

○ **True/False: AIP is the only porphyria that is not associated with cutaneous manifestations.**

False. AIP is one of two acute porphyrias with only neurologic findings. The other is ALA dehydratase deficiency.

○ **What precipitates episodes of the acute porphyrias?**

Prescription or recreational drugs, particularly corticosteroids and derivative hormones. This is why diagnosis is, oftentimes, first made at puberty. Alcohol ingestion, smoking, fasting, infection, stress, and pregnancy are other risk factors.

○ **True/False: All of the heme synthetic enzymes are expressed only in the liver.**

False. Three enzyme deficiencies among the cutaneous porphyrias are expressed in the bone marrow.

○ **What is the most common of the porphyrias?**

Porphyria cutanea tarda (PCT) is the most common of the porphyrias, usually presenting after 10 years of age.

○ **What do AIP and PCT have in common?**

Enzyme expression occurs only in the liver, both have autosomal dominant patterns of inheritance (the former with incomplete penetrance while the latter can be acquired), and both are the most common (the former being acute while the latter being of the cutaneous porphyrias).

○ **What is the typical lesion associated with PCT?**

Photosensitivity-induced vesicles and bullous lesions, or blisters.

○ **PCT is strongly associated with what other disorders?**

Excess alcohol intake, estrogen therapy, systemic lupus erythematosus, diabetes mellitus, chronic renal failure, acquired immunodeficiency syndrome, and chronic hepatitis C. Of note, most patients also have iron overload.

○ **True/False: Patients with acute porphyrias are at increased risk of developing hepatocellular carcinoma.**

True. Even though hepatic involvement is variable and mild.

○ **What two porphyrias are most commonly associated with liver complications?**

PCT and hepatoerythropoietic porphyria (HEP).

○ **What clinical clues should lead to consideration of the diagnosis of porphyria?**

Recurrent bouts of severe abdominal pain, constipation, neuropsychiatric disturbances, and typical dermatologic findings.

○ **How do you treat PCT?**

Avoid precipitating factors (alcohol, sun, etc). Phlebotomy is considered the standard of care. Hydroxychloroquine may also be useful. If possible, HCV treatment should be considered but usually after PCT is adequately treated.

○ **What are the two bile acid transport disorders in which a genetic defect of primary bile acid secretion is believed responsible?**

Byler's syndrome and Alagille's syndrome.

○ **What is the hepatic lesion associated with cystic fibrosis?**

Focal biliary cirrhosis. Over time, focal biliary cirrhosis can progress to multilobular biliary cirrhosis and clinically significant portal hypertension.

○ **True/False: No medical therapy has been shown to be of benefit in patients with cystic fibrosis-related liver disease.**

False. Controlled studies have demonstrated the beneficial effects of ursodeoxycholic acid in terms of improvement in cholestasis and nutritional status.

● ● ● **SUGGESTED READINGS** ● ● ●

Bacon BR, Adams PC, Kowdley KV, Powell LW, Tavill AS. Diagnosis and Management of Hemochromatosis: 2011 Practice Guideline by the American Association for the Study of Liver Diseases. *Hepatology*. 2011;5(1):328-343.

Roberts EA, Schilsky ML. Diagnosis and Treatment of Wilson Disease: An Update. *Hepatology*. 2008;47(6):2098-2111.

CHAPTER 54

Hepatic Tumors and Cysts

Thomas D. Schiano, MD and
M. Isabel Fiel, MD

○ **What is the differential diagnosis of an elevated alpha-fetoprotein (AFP) in a patient with known liver disease?**

Serum AFP levels may be elevated in patients with various liver diseases, most commonly, viral hepatitis. Levels exceeding 1000 ng/mL may be seen in the presence of fulminant hepatitis, teratomas, or in yolk sac/testicular tumors. In patients with chronic hepatitis C virus (HCV), levels may be as high as 300 ng/mL in the absence of hepatocellular carcinoma (HCC). Levels >300–500 ng/mL are almost always consistent with HCC.

○ **True/False: Many patients with HCC may have normal AFP levels.**

True.

○ **What variant of HCC is being demonstrated in the figure below?**

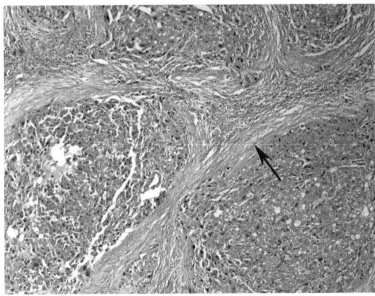

Figure 54-1

The fibrolamellar variant of HCC. Tumor cells are large and contain abundant eosinophilic cytoplasm. This type of liver tumor is characterized by prominent lamellated fibrous tissue (see arrow in Figure 54-1) that dissects through the mass.

431

○   **True/False: The fibrolamellar variant of HCC most commonly manifests with an elevated AFP.**

False. Patients with the fibrolamellar variant of HCC are almost always young, female, and are serum AFP-negative. They do, however, have increased serum concentrations of vitamin B12 binding proteins and neurotensin.

○   **True/False: In a female patient with cirrhosis and ascites, the presence of an elevated CA-125 level strongly suggests the presence of an ovarian tumor.**

False. Although the CA-125 level is elevated in several benign and malignant neoplasms, most commonly ovarian carcinoma, it may be elevated in the presence of ascites from any cause, even in the absence of malignancy.

○   **True/False: An elevated carcinoembryonic antigen (CEA) level in a patient with cirrhosis strongly suggests the possibility of a colonic neoplasm.**

False. Minor elevations of CEA are seen in many patients with HCC and in cirrhosis, in general.

○   **What carcinogens have been linked to the development of angiosarcoma of the liver?**

Previous exposure to Thorotrast, vinyl chloride, arsenic, radium, and inorganic copper.

○   **What are the most common modes of presentation of a hepatocellular adenoma?**

- Intraabdominal catastrophe due to hemorrhage.
- Right upper quadrant abdominal pain.
- Discovery of a palpable liver mass.
- Incidental discovery of a mass on hepatic imaging performed for other reasons.

○   **From what blood vessel does HCC receive its entire blood supply?**

The hepatic artery (the vessel used in therapeutic embolization and chemoembolization) serves as the main blood supply of HCC.

○   **What complications may occur following chemoembolization of an HCC?**

Many patients experience marked right upper quadrant abdominal pain, nausea, vomiting, and high fevers. Additionally, all patients develop transient elevations of liver tests and a minority may develop liver abscess and liver failure. Portal vein thrombosis, cholecystitis, and pancreatitis may also occur.

○   **What unique complications occur with hepatic arterial infusion of chemotherapy for colon cancer metastatic to the liver?**

Gastroduodenal ulceration and inflammation may occur in up to 50% of patients and appears to be related to exposure of the gastroduodenal mucosa to high concentrations of the chemotherapeutic agents. Rarely, patients may develop sclerosing cholangitis-like biliary stricturing that leads to chronic cholestasis and secondary biliary cirrhosis.

○   **True/False: Chemoembolization prolongs survival in HCC.**

False. Chemoembolization is a form of loco-regional therapy for HCC. Gelfoam or other particles along with infusion of chemotherapy are injected into the hepatic arterial system feeding the tumor, producing a temporary reduction in blood flow and more direct exposure to the chemotherapy. Although studies have regularly shown significant reduction in the size of large tumors, there is no consistent increase in patient survival with chemoembolization.

○ **True/False: In the setting of HCC, ascitic fluid cytology almost always reveals malignant cells.**

False. Ascitic fluid cytology is rarely positive in this setting.

○ **Why does Mozambique have the world's highest incidence of HCC?**

The population of Mozambique has a very high incidence of hepatitis B virus (HBV) infection and its soil has one of the world's highest aflatoxin B1 contents. Aflatoxin is an environmental carcinogen and HBV and aflatoxin exposure appear to act synergistically to increase the risk of HCC.

○ **What is the significance of portal vein thrombosis in a liver transplant candidate with known HCC?**

Although portal vein thrombosis may spontaneously occur in the setting of cirrhosis, it may also be due to vascular invasion by the HCC. This would constitute extrahepatic spread of tumor and, thus, preclude liver transplantation (LT).

○ **What nodular liver condition is being shown in the figure and what are its characteristic histologic findings?**

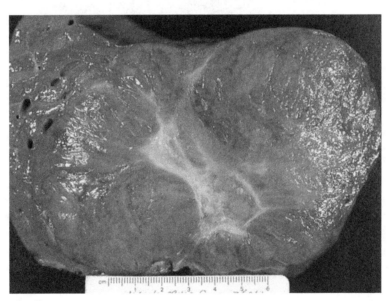

Figure 54-2 See also color plate.

The figure demonstrates the gross appearance of focal nodular hyperplasia. The presence of a central fibrous scar with thin fibrous septa radiating outwards and enclosing nodules, ductular reaction, and abnormal thick-walled vessels embedded within the fibrous tissue are the most characteristic histologic findings.

○ **What predisposing factors are associated with the development of cholangiocarcinoma?**

Primary sclerosing cholangitis, Caroli's disease or Caroli's syndrome, choledochal cysts, chronic hepatolithiasis, recurrent pyogenic cholangitis, and liver fluke (*Clonorchis sinensis*) infection.

○ **True/False: LT is an accepted treatment for polycystic liver disease.**

True. Afflicted patients rarely, if ever, develop complications of portal hypertension and hepatic synthetic dysfunction. However, LT is sometimes needed as a definitive treatment because of the effects on quality of life due to massive hepatomegaly that causes refractory abdominal pain and distention, anorexia, malnutrition, and inanition.

○ **Apart from kidney cysts, do patients with polycystic liver disease have other organ involvement?**

Approximately 5% of patients have cysts in other viscera including the pancreas, spleen, uterus, ovaries, and seminal vesicles. There is also an increased incidence of brain aneurysms.

○ **The most common cause of hepatic cysts worldwide is shown in the figure below. What is the diagnosis?**

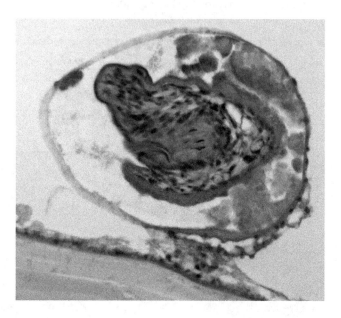

Figure 54-3

Echinococcosis (hydatid disease). The bottom part of the photo shows a non-staining lamellated membrane. Above it is the nucleated germinal membrane and attached to it is a protoscolex with hooklets.

○ **What are CT scan characteristics of an echinococcal cyst?**

Echinococcal cysts are intrahepatic, sharply circumscribed defects with rim enhancement, and usually have calcification within the cyst wall and daughter cysts within them.

○ **What are the complications of hepatic hydatid disease?**

Complications include biliary obstruction from compression of large intrahepatic ducts, cholangitis due to rupture into the biliary tract, secondary infection, and anaphylaxis from peritoneal, pleural, or pericardial rupture.

○ **What is the drug of choice to treat an echinococcal infestation?**

Albendazole, 400 mg BID with meals for 28 days in three successive cycles with a 2-week rest period between cycles.

○ **What risk is associated with traumatic rupture or surgical excision of an hydatid cyst?**

Anaphylaxis. Therefore, appropriate precautions need to be in place.

○ **True/False: The presence of peri-hilar lymphadenopathy in patients with primary sclerosing cholangitis increases the suspicion for a malignancy.**

False. Peri-hilar lymphadenopathy is commonly seen in patients with cirrhosis due to hepatitis C and in most forms of cholestatic liver disease even in the absence of a liver neoplasm.

○ **How does a CT scan differentiate between HCC and a hemangioma?**

HCC appears hyperdense on CT scan with preferential filling during the arterial phase of a dynamic scan, whereas a hemangioma enhances from the periphery inward with additional and persistent enhancement on delayed scans.

○ **What is Stouffer's syndrome?**

Stouffer's syndrome refers to the constellation of constitutional symptoms and nonspecific elevation of liver enzymes in a patient with renal cell carcinoma, even in the absence of metastatic disease to the liver.

○ **What are the most common sites of metastatic spread in patients with HCC?**

In decreasing order of frequency: lung, portal vein, hepatic vein, regional lymph nodes, bone, bone marrow, and peritoneum.

○ **What are the most common tumors metastasizing to the liver?**

Carcinomas of the lung, breast, colon, and pancreas account for the overwhelming majority of hepatic metastases in adults, whereas neuroblastoma, Wilm's tumor, and rhabdomyosarcoma are most common in the pediatric age group.

○ **What is a Klatskin tumor?**

Also termed hilar cholangiocarcinoma, Klatskin tumor occurs at the common bile duct, the main hepatic duct, and at the bifurcation of the right and left main hepatic ducts.

○ **What is Caroli's disease?**

Caroli's disease (type 5 biliary cyst) is a congenital malformation characterized by multifocal intrahepatic bile duct dilation and recurrent episodes of cholangitis. When associated with congenital hepatic fibrosis, it is termed Caroli's syndrome. Despite the absence of cirrhosis, patients may suffer from portal hypertension.

○ **What gastrointestinal and liver complications may occur in a patient with Caroli's disease with congenital hepatic fibrosis (ie, Caroli's syndrome)?**

Portal hypertensive complications such as ascites and variceal bleeding, with the latter occurring much more commonly. Repeated episodes of cholangitis may also occur.

○ **What renal abnormality is associated with Caroli's disease?**

Medullary sponge kidney is present in 60%–80% of cases.

○ **What is Kasabach–Merritt syndrome?**

Thrombocytopenia related to a giant cavernous hemangioma.

○   **The most common benign hepatic tumor is shown in the figure. What is the diagnosis?**

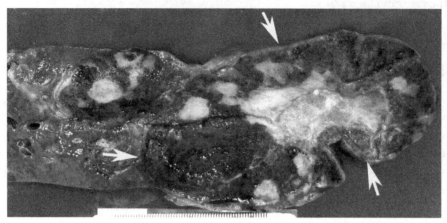

Figure 54-4

The hemangioma, usually an incidental finding, is detected in about 1%–2% of the entire population. The majority of hemangiomas are small. When >4 cm, they are termed cavernous hemangioma. Figure 54-4 shows cut surface of a partial hepatectomy specimen that shows a red brown spongy mass (outlined by white arrows).

○   **What nodular liver condition is shown in the following figure?**

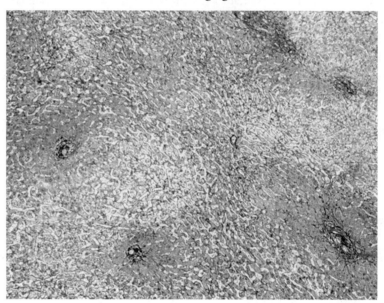

Figure 54-5

Nodular regenerative hyperplasia (NRH) is characterized by diffuse nodularity of the liver in the absence of fibrosis. It is not a tumor but rather a condition that may be associated with a systemic medical condition such as hematologic disorders or collagen vascular disease, as well as the use of certain medications such as ddI, azathioprine, and certain chemotherapeutic agents. Patients may present with complications of portal hypertension. In addition to the nodular configuration being highlighted by the reticulin stain, there is reverse lobulation wherein the portal tract is found in the center of the nodule. This is in contrast to that of a normal lobule where the portal tracts are found at the periphery, and the terminal hepatic venule is present at the center.

○ **Sorafenib is the treatment of far advanced unresectable HCC. What are some of its side effects?**

Systolic hypertension, GI symptoms such as nausea, vomiting, diarrhea, and anorexia, and severe skin rash typically involving the extremities.

○ **What clinical features are associated with hepatic adenomas?**

These lesions tend to occur in women of reproductive age who have history of oral contraceptive use. Adenomas may also be seen in people who are using anabolic steroids and in patients with certain metabolic liver disease (eg, von Gierke's).

○ **True/False: PET scanning is a sensitive and specific imaging modality for the detection of HCC.**

False.

○ **Describe the Milan criteria that are used for patients being listed for LT in the United Network for Organ Sharing (UNOS) system?**

Patients who have a single HCC ≤5 cm or no more than three tumors with the largest diameter ≤3 cm with no gross vascular invasion or metastasis are prioritized to transplantation in the current model for end-stage liver disease (MELD) system. These patients receive a variance of 22 MELD points with the potential for interval increases every 3 months while on the waiting list.

○ **True/False: Preexisting cirrhosis is a prerequisite for the development of HCC.**

False. The presence of HBV infection even in the absence of cirrhosis puts a patient at high risk for the development of HCC. An increasing number of cases of HCC developing in those with hereditary hemochromatosis, nonalcoholic steatohepatitis (NASH), and HCV in the absence of cirrhosis are now being seen.

○ **What is a von Meyenburg complex?**

Von Meyenburg complexes are otherwise known as bile duct hamartomas and arise from remnants of embryonic bile ducts. They are typically discovered incidentally, have nonspecific imaging characteristics, and, when multifocal, can simulate (be confused with) metastases or abscesses.

○ **What is the most common malignant primary hepatic tumor in children?**

Hepatoblastoma. It may occur sporadically or in association with hereditary syndromes such as familial adenomatous polyposis and Beckwith–Wiedemann syndrome.

○ **What pathological features of HCC predict a poor prognosis?**

The presence of gross/macroscopic vascular invasion has a worse prognosis than microvascular invasion. With regards to microvascular invasion, the involvement of many vessels that are large, have thick walls, and are far from the main mass has worse prognosis than microvascular invasion involving small, thin-walled blood vessels present adjacent to the tumor. Poorly differentiated HCC has a worse prognosis than well- or moderately differentiated HCC.

○ **What are some paraneoplastic syndromes associated with HCC?**

Secondary polycythemia, thrombocytosis, hypoglycemia, hypercholesterolemia, and, rarely, hypercalcemia.

○ **How common are simple hepatic cysts?**

Simple hepatic cysts are thought to be congenital in nature and are present in up to 2.5% of the general population. They are almost always asymptomatic and discovered incidentally.

○ **What is an inflammatory pseudotumor?**

Inflammatory pseudotumor is a rare acquired lesion resulting from an inflammatory infectious process. Histologically, it is composed of a mixed population of inflammatory cells such as plasma cells, lymphocytes, and eosinophils in a background of fibrosis. These lesions may be solitary or multiple, are usually well circumscribed, and may spontaneously regress and disappear.

○ **What are the presenting signs of hepatic lymphoma?**

The liver is the one of the most commonly involved organs in lymphoma but primary hepatic lymphomas are rare. They may present as a mass lesion, hepatosplenomegaly, liver disease without lymphadenopathy, fulminant liver failure, or with fever and weight loss. Most are of B-cell origin.

○ **True/False: Biliary papillomatosis may be a risk factor for cholangiocarcinoma.**

True. Although most often benign, malignant transformation to cholangiocarcinoma can occur. These tumors can be solitary or multiple, occurring along the intrahepatic or extrahepatic biliary tree. They are villous and tend to secrete mucin.

○ **True/False: Dysplastic nodules are precursor lesions for cholangiocarcinoma.**

False. These lesions are found to be highly associated with the development of HCC. In particular, the presence of small cell dysplasia and in situ HCC within the dysplastic nodule is often seen in those who have clear-cut HCC elsewhere in the liver.

○ **A patient with advanced HCC develops shortness of breath and evidence of right-sided heart failure. What is the differential diagnosis?**

Patients with HCC can be at risk for the development of deep venous thrombosis and the development of pulmonary emboli. HCC may also involve the hepatic veins with thrombus extension into the right atrium leading to heart failure. A similar type of inferior vena cava thrombosis can be seen in renal cell carcinoma.

○ **What is hepar lobatum?**

Hepar lobatum is diffuse carcinomatosis of the liver from metastatic tumors and can masquerade as cirrhosis.

● ● ● SUGGESTED READINGS ● ● ●

Molina EG, Schiff ER. Benign solid lesions of the liver. In: Schiff ER, Sorrell MF, Maddrey WC, eds. *Schiff's Diseases of the Liver.* 8th ed. Philadelphia, PA: Lippincott-Raven; 1999:1245-1268.

Bruix J, Bru C, Llovet JM. Hepatocellular carcinoma. In: Boyer TD, Wright TL, Manns MP, eds. *Zakim and Boyer's Hepatology: A Textbook of Liver Disease.* 5th ed. Philadelphia, PA: Saunders Elsevier; 2006:1109-1132.

Colombo M, Lencioni R. Benign liver tumors. In: Boyer TD, Wright TL, Manns MP, eds. *Zakim and Boyer's Hepatology: A Textbook of Liver Disease.* 5th ed. Philadelphia, PA: Saunders Elsevier; 2006:1133-1168.

CHAPTER 55

Hepatic Vascular Disorders

Kunal Gupta, MD, MBA and Nicholas Ferrentino, MD

○ **What is the average total blood flow to the liver in mL/min?**

Blood flow normally ranges between 800 and 1200 mL/min. The portal vein supplies the majority of the blood (approximately two-thirds) with the hepatic artery supplying the remainder.

○ **What is the approximate amount of oxygen that the liver is able to extract from the blood and how does this compare to most other gastrointestinal organs?**

The liver is relatively unique in its ability to extract oxygen from the blood—up to 95%—making it much more efficient than most gastrointestinal organs.

○ **What is the proposed mechanism of ischemic reperfusion injury?**

Formation of oxygen-free radicals, predominately by the enzymes NADPH oxidase and xanthine oxidase.

○ **True/False: Ischemic liver diseases are more common in the elderly.**

True. While ischemic liver disease may occur at any age, it most commonly occurs in the older population. This age group is more susceptible to severe cardiac and pulmonary diseases that predispose to ischemia.

○ **What are some causes of ischemic hepatitis?**

Any cause of shock, hemodynamic instability, or "low flow" state (such as with congestive heart failure [CHF]) can cause ischemic injury to the liver. Ischemia can also be caused by local disruption of the hepatic blood flow such as in hepatic sickle cell crisis and hepatic artery thrombosis.

○ **What are the common symptoms of ischemic hepatitis?**

Ischemic hepatitis is usually detected because of extreme elevations in liver biochemical tests (aminotransferase levels, particularly) following a hypotensive episode. Occasional patients have symptoms suggesting acute hepatitis including nausea, vomiting, anorexia, malaise, and right upper quadrant (RUQ) pain.

○ **What is the classic pattern of liver biochemical tests of ischemic hepatitis?**

The typical pattern consists of a stark rise in serum aminotransferase levels also associated with a large rise in lactate dehydrogenase levels. Peak aminotransferase levels are typically 25–250 times the upper limit of normal and are reached within 1 to 3 days of the hemodynamic insult. Following recovery from the hypotensive episode, the liver tests rapidly return to normal.

○ **What is the hallmark histopathologic finding in ischemic disorders of the liver?**

Necrosis of hepatocytes in zone 3 of the hepatic acinus associated with a variable degree of architectural collapse around the central vein.

○ **How does hepatic veno-occlusive disease typically present clinically?**

Nonthrombotic, fibrous, obliterative endophlebitis of small intrahepatic veins, originally described by Chiari, is now referred to as hepatic veno-occlusive disease. Hepatic veno-occlusive disease typically presents with hepatomegaly, ascites, and weight gain.

○ **Name the classic etiology of hepatic veno-occlusive disease.**

Pyrrolizidine alkaloid ingestion typically from plants used to make some herbal teas. Other etiologies include irradiation and high-dose chemotherapy prior to bone marrow transplantation, systemic lupus erythematosus, and agents such as azathioprine, cytosine arabinoside, 6-mercaptopurine, urethane, and possibly oral contraceptives.

○ **What is the mainstay of treatment for hepatic veno-occlusive disease secondary to pyrrolizidine alkaloid ingestion?**

One-half of patients recover completely with fluid and sodium restriction.

○ **True/False: Serum aminotransferases are typically elevated in hepatic veno-occlusive disease.**

True (80%–85%). Hyperbilirubinemia (bilirubin 15–20 mg/dL) and elevated alkaline phosphatase (250–300 IU/L) may also occur.

○ **What percentage of bone marrow transplant patients are thought to acquire hepatic veno-occlusive disease?**

10%–20%.

○ **What is the reported mortality rate from hepatic veno-occlusive disease in bone marrow transplant patients?**

20%–40%.

○ **What is the classic order of manifestation of signs and symptoms in hepatic veno-occlusive disease in the bone marrow transplant setting?**

Weight gain occurring 8 or 9 days following the transplant, hyperbilirubinemia in 11–12 days, elevated aspartate aminotransferase and alkaline phosphatase in 13–15 days, and hepatomegaly and ascites within 1–2 weeks of bone marrow transplantation.

○ **How is the diagnosis of hepatic veno-occlusive disease made?**

If the patient is status post bone marrow transplant and the clinical syndrome typical, presumptive diagnosis can be made without further studies. In less clear cases, liver biopsy is warranted. Unfortunately, these patients are usually severely thrombocytopenic complicating the performance of any invasive procedure. The transjugular approach to liver biopsy may be a less risky alternative in this situation. Ultrasound with Doppler flow study, CT scan, and MRI are all options to determine hepatic vein patency to rule out Budd–Chiari syndrome.

◯ **What are the characteristics of liver biopsy that suggest hepatic veno-occlusive disease?**

The hepatic venule is typically obliterated, hepatocyte dropout is noted, and sinusoidal dilation is present.

◯ **What etiology of hepatic veno-occlusive disease is associated with a higher incidence of severe, chronic, and often fatal disease progression?**

Bone marrow (peripheral stem cell) transplantation.

◯ **What disease is associated with "atrophic infarcts of Zahn"?**

Nodular regenerative hyperplasia.

◯ **Name three processes associated with peliosis hepatis.**

Tuberculosis, AIDS, and drugs.

◯ **How many major hepatic veins drain into the inferior vena cava?**

Three.

◯ **What are the causes of Budd–Chiari syndrome?**

Hypercoagulable states and neoplasms are common causes in the Western world. Examples include myeloproliferative disorders, paroxysmal nocturnal hemoglobinuria, antithrombin III deficiency, protein C and S deficiencies, neoplasms, infections, collagen vascular diseases, Behcet's disease, sarcoidosis, oral contraceptives, pregnancy, inflammatory bowel disease, cirrhosis, polycystic liver disease, and idiopathic. Membranes or webs are important causes of outflow obstruction in Asia and South Africa.

◯ **Name neoplasms associated with Budd–Chiari syndrome.**

Primary hepatocellular, renal, adrenal, pulmonary, pancreatic, and gastric carcinomas. Benign and malignant vascular neoplasms (leiomyomas, leiomyosarcomas, and rhabdomyosarcomas) arising within the hepatic veins or vena cava have also been associated with Budd–Chiari syndrome and hepatic failure.

◯ **What is the typical clinical presentation in Budd–Chiari syndrome?**

A spectrum of disease is possible, ranging from an asymptomatic state to fulminant hepatic failure or cirrhosis with associated complications. Acute obstruction is associated with RUQ pain, nausea and vomiting, hepatomegaly, and ascites. Jaundice and splenomegaly may be noted but are usually mild.

Most patients present with a subacute course of less than 6 months and complain of vague RUQ discomfort, hepatomegaly, mild-to-moderate ascites, and splenomegaly. Jaundice is either absent or mild. Symptomatic disease of more than 6 months presenting as fatigue, bleeding varices, encephalopathy, coagulopathy, hepatorenal syndrome, and/or malnutrition suggests chronic obstruction. Massive hepatocellular necrosis with fulminant hepatic failure is a rare manifestation of Budd–Chiari syndrome and typically follows rapid and complete occlusion of all hepatic veins. Progressive encephalopathy, coagulopathy, and death are inevitable within 8 weeks of occlusion if treatment is not provided.

◯ **What three symptoms characterize acute, rapidly progressive Budd–Chiari syndrome?**

Hepatomegaly, RUQ pain, and ascites.

○ **An enlarged spleen is often found in patients with Budd–Chiari syndrome. Name two possible causes of an enlarged spleen in this disorder.**

Portal hypertension and an underlying myeloproliferative disorder.

○ **What is the prognosis for symptomatic, untreated patients with Budd–Chiari syndrome?**

Poor. The average life span is from 3 months to 3 years after initial diagnosis. The patients often develop renal failure, variceal bleeding, hepatic encephalopathy, and jaundice.

○ **What is the prognosis for asymptomatic individuals with Budd–Chiari syndrome?**

Excellent. This suggests thrombosis of only two of the three hepatic veins or adequate collateral compensation.

○ **Patients often do not present acutely with Budd–Chiari syndrome. If an obstruction is established in this case, what is the treatment of choice?**

Surgical decompression of the liver via shunt surgery. In those with advanced fibrosis or cirrhosis, liver transplantation may be considered.

○ **Describe the histological appearance of the liver in Budd–Chiari syndrome.**

Acute obstruction reveals significant centrilobular congestion and dilation of sinusoids. Atrophy, necrosis, and dropout of centrizonal hepatocytes with extension to periportal regions are present with severe injury. With chronic disease, complete obliteration of central veins associated with midzonal and centrilobular fibrosis with or without cirrhosis is noted.

○ **What laboratory abnormalities are usually present in Budd–Chiari syndrome?**

Standard laboratory investigations are rarely helpful. Twenty-five percent to 50% of patients with venous outflow obstruction present with either normal or mildly abnormal aspartate and alanine aminotransferases. However, patients presenting with acute disease or fulminant hepatic failure may display values greater than 1000 IU/L, especially if there is accompanying portal vein thrombosis. In addition, serum bilirubin, alkaline phosphatase, and prothrombin time are usually normal or mildly elevated.

○ **What tests are helpful in the diagnosis of Budd–Chiari syndrome?**

Radiologic imaging and liver biopsy.

○ **What is the sensitivity of ultrasound in the evaluation of Budd–Chiari syndrome?**

85%–95%. The addition of Doppler to conventional ultrasound is more sensitive than real-time investigation alone.

○ **What is the role of the CT scan in the evaluation of Budd–Chiari syndrome?**

The CT scan is helpful in evaluating abnormalities of the hepatic veins and vena cava including membranes, the extent of hepatic parenchymal disease, and the presence of ascites and splenomegaly.

○ **What is the gold standard in the diagnosis of Budd–Chiari syndrome?**

Angiography. It not only provides information regarding cause and location of obstruction but is also helpful in obtaining pressure measurements, which are important for surgeons before decompression. Ideally, all patients considered for surgery should undergo angiography in addition to liver biopsy.

○ **What medical options exist for the treatment of Budd–Chiari syndrome?**

Medical therapies, while generally ineffective, include sodium restriction, diuretics, and therapeutic paracentesis. In patients who present with acute incomplete thrombotic obstruction, anticoagulation, and thrombolysis are alternatives.

○ **Discuss the role of interventional radiology in the treatment of Budd–Chiari syndrome.**

Percutaneous transluminal balloon angioplasty and stent placement is an effective therapy for hepatic outflow obstruction secondary to caval webs or hepatic venous stenosis. Often when angioplasty and stenting is ineffective, the transjugular intrahepatic portosystemic shunt (TIPS) can also be used to decompress congested segments in the liver by creation of an alternative venous outflow tract.

○ **What surgical shunts are useful in the treatment of Budd–Chiari syndrome?**

Decompressive shunts should be considered the standard of care for patients with acute or subacute venous occlusion. Options include 1) side-to-side portocaval shunts, 2) mesocaval shunts (for patients with compression of the retrohepatic cava by caudate lobar hypertrophy), and 3) mesoatrial shunts (for patients with caval obstruction and a significant gradient between the cava and right atrium). After surgery, long-term anticoagulation is recommended to minimize the chance of recurrent thrombosis.

○ **When should liver transplantation be considered in patients with Budd–Chiari syndrome?**

- Fulminant liver failure
- End-stage liver disease
- Patients with significant liver disease who decompensate after receiving decompressive shunts
- Shunt failure
- Venous thrombosis attributable to protein C, protein S, or antithrombin III deficiency

○ **What is the leading cause of portal hypertension?**

Thirty percent of the cases of portal hypertension in children and 75% of the cases in adults are caused by portal vein thrombosis.

○ **What are the "local" risk factors for portal vein thrombosis?**

Cancer, focal inflammatory lesions, injury to the portal venous system, and cirrhosis.

○ **What three Philadelphia-negative myeloproliferative diseases are considered "general" risk factors for portal vein thrombosis?**

Polycythemia rubra vera, essential thrombocythemia, and myelofibrosis.

○ **What is the difference between acute and chronic portal vein thrombosis?**

Acute portal vein thrombosis is the sudden formation of a partial or complete thrombus in the portal vein, whereas chronic portal vein thrombosis (also known as portal cavernoma) is a thrombus in the portal vein, which involves the formation of hepatopetal collateral veins.

● ● ● SUGGESTED READINGS ● ● ●

Plessier A, Valla DC. Budd–Chiari syndrome. *Semin Liver Dis*. 2008;28(3):259-269.

Crawford JM. Vascular disorders of the liver. *Clin Liver Dis*. 2010;14(4):635-650.

Senzolo M, Riggio O, Primignani M; Italian Association for the Study of the Liver. Vascular disorders of the liver: recommendations from the Italian Association for the Study of the Liver (AISF) ad hoc committee. *Dig Liver Dis*. 2011;43(7):503-514.

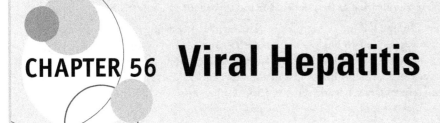

CHAPTER 56 Viral Hepatitis

Marco A. Olivera-Martínez, MD and Sandeep Mukherjee, MD

○ **What are the antiviral actions of interferons?**

Interferons are naturally occurring glycoproteins produced by cells in response to a variety of stimuli including viral infection. Interferons have direct antiviral effects postulated to occur through induction of cellular enzymes that interfere with viral synthesis such as up-regulation of the mitogen activated protein kinase (MAPK) that enhances some signaling pathways. Inhibition of viral RNA and DNA transcription and translation is likely but unproven. Interferons are also antiproliferative and might induce suppression of the necro-inflammatory response. In addition, interferons have immunomodulatory properties and may exert antiviral actions through augmentation of cellular immune function.

○ **What is the risk of interferon precipitating autoimmune phenomena?**

Hyperthyroidism (5%), hypothyroidism (3%), autoimmune thrombocytopenia (<1%), erythema multiforme (<1%), interstitial nephritis (<1%), interstitial pneumonitis (<1%), lupus-like syndrome (<1%), and psoriasis (<1%). Interferon has also been associated with exacerbation of rheumatoid arthritis (<1%), ulcerative colitis (<1%), and vasculitis (<1%).

○ **True/False: It can be challenging to differentiate autoimmune hepatitis from chronic hepatitis C virus (HCV).**

True. Low titers of antinuclear antibodies (ANA) occur in 40%–70% of patients with chronic HCV. ANA titers over 1:160 occur in 20% of patients with chronic HCV. Hypergammaglobulinemia is associated with a false-positive enzyme-linked immunosorbent assay (ELISA) test for HCV in 20% (predominantly young women). Steroid therapy in chronic HCV will decrease alanine aminotransferase levels but elevate HCV RNA levels. Severe hepatitis may occur when autoimmune hepatitis is treated with interferon due to its immunomodulatory effect. Unless the diagnosis of HCV infection is supported by the presence of HCV RNA, steroid therapy should be the primary initial treatment choice.

○ **A patient with chronic hepatitis B virus (HBV) develops a rise in aminotransferases 4 weeks after initiation of pegylated interferon therapy. What should be the response of the treating gastroenterologist?**

During or immediately after interferon therapy for HBV, patient responders (those that lose HBeAg and HBV DNA) frequently will develop increased alanine aminotransferase (ALT) levels. Continued interferon therapy with close monitoring of the patient and symptomatic treatment of side effects is indicated. Because of the cost, side effects, and toxicity of interferon therapy for chronic HBV, patients selected for therapy should exhibit elevated ALT and low HBV DNA, and have no evidence of decompensated liver disease.

○ **What oral antiviral should be recommended as first choice for the treatment of hepatitis B?**

Tenofovir was approved by the FDA in 2008. It is currently recommended as a first-line treatment for chronic hepatitis B. Its efficacy was demonstrated in two double-blind, placebo-controlled trials. In these trials, a higher proportion of patients taking tenofovir showed undetectable HBV DNA when compared to patients receiving adefovir (76% versus 13%, respectively) and similar results were found when ALT and HB surface antigen (HBsAg) were evaluated. No resistance to tenofovir has been detected in patients after 72 weeks of treatment. An alternative first-line treatment is entecavir. Adefovir is now considered a second-line treatment for HBV.

○ **What is the mechanism of the antiviral action of tenofovir in the therapy of chronic HBV?**

Tenofovir is an acyclic nucleotide analog that inhibits HBV viral DNA polymerase-reverse transcriptase.

○ **What is the incidence of the appearance of YMDD mutants in HBV patients undergoing therapy with lamivudine?**

Fifteen percent to 35% of patients treated with lamivudine (100 mg/day) for 12 months develop escape mutations in the active site of the HBV polymerase gene (YMDD locus). After 5 years of treatment, up to 66% of the patients receiving lamivudine might develop YMDD mutation. This molecular virologic event is associated with an increase in ALT and reappearance of HBV DNA.

○ **What are the possible clinical presentations of acute hepatitis A viral (HAV) infection in adults?**

Rarely, jaundice can persist for weeks to months in adults with HAV. This syndrome is known as prolonged cholestasis and can persist for 3 to 5 months. Relapsing hepatitis can also occur in as many as 10% of HAV patients. This syndrome is characterized by a secondary elevation and peak of aminotransferase levels once they were already trending toward normal and, in some instances, even after they reach the normal range. Cholestatic and relapsing HAV infections do not result in increased mortality.

○ **What is the clinical significance of hepatitis B core antibody (anti-HBc)?**

To understand the anti-HBc, it is important to understand first that the core antigen is the only HBV antigen that cannot be quantified in peripheral blood since it is located in the nuclei of infected cells. HBsAg and HBeAg can both be measured in peripheral blood. On the other hand, the antibody directed against the core antigen can be detected in blood. Anti-HBc can be detected in its two forms: IgM and IgG. In acute HBV infection, IgM anti-HBc appears approximately 1 month after HBsAg becomes positive and shortly before the ALT rises. IgM anti-HBc usually indicates acute HBV infection and declines before anti-HBs appears. IgG anti-HBc persists in patients with anti-HBs and patients that develop chronic HBV with HBsAg. The clinical significance of an isolated IgG anti-HBc is unknown; however, affected individuals are not allowed to donate blood, and their organ donation may be associated with transmission of HBV infection.

○ **What is the significance of an HBV precore mutant?**

Mutations of HBV DNA replication are not unusual. The precore mutation involving a G to A change at nucleotide 1896 is well described. This mutation prevents synthesis of HBeAg. The presence of the A1896 mutant should be suspected in patients with elevated ALT, presence of HBsAg, absence of HBeAg, and positive anti-HBe. HBV DNA should be present. In other words, the precore mutant confers the possibility to the HBV to achieve replication despite the absence of HBeAg, which was traditionally described as a replication marker. Patients with precore mutant (e antigen negative) have higher risk of developing chronic hepatitis, cirrhosis, and hepatocellular carcinoma compared to patients with HBeAg positive viral infection.

○ **What is the clinical significance of an "HBsAg carrier"?**

Classically, in these patients, HBV DNA persists at levels that are undetectable by current technology/assays. HBeAg is negative, no hepatic inflammation is present, and ALT is persistently in the normal range; all this occurs despite the presence of HBsAg. However, if replication increases, then the HBV DNA might become detectable triggering liver tissue inflammation with secondary elevation of ALT.

○ **What percentage of patients with hepatocellular carcinoma have HBV or HCV infection?**

The prevalence of HBsAg in patients with hepatocellular carcinoma varies from country to country and ranges from 7% (United States) to 87% (Korea). Over 80% of all hepatocellular carcinoma patients have cirrhosis. In the case of hepatitis B, some patients might develop hepatocellular carcinoma even in the absence of cirrhosis. Nevertheless, cirrhosis is a risk factor for the development of hepatoma when patients have HCV or HBV. Cirrhotic patients with HCV have a 7% risk of hepatoma at 5 years and a 14% at 10 years after diagnosis.

○ **How is chronic hepatitis D prevented and who is at risk of acquiring it?**

Hepatitis D (or delta) is caused by a small circular, enveloped RNA, hepatotropic virus. Hepatitis D virus (HDV) is considered a satellite or "incomplete" virus since it requires the presence of HBV to infect and propagate within the host. The single stranded RNA virus has an outer coat conformed by HBsAg. Its pathophysiology is incompletely understood, but it seems that the hepatocyte HBV surface receptor also recognizes the HDV through the HBsAg and this is the same reason for which HBV vaccination protects against HDV infection. The same populations at risk to acquire HBV are also at risk of acquiring HDV.

○ **True/False: Coinfection with hepatitis D and hepatitis B is associated with a better prognosis.**

True. Hepatitis D can be acquired as a coinfection (patients infected at the same time with HBV and HDV) and as a superinfection (patients that have chronic hepatitis B and are then infected with hepatitis D). Coinfection is associated with a better prognosis, whereas superinfection is associated with a poorer prognosis.

○ **What is the difference in the natural history of HDV infection between coinfection with HBV versus superinfection of HBV?**

Only 2% of coinfections become chronic compared to 90% of superinfected patients.

○ **What subsets of patients with end-stage HBV infection would be expected to have improved survival after liver transplantation?**

Patients with fulminant hepatitis (acute liver failure) from HBV, HDV coinfection, or undetectable HBV DNA would have a lower incidence of graft reinfection than patients that are HBeAg positive and have HBV DNA. Patients that have no history of drug resistance to nucleotide or nucleoside analogs also carry a better prognosis than those patients with a positive history of drug resistance. Immunoprophylaxis with a combination of hepatitis B immunoglobulin and oral antivirals (nucleotide or nucleoside analogs) decreases the incidence of HBV graft reinfection and enhances survival in patients with evidence of pretransplant HBV DNA.

○ **Describe the pathological grading and staging scoring system for chronic hepatitis.**

One of the most common classifications used in the United Stated is the Ludwig–Batts classification (Mayo Clinic) and is as follows:

Grade (inflammation)	Stage (fibrosis)
1. Minimal activity	1. Mild expansion of portal tracts
2. Mild piecemeal necrosis	2. Periportal fibrosis
3. Moderate activity with spotty lobular necrosis	3. Bridging fibrosis
4. Severe activity with piecemeal and lobular necrosis	4. Cirrhosis

○ **Describe the unique clinical manifestations of hepatitis E virus (HEV) infection.**

HEV is a single-stranded RNA virus that was originally classified as a Calicivirus and later reclassified. Now it is considered a Hepevirus. The transmission of this virus is through the fecal-oral route and the symptoms are very similar to those of hepatitis A. This virus, like HAV, only causes acute hepatitis. There are no reported cases of chronic hepatitis E. Fulminant hepatitis may occur in as many as 1%–2% and there is a remarkable increase in mortality for infected pregnant women in the third trimester.

○ **What percentage of patients with infectious mononucleosis have liver involvement?**

Approximately 50%–80% have aminotransferase elevations while 5% become icteric.

○ **Describe the clinical spectrum of cytomegalovirus (CMV) hepatitis.**

In general, 50%–80% of individuals have serum antibodies to CMV by age 35. CMV hepatitis in healthy children and adults is usually asymptomatic and subclinical. Neonates may develop jaundice and liver failure. Primary and secondary (reactivation) CMV infections may occur in immunosuppressed patients. The diagnosis of CMV hepatitis used to require IgM antibody or a rise in IgG titer and a liver biopsy. Currently, more accurate biological markers include a CMV quantitative viral load, which specifically measures the viral DNA (obtained by polymerase chain reaction [PCR]). Liver pathology classically shows giant cells with intranuclear inclusions. The virus may be identified from culture of liver tissue or body fluid.

○ **What populations are at risk of developing fulminant herpes simplex hepatitis?**

Neonates, pregnant women in the third trimester, and immunocompromised patients.

○ **What are the possible extrahepatic manifestations of HCV infection?**

Most likely	*Possible*
Cryoglobulinemia	B-cell lymphoma
Vasculitis	Sjogren's syndrome
Glomerulonephritis	Idiopathic thrombocytopenic purpura
Porphyria cutanea tarda	Lichen planus
Thyroiditis	

○ **What are the most common genotypes of HCV infection in the United States?**

HCV has a high mutation rate during replication. The accumulation of mutations during the evolution of HCV worldwide has led to genetic heterogeneity among isolates and at least six major genotypes (1 to 6).

The most common genotypes infecting patients in North America (about 70% of the cases) are genotype 1a and less commonly 1b. Genotype 1 is considered "hard to treat" since it requires 48 weeks of treatment with pegylated interferon and ribavirin.

○ **What are the major etiologies of chronic liver disease in the United States?**

HCV	26%	Alcohol	21%
Fatty liver disease	17%*	HCV + Alcohol	15%
HBV	11%	Other	5%**
HBV + Alcohol	3%		

Note: *Includes most of the cases known previously as cryptogenic.
**Includes autoimmune hepatitis, PBC, and PSC as well as metabolic and inborn errors of metabolism.

○ **How is hepatitis A transmitted and what is its prevalence in the United States?**

Although the primary route is fecal-oral, through contaminated food or water, and in endemic areas by contaminated food handlers, transmission of HAV has been documented by parenteral and sexual means via blood transfusion and homosexual activity, respectively. The parenteral and sexual transmission of HAV takes place when the blood donor or the sexual partner is actively (acutely) infected since there is no chronic form of hepatitis A. The prevalence of IgG antibody to HAV is 10% in children and 37% in adults.

○ **True/False: The standard therapy of hepatitis A is supportive/symptomatic.**

True. Other than supportive symptomatic therapy, there is no defined protocol. There is no evidence that corticosteroids are helpful. Postexposure prophylaxis is accomplished by serum immunoglobulin (0.02 mL/kg) administered by intramuscular injection. There is also evidence to suggest that immediate HAV vaccination, by itself, may be effective in the setting of postexposure prophylaxis.

○ **What are the phases of perinatally acquired chronic HBV?**

Initial phase: Immune tolerance—HBeAg positive, high HBV DNA level, normal ALT.

Second phase: Immune clearance—between the ages of 15 and 35, HBeAg clearance, elevated ALT, mostly asymptomatic, rare hepatic failure, or cirrhosis.

Third phase: Nonreplicating—HBsAg negative, loss of or very low HBV DNA, normal ALT.

The fourth and fifth phases have also been recently described. The fourth phase is called reactivation and might occur in the presence of immunocompromised states such as chemotherapy. The fifth phase is the development of hepatocelluar carcinoma.

○ **How is the diagnosis of acute HCV infection made?**

Because anti-HCV by ELISA is often undetectable for 5 or 6 weeks, testing for HCV RNA is necessary.

○ **What is the major side effect of oral ribavirin therapy for HCV?**

A dose-dependent hemolytic anemia occurs within 2 to 6 weeks after beginning ribavirin with 15% of hemoglobin tested falling 4 g when 1200 mg/day is administered. Teratogenicity is another important side effect. A patient in the reproductive age receiving ribavirin as part of HCV treatment should practice contraception. If the patient happens to be a male, contraception should be practiced by his sexual partner since ribavirin is secreted in semen.

○ **What is the current state-of-the-art treatment of chronic hepatitis C infection in the United States?**

In June 2011, the FDA approved two new drugs (protease inhibitors) to be used in combination with the previous standard of care (pegylated interferon + ribavirin) in the treatment of genotype 1 chronic hepatitis C infection (so-called "triple therapy"):

1. Telaprevir + Pegylated Interferon α 2A + Ribavirin

2. Boceprevir + Pegylated Interferon α 2B + Ribavirin

The other hepatitis C genotypes should continue to be treated with pegylated interferon + ribavirin alone.

○ **What are the most common side effects of telaprevir therapy for HCV?**

Cutaneous manifestations (rashes) and pruritus may occur in up to 50% but are usually mild to moderate in severity.

○ **What are potential side effect of oral boceprevir therapy for HCV?**

The most common side effects include fatigue, anemia, nausea, headache, and dysgeusia. The addition of boceprevir to peginterferon and ribavirin has been associated with decreases in hemoglobin concentration (and neutropenia and thrombocytopenia also) beyond those with peginterferon and ribavirin alone.

○ **True/False: Individuals at risk of HIV infection are also at risk for HBV and HCV infection.**

True. These viruses are blood-borne pathogens that can be transmitted through the same routes: IV drug use, sexual contact, and vertical transmission from mother to child during pregnancy or birth. Coinfection with HBV or HCV has emerged as a major cause of morbidity and mortality among patients with chronic HIV infection receiving highly active antiretroviral therapy (HAART). A recent meta-analysis has demonstrated that HCV—HIV coinfection is more frequent than HBV–HIV coinfection.

○ **How does coinfection with HIV affect hepatitis B infection and its treatment?**

Effects of coinfection of HIV with hepatitis B:
- Increased risk of reactivation of hepatitis B.
- Increased development of chronic disease (~20%) after acute infection.
- Attenuation of the severity of biochemical and histological liver disease.
- Immune reconstitution with HAART therapy may cause a flare of the hepatitis B resulting in fulminant hepatic failure.

Effects on hepatitis B treatment:
- Because emtricitabine (FTC), lamivudine (3TC), and tenofovir (TDF) have activity against both HIV and HBV, if HBV or HIV treatment is needed, HAART should be initiated with the combination of TDF + FTC or TDF + 3TC as the nucleoside reverse transcriptase inhibitor (NRTI) backbone of HAART and for treatment of active Hepatitis B.
- If HBV treatment is needed and TDF cannot safely be used, the alternative recommended HBV therapy is entecavir in addition to a fully suppressive HAART regimen. Of importance, entecavir should not be considered to be a part of the HAART.
- Use of entecavir or lamivudine alone leads to rapid development of HIV drug resistance at M184V position of the reverse transcriptase.

○ **How does coinfection with HIV affect hepatitis C disease course and treatment?**

Effect on Hepatitis C disease course:
- HCV viral load is much higher than in HIV-negative patients.
- Rapid progress of liver fibrosis and an accelerated progression to cirrhosis, 10 years compared to 20 years in immunocompetent hosts.
- Higher liver-related toxicity rates with antiretroviral therapy.
- HAART is also associated with a rise in HCV RNA and aminotransferases.
- Increases of CD4 cell counts with HAART associated with better hepatic outcomes.

Effect on hepatitis C treatment:
- Lower sustained viral response (SVR) with peg-interferon and ribavirin, 14%–44% in genotype 1 compared to ~55% in normal host.
- If CD4 counts < 200 cells/mm^3, it may be preferable to initiate HAART and delay HCV therapy until CD4 counts increase as a result of HIV treatment.
- Patients receiving or considering therapy with ribavirin should avoid didanosine, stavudine, and zidovudine.

○ **What are the time landmarks used to predict response and determine length of treatment in the management of chronic hepatitis C?**
- Rapid viral response (RVR): HCV-RNA is *non-detectable* at week 4 of treatment.
- Early viral response (EVR): HCV-RNA decreased *at least* 2 logarithms from the baseline viral load.
- Partial response at 12 weeks is considered the decrease of viral load of less than 2 logarithms.
- Delayed response is a decrease of less than 2 logarithms at week 12 of treatment that is followed by a negative viral load (nondetectable HCV-RNA) at 24 weeks of treatment.
- End of treatment response (ETR): HCV-RNA is *non-detectable* at the end of the treatment.
- SVR: HCV-RNA is *non-detectable*, 6 months after the end of the treatment.
- Nonresponder: A nonresponder is the individual that, despite adequate treatment, does not present with decreased viral load during treatment.
- Relapse: A relapse presents as a positive viral load after developing viral response to treatment, most commonly a relapse presents after a partial EVR or a delayed response.
- Recurrence: A recurrence presents as a positive or detectable HCV-RNA after developing ETR.

Among these landmarks, the presence of RVR is the best prognostic factor of an SVR.

○ **What viral factors are associated with an SVR?**

Viral factors that are considered prognostic of a poor viral response or nonresponse to antiviral treatment include:

- Genotype: HCV genotypes 1 and 4 are considered "hard to treat." They require 48 weeks of treatment and the possibilities of SVR are around 50%–60% compared to genotype 2 that requires 24 weeks of treatment and can reach an SVR around 80%.
- Genotype 3 is considered separately since the response to treatment also has a relationship to the amount of steatosis present in the liver. It has been considered that semiquantitative steatosis of less than 30% carries a better prognosis than higher quantitation.
- HCV-RNA: Viral load is an important prognostic factor. The threshold to define a high viral load has changed as the assays to measure viral RNA have evolved. Currently, a viral load of 400,000 IU or less is considered a low viral load and carries a better prognosis to develop SVR than higher viral loads.
- Core and NS5 gene amino-acid substitutions: There is evidence pointing to substitutions in the NS5 and core regions of the virus as involved in the viral response to interferon treatment.
- The presence of interleukin 28B polymorphisms (see next question).

○ **True/False: Interleukin 28B (IL-28B) polymorphisms are associated with response to interferon therapy.**

True. The single nucleotide polymorphisms (SNPs) of interleukin 28B are significantly associated with the outcome of interferon treatment of hepatitis C. These SNPs are rs 2979860 and rs 8099917 and are characterized by alleles TT, TG, and GG. SVR is achieved in approximately 14% of patients infected by genotype 1 HCV who carry the TG or GG alleles. Patients with the TT allele carry up to 58% of SVR rate when treated with pegylated interferon and ribavirin.

• • • SUGGESTED READINGS • • •

Marcellin P, Heathcote J, Buti M, et al. Tenofovir disoproxil fumarate versus adefovir dipivoxil for chronic hepatitis B. *N Engl J Med.* 2008;359:2442-2455.

Poordad F, McCone J, Bacon BR, et al. Boceprevir for untreated chronic HCV genotype 1 infection. *N Engl J Med.* 2011;364: 1195-1217.

Carneiro de Moura M, Marinho R. Natural history and clinical manifestations of chronic hepatitis B virus. *Enferm Infec Microbiol Clin.* 2008;26(Suppl)7:11-18.

Zeuzem S, Andreone P, Pol S, et al. Telaprevir for retreatment of HCV infection. *N Engl J Med.* 2011;364:2417-2428.

Berg T, Sarrazin C, Herrmann E, et al. Prediction of treatment outcome in patients with chronic hepatitis C: significance of baseline parameters and viral dynamics during therapy. *Hepatology.* 2003;37:600-609.

Chen JJ, Yu CB, Du WB, Li LJ. Prevalence of hepatitis B and C in HIV-infected patients: a metaanalysis. *Hepatobiliary Pancreat Dis Int.* 2011;10:122-127.

National Institutes of Health Consensus development conference statement: Management of hepatitis C: June 10-12, 2002. *Hepatology.* 2002;36(Suppl)1:S3-S20.

Hayashi K, Katano Y, Honda T, et al. Association of interleukin 28B and mutations in the core NS5A region of hepatitis C virus with response to peg-interferon and ribavirin therapy. Liver International (Web ahead of printing). DOI: 10.1111/j 1478-3231. 2011.02571.x

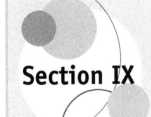

Section IX

MISCELLANEOUS TOPICS

| CHAPTER 57 | # Biostatistics for the Gastroenterologist |

Kendra K. Schmid, PhD and Elizabeth Lyden, MS

○ **The two most common measures of central tendency are the mean and median. Describe how to calculate each and explain the major difference between them.**

To calculate the mean (average), add up all of the observations and divide by the number of observations. The median is the middle observation when all of the observations have been ordered. The mean can be influenced by extreme data values while the median is not.

○ **For a skewed distribution, which is a better choice as a measure of central tendency, the mean or the median? Why?**

The median, since the mean can be influenced by extreme values.

○ **Describe how the mean and median would compare for skewed distributions.**

For a distribution that is skewed to the right (positively skewed), the mean will be greater than the median. For a distribution that is skewed to the left (negatively skewed), the mean will be less than the median. For symmetric distributions, the mean and the median will be similar.

○ **Name and describe three measures of dispersion.**

The most common measure of dispersion is the standard deviation, which measures the average distance between observations and the mean. Other measures of dispersion are range (maximum − minimum), coefficient of variation (standard deviation/mean × 100%) and the interquartile range (75th percentile − 25th percentile).

○ **Which measure of dispersion is most appropriate to present with each measure of central tendency?**

The standard deviation should be reported with the mean as it measures the average distance between observations and the mean. The interquartile range can be reported with the median. Range is often reported with either mean or median. It is not appropriate to report standard deviation with the median.

○ **An investigator is interested in comparing two numerical distributions that are measured on different scales. Should the researcher use the standard deviation or the coefficient of variation? Why?**

The investigator should use the coefficient of variation since the coefficient of variation adjusts for the scales of the variables by dividing the standard deviation by the mean.

○   **Explain the difference between standard deviation and standard error.**

The standard deviation summarizes the variability of a group of observations. The standard error summarizes the expected variability of a sample statistic based on taking repeated samples of the same size.

○   **What statistic is most often used to describe the relationship between two numerical variables?**

Correlation coefficient.

○   **For two variables X and Y, the correlation coefficient is $r = .89$. How does this describe the relationship between X and Y?**

Since r is positive and close to 1, as the values of X increase, the values of Y also tend to increase. In this case, we say that X and Y are positively correlated and the relationship between them is strong.

○   **True/False: A correlation coefficient is $r = .05$. This means that X and Y are not related.**

False. The correlation coefficient r measures the *linear* relationship between X and Y. Since r is close to 0, we can only say that X and Y are not *linearly* related. They may, however, be related in some manner which is not linear.

○   **True/False: The correlation between two variables, X and Y, is $r = .70$. The correlation between two other variables, Z and W, is $r = -.79$. Variables Z and W demonstrate a stronger linear relationship.**

True. Z and W have a stronger linear relationship because the correlation between the two is larger. The sign of the correlation coefficient tells the direction of the relationship while the magnitude gives information on the strength.

○   **True/False: The equation of the regression line for two variables X and Y is: $Y = 1.34 - .7X$. X and Y are positively correlated.**

False. X and Y are negatively correlated. You can tell by examining the slope of the regression equation to see that as X increases, Y decreases.

○   **Describe the coefficient of determination.**

The coefficient of determination, or r^2, is the squared correlation. It describes the proportion of the variation in the dependent variable (Y) that is explained by the independent variable (X).

○   **Name a distribution that has a bell shape and a distribution that is skewed.**

The normal distribution and t-distribution are bell shaped. The chi-square distribution and F distribution are skewed.

○   **Name a distribution typically used to describe count data and one typically used to describe success-failure data.**

The Poisson distribution is often used to model count data and the binomial distribution can be used for success-failure data.

○   **According to The Surveillance, Epidemiology, and End Results (SEER) Program of the National Cancer Institute (NCI), the probability that a newly diagnosed patient with colon cancer has Stage I disease (confined to the primary site) is .39 and Stage IV disease (metastasized) is .20. What is the probability that a newly diagnosed patient with colon cancer has either Stage I or Stage IV disease?**

$.39 + .20 = .59$. In contrast, the probability that a newly diagnosed person has neither Stage I nor Stage IV is .41 $(1 - .59 = .41)$.

○ **True/False: The events described in the previous question are mutually exclusive.**

True. Mutually exclusive events are events that cannot occur simultaneously. These two events are mutually exclusive since a newly diagnosed patient with colon cancer cannot be classified with both Stage I and Stage IV diseases.

○ **Describe what it means for two events to be independent.**

Two events are independent if the outcome of the first event does not affect the outcome of the second event.

○ **In tests used for screening purposes, differentiate between sensitivity and specificity.**

Sensitivity indicates how good a screening test is at identifying the disease for which it is testing. It refers to the proportion of patients with the disease who test positive. Sensitivity can be calculated as follows: True positive/(True positive + False negative) × 100%.

Specificity indicates how good a screening test is at identifying the nondiseased group. It refers to the proportion of patients without the disease who test negative. Specificity can be calculated as follows: True negative/(True negative + False positive) × 100%.

○ **Define positive predictive value of a screening test and indicate when it is most predictive of the disease in question.**

The positive predictive value of a screening test is the probability that the patient has the disease if the patient tested positive for the disease. The higher the prevalence of the disease in the population being tested, the more likely a positive test is a true positive.

○ **Calculate the sensitivity, specificity, positive predictive value, negative predictive value, and prevalence from the following 2 × 2 table, which shows the results of screening for IgA antigliadin (AGA) for diagnosing celiac disease (*Gastroenterology*. 2001 Apr;120[5,1]:A395).**

	Celiac Disease	*Control*
Elevated AGA	99	20
Normal AGA	31	389

Sensitivity: 99/(99 + 31) = .762 or 76.2%
Specificity: 389/(20 + 389) = .951 or 95.1%
Positive predictive value: 99/(99 + 20) = .832 or 83.2%
Negative predictive value: 389/(31 + 389) = .926 or 92.6%
Prevalence: (99 + 31)/(99 + 20 + 31 + 389) = .241 or 24.1%

○ **Define odds.**

Odds are used to compare one outcome to another outcome. For example, if in a certain population the odds of having a specific disease are 1:3, we would expect one person to have the disease for every three who do not.

○ **Define odds ratio.**

The odds ratio measures the association between a risk factor and a disease. It is defined as the odds of disease among individuals exposed to a risk factor divided by the odds of disease among individuals not exposed to that risk factor.

○ **What does an odds ratio of 1 indicate?**

An odds ratio of 1 indicates no association between a potential risk factor and the disease of interest. In other words, the odds of disease among exposed individuals are similar to the odds of disease among unexposed individuals.

○ **True/False: The odds of having disease A are twice as high in vegetarians as in nonvegetarians (ie, odds ratio = 2). The corresponding odds ratio for disease B is 0.5. Disease A is more strongly associated with eating habits.**

False. The strength of the association is the same, only the direction of the association differs. The odds of disease A are twice as high in vegetarians as in nonvegetarians, while the odds of disease B are twice as high in nonvegetarians as in vegetarians.

○ **Distinguish between relative risk reduction (RRR) and absolute risk reduction (ARR).**

RRR is the reduction of adverse outcomes achieved by a treatment expressed as a proportion of the adverse outcomes in the control group.

$$RRR = \frac{(\% \text{ of control patients with adverse outcome}) - (\% \text{ of treatment patients with adverse outcome})}{(\% \text{ of control patients with adverse outcome})}$$

ARR is the difference in the rates of adverse outcomes between the control and treated groups.

$$ARR = (\% \text{ of control patients with adverse outcome}) - (\% \text{ of treatment patients with adverse outcome})$$

○ **Define what is meant by the number needed to treat (NNT).**

NNT is the number of patients that need to be treated with a new therapy to prevent one additional adverse outcome. It is the inverse of the ARR.

$$NNT = \frac{1}{ARR}$$

○ **True/False: The odds ratio estimates the relative risk when the disease of interest is common in the study population (>10%).**

False. The more prevalent the disease of interest, the more the odds ratio overestimates the relative risk when it is >1 or underestimates it when it is <1. The odds ratio provides a good estimate of the relative risk when the disease of interest is rare in the study population (<10%).

○ **In a study designed to demonstrate that giving a proton pump inhibitor (PPI) prior to eradication therapy of *Helicobacter pylori* (HP) provides better patient adherence to therapy and therefore improved successful eradication rates than immediate triple therapy (TT), 33.33% of the TT group (controls) failed to achieve HP eradication and 18.42% of the PPI prior group (treated) failed to achieve HP eradication. (*Gastroenterology*. 2010 May;138[5,1]:S 338). Calculate the ARR, RRR, and NNT (with the TT group considered to be the control).**

ARR = 33.33% − 18.42% = 14.91% or .15
RRR = (33.33% − 18.42%)/33.33% = 44.73% or .45
NNT = 1/.15 = 6.7 or 7 patients.

○ **Differentiate between point estimation and interval estimation. Which type is preferred?**

Point estimation involves using a summary statistic obtained from a sample as an estimate of a population parameter (for example, the sample mean is used as an estimate of the population mean, μ Interval estimation involves creating an interval around the point estimate that contains reasonable values for the population parameter (also known as a confidence interval). Interval estimation is almost always preferred to point estimation as it provides information on the variability of the estimate.

○ **What does a 95% confidence interval imply?**

It implies that if we repeatedly select random samples from the same population as our data and construct interval estimates for each sample, 95 out of 100 of the intervals would be expected to contain the true parameter.

○ **Explain the meaning of the 95% confidence interval: (23 < μ < 35).**

If a large number of such confidence intervals are constructed, about 95% of them will contain the true mean; therefore, we can be 95% confident that the true mean is between 23 and 35. It does not mean that the probability that μ is between 23 and 35 is 95%.

○ **Differentiate between type I and type II errors in hypothesis testing.**

Type I error (false-positive) is rejecting the null hypothesis when it is true; the probability of a type I error is denoted by α.

Type II error (false-negative) is failing to reject the null hypothesis when it is false; the probability of a type II error is denoted by β. The power of a statistical test is $1 - \beta$.

○ **Differentiate between a two-tailed and a one-tailed test.**

A two-tailed (or nondirectional) test occurs when researchers do not know *a priori* the direction of the value they expect to observe in the sample. For example, they want to know if the sample mean differs from the population mean.

A one-tailed (or directional) test occurs when researchers know *a priori* the direction of any true difference between the value observed in the sample and the population parameter. For example, they want to know if the sample mean is larger (or smaller) than the population mean.

○ **True/False: The *P*-value is the probability of obtaining a result as extreme or more extreme than the result obtained from the sample when the null hypothesis is assumed to be true.**

True.

○ **A researcher is interested in the following hypothesis test:**
   $H_0: \mu \leq 0$
   $H_1: \mu > 0$

Is this a one-tailed or a two-tailed test?

This is a one-tailed test. This can be determined by examining the alternative hypothesis. For this test, the null hypothesis is rejected only if μ is sufficiently *greater* than zero. The hypothesis test $H_0: \mu = 0$ versus $H_1: \mu \neq 0$ is an example of a two-tailed test since the null hypothesis is rejected if μ is sufficiently greater than zero *or* if μ is sufficiently less than zero.

○ **A researcher is interested in the following hypothesis test with a .05 level of significance ($\alpha = .05$):**
   $H_0: \mu \leq 0$
   $H_1: \mu > 0$

The *P*-value is found to be .03. What is the conclusion of the test?

The *P*-value rule is to reject H_0 if the *P*-value is less than α and do not reject H_0 if the *P*-value is greater than or equal to α. Since the *P*-value is .03 and $\alpha = .05$, the conclusion is reject H_0 (the null hypothesis).

○ **How is the power of this type of test defined?**

The power of a test is the probability of rejecting the null hypothesis when in fact the null hypothesis is false. Typically, at least 80% power to detect an effect is desired.

○ **In a study designed to look at antibiotic prophylaxis in necrotizing pancreatitis, a total sample size of 200 patients was calculated to demonstrate with a power of 90% that antibiotic prophylaxis reduces the proportion of patients with infected pancreatic necrosis from 40% placebo (PLA) to 20% ciprofloxacin/ metronidazole (CIP/MET) (*Gastroenterology.* 2004 Apr;126[4]:997-1004.). If the researcher decides that a difference between groups of 10% is more clinically relevant, how will the required number of patients be affected?**

To detect a smaller effect (10% versus 20% difference), more patients will be needed. If we want to distinguish groups based on a finer scale, more information about the groups is needed. Larger effects are easier to see, so they require fewer subjects.

○ **A researcher is interested in the following hypothesis test with significance level .05 ($\alpha = .05$):**
$$H_0: \mu = 0$$
$$H_1: \mu \neq 0$$

The 95% confidence interval for μ is: ($-2.3 \leq \mu \leq 1.5$). What is the conclusion of the hypothesis test?

Since zero is included in the above confidence interval, zero is included as one of the reasonable values for μ. In other words, it is possible that in fact $\mu = 0$. Therefore, the conclusion is do not reject H_0.

○ **What is meant by a nonparametric test?**

Nonparametric tests do not specify the distribution of the data. In other words, they are distribution-free tests. Nonparametric tests should be used when the data are not normally distributed or the distribution is unknown.

○ **Explain the difference between an observational study and an experimental study.**

In an observational study, patients are observed (no intervention is applied) and the characteristics of interest are recorded. In an experimental study, an intervention is applied and the effect of the treatment on the subjects is analyzed.

○ **Explain the difference between a case-control study and a cohort study.**

A case-control study compares a group of individuals with the disease of interest (cases) with a group of individuals without the disease of interest (controls), and looks back in time to see how the characteristics of the two groups differ. A cohort study identifies a group of individuals exposed to risk factor and a group of individuals unexposed to a risk factor, and follows the groups over a period of time to see if the risk factor affects disease development.

○ **What is a double-blind trial and what is its purpose?**

A double-blind trial is when neither the experimenter nor the subject knows whether they are in the control group or the treatment group. The purpose is to reduce the chance for bias by preventing the researcher from interpreting the results in a manner that supports the researcher's goals. This is especially important in a trial with a subjective outcome.

○ **What does concealment of allocation mean with respect to clinical trials?**

Concealment of allocation means that the researcher who enrolls patients into a trial (ie, attempts to get informed consent from the patient) does not know if the next patient to enter the trial will get the experimental treatment or a placebo.

○　**Differentiate between an intention-to-treat analysis and per protocol analysis.**

Intention-to-treat analysis is when all patients who enrolled in a clinical trial are included in the final data analysis, regardless of whether or not the patient completed the trial.

Per protocol analysis is when only patients who properly complete the clinical trial are included in the final data analysis.

○　**A study is designed so that every member of the population has an equal probability of being selected for the study. What sampling method is being used?**

Simple random sampling.

○　**Differentiate between the life-table method and the Kaplan–Meier method of calculating estimates of the survival distribution.**

Life-table method: The time axis showing the total observation period or follow-up time is divided into distinct intervals (not necessarily of equal length) and the numbers of deaths and withdrawals (censored patients) are shown for each interval. This method is useful when the exact times of death or withdrawal are unknown.

Kaplan–Meier method: Exact times of death and withdrawal must be known as calculations are made at each time of death. Similar to the life-table method, the survival curve will resemble a step function; curves constructed by the Kaplan–Meier estimate will step down at each time of death.

○　**Define median survival.**

Median survival is defined as the time at which 50% of the population under study has "failed" (died, progressed, relapsed, etc).

○　**Explain what is meant by censored observation.**

Censored observation refers to patients who do not reach a disease endpoint (died, progressed, relapsed, etc) during their period of follow-up. A patient is censored at time t if the patient has been followed up to time t and has not "failed" (died, progressed, relapsed, etc).

● ● ●　SUGGESTED READINGS　● ● ●

Petrie A, Sabin C. *Medical Statistics at a Glance.* 3rd ed. West Sussex, UK: John Wiley & Sons; 2009.

Altman DG. *Practical Statistics for Medical Research.* London: Chapman & Hall; 1991.

CHAPTER 58

Gastrointestinal and Liver Dermatoses

Michelle O. DiBaise, PA-C, MPAS, DFAAPA

○ **What are the four D's of pellagra?**

1. Dermatitis (photosensitive)
2. Diarrhea
3. Dementia
4. Death

○ **A deficiency in what nutrients may cause pellagra?**

- Niacin (most commonly)
- Tryptophan

○ **What other causes of pellagra exist?**

- Alterations in tryptophan metabolism secondary to carcinoid
- Chronic alcoholism
- Chronic colitis
- Chronic dialysis
- Cirrhosis of the liver
- Prolonged diarrhea
- Tuberculosis of the GI tract
- HIV infection
- Hartnup's disease
- Use of isoniazid, 5-fluorouracil, 6-mercaptopurine, or sulfapyridine

○ **Vitiligo has been associated with what nutritional deficiencies?**

- Vitamin B12
- Folic acid
- Vitamin C

○ **What disease/nutritional deficiency leads to perifollicular purpura?**

Scurvy/vitamin C deficiency. Other findings include poor wound healing, corkscrew hairs, and gingival bleeding.

○   **What percent of patients with the type of neurocutaneous porphyria shown in the figure will develop hepatic cirrhosis?**

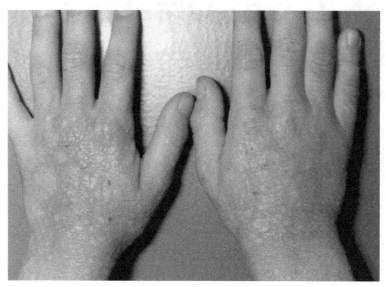

Figure 58-1

Two to five percent of patients with erythropoeitic protoporphyria (EPP) will develop cirrhosis. The enzyme defect responsible for EPP is ferrochelatase.

○   **Plummer–Vinson syndrome is associated with what findings?**

- A postcricoid web
- Koilonychia ("spoon nails")
- Angular stomatitis
- Sore tongue
- Iron deficiency

○   **What percent of patients with Plummer–Vinson syndrome are at risk of developing a carcinoma?**

Between 3% and 15% will develop squamous cell carcinoma at the site of the postcricoid web. Patients with coexisting celiac disease may be at an even greater risk. There is a rare association of Plummer–Vinson syndrome with gastric carcinoma particularly in patients with previous gastric surgery.

○   **What is the classical dermatologic finding in patients with hemochromatosis?**

Bronze to metallic gray pigmentation of the skin.

○   **What autosomal recessive condition leads to a perioral, acral and genital eczematous eruption, alopecia, glossitis, and diarrhea?**

Acrodermatitis enteropathica.

○   **What is the underlying nutritional cause of acrodermatitis enteropathica?**

Zinc deficiency.

○   **What skin reactions are found in PCT?**

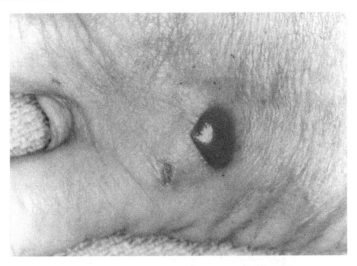

Figure 58-2

- Vesicles/bullae on dorsa of hands/feet
- Skin fragility/scarring
- Hyperpigmentation
- Sclerodermoid plaques
- Milia on fingers/hands
- Hypertrichosis

The enzyme defect responsible in PCT is uroporphyrinogen decarboxylase.

○   **A 39-year-old man with a long history of recurrent epistaxis presents with melena. The oro-labial lesions demonstrated in the figure are noted. What is the most likely diagnosis?**

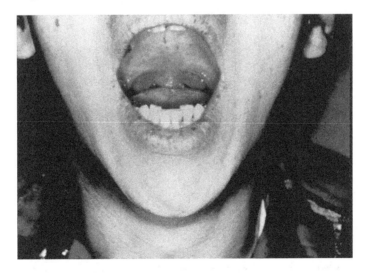

Figure 58-3

Hereditary hemorrhagic telangiectasia (Osler–Weber–Rendu syndrome).

○   **Treatment for the condition illustrated in the figure includes what modalities?**

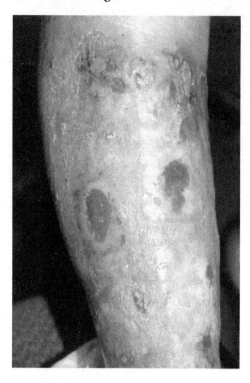

Figure 58-4

The lesion is pyoderma gangrenosum. Treat the underlying disorder, if one exists (40%–50% of cases are idiopathic). Surgical debridement should be avoided as it can stimulate the development of new lesions. Other treatment options include:

- Systemic glucocorticoids
- Dapsone
- Sulfapyridine
- Sulfasalazine
- Cyclosporine
- Tacrolimus
- 6-mercaptopurine
- Azathioprine
- Methotrexate
- Cyclophosphamide
- Chlorambucil
- Clofazimine
- Minocycline
- Colchicine
- Plasmapheresis
- Thalidomide

○   **What genetic mutation is responsible for inherited acrodermatitis enteropathica?**

SLC39A4 gene located on band 8q24.3 that encodes a transmembrane protein required for zinc uptake and is expressed on the enterocytes of the duodenum and jejunum.

○   A 59-year-old woman with diabetes mellitus presents with bilateral, symmetrical, pruritic vesicles on the elbows, knees, buttocks, and lower back. A skin biopsy reveals granular dermal papillary deposits of IgA. What is the diagnosis?

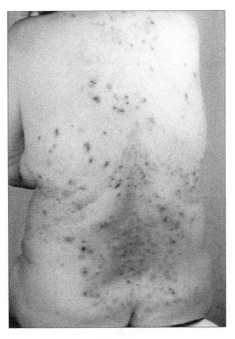

Figure 58-5

Dermatitis herpetiformis.

○   A 27-year-old man presented for sigmoidoscopy because of intermittent hematochezia. Numerous polyps were seen. A peculiar freckling pattern on his lips was also noted. What is the most likely diagnosis?

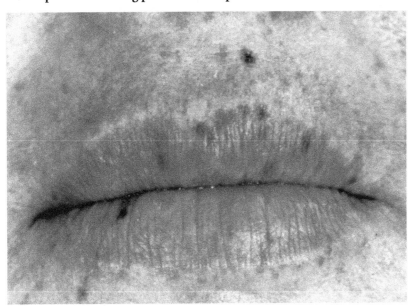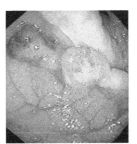

Figure 58-6

Peutz–Jeghers syndrome.

○ **A 72-year-old woman presents with periorofacial, intertriginous, and perigenital circinate lesions with vesicles, crusting, and postinflammatory pigmentation in association with glossitis, weight loss, diarrhea, and diabetes. The rash is shown below. What is the diagnosis?**

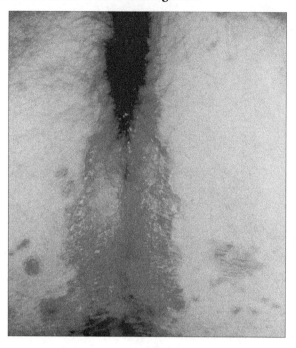

Figure 58-7

Glucagonoma. It arises in the islet cells of the pancreas and is associated with a distinctive dermatitis referred to as necrolytic migratory erythema (NME), which is histologically similar to acrodermatitis enteropathica. Since the rash of NME may be an early sign in slow-growing tumors, this differential should be kept in mind.

○ **What gastrointestinal (GI) conditions may lead to acquired zinc deficiency?**

- Chronic inflammatory bowel disease (IBD) with diarrhea and/or malabsorption
- Steatorrhea
- Pancreatic insufficiency
- Cirrhosis
- Surgically induced conditions such as short bowel syndrome

○ **What are the cutaneous manifestations of hepatitis C?**

- Lichen planus
- Porphyria cutanea tarda (PCT)
- Leukocytoclastic vasculitis/cryoglobulinemia
- Sialadenitis/sicca syndrome
- Corneal ulceration
- Pruritis with excoriations
- Urticaria
- Jaundice
- Erythema nodosum (EN)
- Erythema multiforme (EM)
- Polyarteritis nodosa

○   **What condition is associated with the nail changes illustrated in the figure below?**

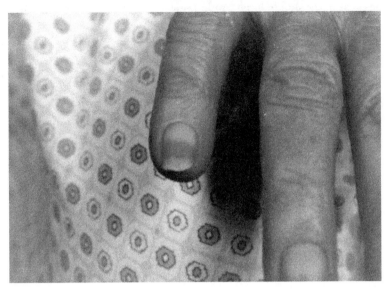

Figure 58-8

Cirrhosis. Skin and nail findings associated with cirrhosis include:
- White nails referred to as Terry's nails
- Spider nevi
- Diffuse muddy gray color of the skin or a blotchy brown pigmentation
- Linear pigmentation in skin creases
- Perioral and periorbital hyperpigmentation (chloasma hepaticum)
- Guttate hypomelanosis
- Palmar erythema
- Portal-systemic collaterals over the abdomen
- Purpura
- Decrease in facial and body hair growth

○   **What percent of PCT patients have associated chronic hepatitis C?**

Approximately 70%.

○   **What cutaneous side effects are seen with interferon-α therapy?**

- Urticaria
- Lupus-like illness
- Psoriasis
- Vitiligo
- Systemic sclerosis
- Idiopathic thrombocytopenic purpura

○   **What diagnoses should be considered when there are skin findings consistent with PCT in addition to acute episodes of abdominal pain, nausea, vomiting, paralysis, and seizures?**

- Variegate porphyria (VP) (most common in South Africans of Dutch ancestry)
- Hereditary coproporphyria (HCP)

○   **A 32-year-old man with AIDS presents with melena. The skin lesions illustrated in the figure below are noted. What is the cause of the skin lesions? Could these lesions be responsible for the GI bleeding?**

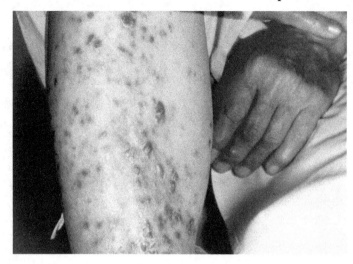

Figure 58-9

Kaposi's sarcoma (KS). It is found in up to 10%–15% of HIV-infected individuals.

In the alimentary tract, KS typically occurs as bulky gingival or palatal lesions, or GI lesions resulting in difficulty with chewing, swallowing, and obstruction to flow, respectively.

Rarely, it is a cause of GI bleeding.

○   **A 19-year-old man presents with massive hematochezia and hemodynamic instability. He has no other health problems but does experience recurrent painless skin lesions as shown in the figure below. What is the diagnosis?**

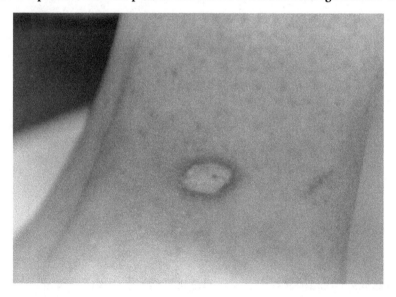

Figure 58-10

Degos' disease or malignant atrophic papulosis. This is a very rare disorder that affects the skin, GI tract, and central nervous system, and may lead to massive bleeding and death.

○ **What drugs can precipitate an attack of VP?**

Inducers of hepatic cytochrome P450 such as barbiturates, dapsone, and estrogens.

○ **What diagnosis should be considered in a patient with dysphagia, heartburn, and fibrotic skin with beaking of the nose, cutaneous telangiectasia, and thinning of the lips?**

Systemic sclerosis.

○ **What does CREST stand for?**

- **C**alcinosis cutis
- **R**aynaud's phenomenon
- **E**sophageal dysmotility
- **S**clerodactyly
- **T**elangiectasias

○ **Patients with Ehlers–Danlos syndrome (EDS) are at high risk for what GI problems?**

Patients with type IV (arterial subtype) EDS that exhibit hyperextensibility, skin fragility, and the formation of hypertrophic scars are at risk for rupture of the large intestine and/or rupture of the mesenteric arteries in the abdomen. Hernias and diverticula with associated GI bleeding may also be seen.

○ **Yellowish papules in flexural skin and rectal mucosa giving a "plucked chicken" appearance, ocular angioid streaks, hypertension, and GI hemorrhage are suggestive of what disorder?**

Pseudoxanthoma elasticum. Other findings may include retinal hemorrhage and detachment, claudication, angina pectoris, abdominal angina, and urinary tract bleeding.

○ **What GI symptoms are commonly seen in patients with cutis laxa?**

Hernias (inguinal, umbilical, and obturator), diverticula of the GI tract, and chronic diarrhea.

○ **What conditions with dermatologic manifestations are associated with GI bleeding?**

- Hereditary hemorrhagic telangiectasia
- Blue rubber bleb nevus syndrome
- Ehlers–Danlos syndrome
- Pseudoxanthoma elasticum
- Kaposi's sarcoma (human herpes virus 8)
- Vasculitides (Henoch–Schoenlein disease and polyarteritis nodosa)
- Dego's disease (malignant atrophic papulosis)

○ **What conditions are associated with both GI polyps and dermatologic manifestations?**

- Gardner's syndrome (associated with multiple epidermal inclusion cysts, lipomas, osteomas of the face, GI adenomas)
- Peutz–Jegher's syndrome (associated with freckling around the mouth and on the lips, benign GI hamartomas)
- Cronkhite–Canada syndrome (associated with patchy alopecia, nail changes and inflammatory polyps of the stomach and bowel)
- Neurofibromatosis or Von Recklinghausen's syndrome, type I (associated with axillary and inguinal freckling, café au lait spots, and neurofibromas of the skin and gut)
- Cowden's disease (an autosomal disorder associated with multiple tricholemmomas [resembling warts] around the mouth, nose and ears, colon polyps, abnormalities of the thyroid, and breast)

○ **What skin signs may aid in the diagnosis of acute hemorrhagic pancreatitis?**

- Cullen's sign (periumbilical ecchymosis)
- Grey Turner's sign (flank ecchymosis)

○ **What cutaneous signs may herald an underlying GI malignancy?**

- Dermatomyositis in adults over 50—associated with gastric and colonic carcinomas.
- Acanthosis nigricans—paraneoplastic variant presents with warty thickening of mouth and palms ("tripe hands") and is associated with adenocarcinoma of the stomach and bowel.
- Sister Mary Joseph nodule (umbilical metastasis)—associated with carcinoma of the stomach, colon, and ovary.
- Muir–Torre syndrome—autosomal dominant disorder presenting with multiple sebaceous tumors is associated with colon cancer.
- The sign of Leser–Trélat (controversial)—sudden onset of multiple, pruritic seborrheic keratoses has been reported to occur with malignancy of the stomach, breast, prostate, lung, and colon.
- Acrokeratosis of Bazex—symmetrical psoriaform eruption affecting the hands, feet, ears, and nose, seen predominantly in males, and is associated with tumors of the pharynx, esophagus, tongue, and lungs.
- Erythema gyratum repens—a raised, erythematous, concentric eruption that migrates on the skin and is likened to a "wood grain" pattern has been associated with tumors of the breast, lung, bladder, prostate, cervix, stomach, esophagus, and multiple myeloma.
- Ataxia telangiectasia—oculocutaneous telangiectasia, xerosis, gray hair, atrophic or sclerotic skin, recurrent impetigo with progressive cerebellar ataxia and an increased incidence of tumors of the oral cavity, breast, stomach, and pancreas.
- Sweet's syndrome (acute febrile neutrophilic dermatosis)—erythematous to bluish papules or nodules that coalesce to form well-demarcated plaques, likened to a "relief of a mountain range." Twenty percent of cases are associated with malignancy. Most commonly seen with acute myelocytic leukemia, it has also been reported to occur with gastric carcinoma and adenocarcinoma of the rectum.
- Acquired ichthyosis—excessively dry skin with tessellated or tile-like scale predominantly on the lower extremities can be seen in many underlying gut tumors but most commonly is associated with lymphoma.

○ **What cutaneous differences occur in the carcinoid syndrome depending on where the tumor originates in relation to the embryologic foregut, midgut, and hindgut?**

- Foregut tumors (bronchus, stomach, pancreas) produce serotonin and histamine leading to peptic ulcer disease, brighter and more persistent flushing reactions, lacrimation, sweating, vomiting, and asthma.
- Midgut tumors (small intestine to midcolon) are associated with a bluish flushing with mixed erythema and pallor, hypotension, and bronchoconstriction.
- Hindgut tumors (descending colon and rectum) are not associated with flushing or other manifestations of carcinoid syndrome.

○ **What conditions should be considered in a patient with a painful, erythematous nodule of the lower extremity and known IBD?**

- Pyoderma gangrenosum (PG) begins as a painful nodule or pustule then develops into an ulcer with a serpiginous, erythematous to violaceous border and boggy, necrotic base and may not resolve once the bowel disease is under control. PG is more common in patients with ulcerative colitis than Crohn's disease and may also occur in patients with chronic active hepatitis, diverticulitis, primary biliary cirrhosis, gastric and duodenal ulcers, rheumatoid arthritis, myeloma, and collagen-vascular diseases.
- Erythema nodosum lesions are erythematous, painful nodules that occur predominantly on the extensor surfaces of the lower extremities and may precede the onset of IBD. EN is more common in patients with ulcerative colitis than Crohn's disease and may also be seen in patients with sarcoidosis, bacterial, viral, acid fast bacilli (AFB) and fungal infections, Behçet's, oral contraceptive use, and lymphoma.

○ **What GI condition is associated with dermatitis herpetiformis?**

Gluten-sensitive enteropathy (ie, celiac disease).

○ **What treatment options are available for dermatitis herpetiformis?**

- Gluten-free diet (will resolve intestinal and skin lesions)
- Dapsone (skin lesions respond more rapidly to medications)
- Sulfapyridine (in dapsone-intolerant patients)

○ **What GI manifestations may be seen in patients with urticaria pigmentosa?**

Gastric hypersecretion due to elevated plasma histamine leading to gastritis, peptic ulcer disease, diarrhea, abdominal pain, malabsorption in 30% of patients, and abnormal liver tests, in particular alkaline phosphatase.

○ **What skin changes may be seen in patients with primary biliary cirrhosis?**

- Melanosis, predominantly in exposed areas
- Clubbing
- Scleroderma-associated features
- Lichen planus
- Jaundice
- Excoriations from itching
- Xanthomas on the hands feet and trunk, xanthelasma, and occasionally tuberous xanthomas

○ **What skin changes may be seen in patients with Wilson's disease?**

- Azure lunulae or bluish color of the lunular area of the nails
- Kayser–Fleischer rings of the cornea

○ **Where is the most common GI site of involvement in metastatic malignant melanoma?**

Small bowel. Nevertheless, malignant melanoma may metastasize anywhere in the GI tract, pancreas, and liver. Primary melanoma may also arise anywhere along the GI tract, often presenting with GI bleeding.

○ **What cutaneous side effects have been seen with anti-TNF-α therapy?**

- Urticaria
- Erythema
- Lichenoid skin eruptions
- Psoriasis
- Atopic dermatitis

○ **What GI manifestations may be seen in primary systemic amyloidosis?**

- Petechiae, purpura, ecchymoses spontaneously or after minor trauma on the skin, and oral cavity (most common)
- Waxy, smooth papules, nodules, and plaques (skin and oral cavity)
- Xerostomia
- Macroglossia with or without nodularity
- Chronic intestinal pseudoobstruction
- GI hemorrhage
- Hepatomegaly
- Gastric carcinoma
- Diarrhea, malabsorption, and protein-losing enteropathy

○   **What potentially fatal dermatologic condition can occur in a patient with a glomerular filtration rate (GFR) <30 mL/min who has a magnetic resonance imaging study with contrast?**

Nephrogenic systemic fibrosis typically presents with progressive fibrosis of the skin that is both pruritic and painful. It can involve multiple organs including the liver, lung, skeletal muscle, and heart, and is associated with gadolinium use in patients with renal failure.

○   **What GI disorder has been linked to the use of isotretinoin (Accutane)?**

IBD. A true causal link has not yet been proven; however, recent epidemiological evidence suggests a strong association between the use of isotretinoin and ulcerative colitis. The association between isotretinoin and Crohn's disease appears to be less strong. While the potential causal relationship is controversial, large jury settlements have been made to isotretinoin users who developed IBD.

● ● ● **SUGGESTED READINGS** ● ● ●

Marks J. The Relationship of Gastrointestinal Disease and the Skin. *Clinics in Gastroenter.* 1983;12(3):693-712.

Johnston GA, Graham-Brown RAC. The Skin and Disorders of the Alimentary Tract, the Hepatobiliary System, Kidney, and Cardiopulmonary System. In: Wolff K, Goldsmith L, Katz S, et al, eds. *Fitzpatrick's Dermatology in General Medicine.* 7th ed, Vol 2. New York: McGraw-Hill; 2007.

CHAPTER 59

Gastrointestinal and Hepatobiliary Manifestations of HIV and AIDS

Humberto Sifuentes, MD, Parakkal Deepak, MD, and Eli D. Ehrenpreis, MD

○ **What is the basic management of opportunistic infections occurring in human immunodeficiency (HIV) and acquired immune deficiency syndrome (AIDS)?**

Because of highly active antiretroviral therapy (HAART), when opportunistic infections are diagnosed, both the opportunistic infection and the underlying HIV infection are treated at the same time.

○ **Which HAART medications are associated with pill-induced esophagitis?**

Zidovudine (AZT) and zalcitabine (ddC).

○ **What is the most common opportunistic infection involving the esophagus in HIV-infected patients?**

Candida is the most common fungal infection and cytomegalovirus (CMV) is the most common viral infection.

○ **What causes oral hairy leukoplakia?**

Epstein–Barr virus (EBV). Oral hairy leukoplakia appears as white plaques that coat the lateral aspects of the tongue.

○ **What area of an ulcer would you biopsy to detect herpes simplex virus (HSV)? CMV?**

Biopsy the edge (area of viral replication) of the ulcer to detect HSV and the ulcer base (CMV does not invade squamous epithelium) to detect CMV.

○ **What name is given to an ulcer seen on endoscopy in an HIV-infected patient with histopathology showing no viral cytopathic effect and no clinical or endoscopic evidence of reflux or pill-induced ulceration?**

Idiopathic esophageal ulcer. These ulcers often present with odynophagia and substernal chest pain and may be deep and multiple in number. Ninety percent respond to oral or intralesional steroids. They also appear to be responsive to thalidomide.

○ **True/False: Empiric treatment with an antifungal agent such as fluconazole should be administered to a patient with HIV who is complaining of dysphagia without odynophagia and who has oral thrush on exam.**

True. The presumptive diagnosis is esophageal Candidiasis. Up to two-thirds of patients with *Candida* esophagitis have oral thrush. Odynophagia is usually not severe with candidiasis and if present should prompt an endoscopic evaluation for possible mucosal ulceration.

○ **Why is ketoconazole less effective than fluconazole in the treatment of Candidiasis?**

The absorption of ketoconazole and itraconazole is pH dependent—requiring an acidic pH for absorption. Achlorhydria has been well described in association with HIV infection. Concomitant use of H_2 blockers or proton pump inhibitors is also common in HIV-infected patients. Absorption of fluconazole is not pH dependent.

○ **What is the most common gastrointestinal symptom in HIV-infected patients?**

Diarrhea. Prevalence rates of 50%–90% have been recorded.

○ **What is the most common infection of the small bowel in patients with AIDS?**

Cryptosporidiosis. This protozoa causes a self-limited diarrheal illness in normal hosts. However, in patients with AIDS, this infection can cause high volume, watery diarrhea often without the presence of fecal leukocytes and usually with malabsorption and weight loss. The disease course is worse with increasing degrees of immunodeficiency. Nitazoxanide is approved by the U.S. Food and Drug Administration for the treatment of cryptosporidiosis in non-HIV infected patients but, to date, this agent has not been effective for the treatment of HIV-infected patients. The treatment of choice in HIV-infected patients with cryptosporidiosis is HAART. Paromomycin is no more effective than placebo in HIV-associated cryptosporidiosis.

○ **What measure can patients with CD4 counts < 200 take to decrease infection with *Cryptosporidium*?**

Boil or filter the water. This eliminates oocytes. They should also minimize oral exposure of water from lakes, streams, and public swimming pools.

○ **In HIV-infected patients, name a protozoal infection of the small bowel that responds well to antibiotic therapy.**

Isospora belli. This infection is endemic in developing countries (Haiti and Africa). The treatment of choice is trimethoprim-sulfamethoxazole. Patients intolerant to sulfonamides can use pyrimethamine. Relapses can occur and require maintenance therapy.

○ **An HIV-positive patient with chronic diarrhea undergoes small bowel biopsy. On electron microscopy, a "cat's eye" appearance of the enterocyte nucleus with a supranuclear indentation is noted. What is the cause of the diarrhea?**

The appearance of the nucleus is caused by a merozite indicating infection with microsporidium, probably the species *Enterocytozoon bieneusi*. This species accounts for about 80% of all microsporidial infections and is often refractory to treatment. *Encephalitozoon intestinalis* makes up the other 20% of microsporidial infections. Albendazole is treatment of choice for *E. intestinalis*. No consistent therapy exists for *E. bieneusi*. Although albendazole has been reported to reduce frequency and volume of diarrhea, it does not clear the organism on stool specimens or duodenal biopsy specimens.

○ **What is the most common viral infection that causes diarrhea in AIDS?**

Cytomegalovirus. The infection may be limited to the right side of the colon in up to 18%–30% of patients. Hence, patient should undergo a full colonoscopy particularly if the distal colon is endoscopically normal.

○ **What are the serious complications of CMV enteritis and colitis?**

Severe abdominal pain, mucosal ischemic ulcerations, bleeding, fistula, and perforation. Patients may present with an acute abdomen. CMV enteritis or colitis should be suspected in this clinical setting in a patient with AIDS and a very low CD4 count.

○ **What is the initial treatment of choice for intestinal CMV infection?**

Ganciclovir or valganciclovir. Although effective, cidofovir and foscarnet are considered second-line treatments because of the limited studies in GI disease and associated toxicities. Prior to treatment, the patient should undergo ophthalmologic examination to evaluate for CMV retinitis.

○ **What is the most significant side effect of treatment with ganciclovir and valganciclovir?**

Neutropenia. These drugs cause neutropenia in 20%–40% of patients and thrombocytopenia in 5% of patients. Zidovudine has potentiating effects on drug-induced neutropenia. Hence, other HAART medications are recommended.

○ **What is the most common bacterial cause of diarrhea in HIV-infected patients?**

Clostridium difficile associated diarrhea. The incidence of *C. difficile* in this population is increased due to the frequent use of antibiotics and increased amount of time spent hospitalized. The clinical presentation, response to therapy, and relapse rates are similar to immunocompetent patients.

○ **How do the presentations of gastrointestinal *Mycobacterium avium* complex (MAC) and *Mycobacterium tuberculosis* (MTB) in HIV-infected patients differ?**

MAC is the most common mycobacterial infection in patients with AIDS. MAC usually presents as an asymptomatic infection, most commonly in the duodenum and can appear as patchy areas of edema, erythema, friability, erosions, nodularity, a frosted appearance, or yellowish nodules or plaques on endoscopy. Alternatively, massive small intestinal infiltration with MAC may cause diarrhea and malabsorption. Concomitant hepatomegaly or splenomegaly with anemia is often present. Treatment includes 2 or 3 antimicrobials for at least 12 months. Commonly used first-line drugs include macrolides (clarithromycin or azithromycin), ethambutol, and rifamycins (rifampin, rifabutin). Aminoglycosides, such as streptomycin and amikacin, are also used as additional agents. Prophylaxis is recommended for all patients with CD4 cell count less than 50/mm³. Effective drugs include macrolides and rifabutin.

MTB usually causes symptomatic illness and generally affects the ileocecal region. MTB has been associated with the formation of bulky mesenteric or retroperitoneal adenopathy with areas of central necrosis seen on computed tomography. MTB infection responds well to multidrug antitubercular therapy.

○ **True/False: Octreotide plays a major role in the management of chronic diarrhea in patients with AIDS.**

False. Octreotide is a somatostatin analogue that acts as an antisecretory and antimotility agent. Some research suggests that HIV shares amino acid sequences with vasoactive intestinal peptide (VIP), thus upregulating the VIP receptors and contributing to chronic HIV-associated diarrhea. Octreotide has been postulated to interfere with this mechanism. Nevertheless, a randomized, placebo-controlled trial failed to show any benefit of octreotide as treatment of HIV-infected patients with chronic diarrhea.

○ **What malabsorptive disease can mimic MAC infection of the gastrointestinal tract?**

Whipple's disease. After the atypical mycobacteria are ingested from contaminated water, they are phagocytosed by macrophages but are not killed. They invade tissues causing lymphadenopathy and organomegaly. In the gut, they invade the wall impairing lymph flow and causing fat malabsorption and exudative enteropathy. Histologically, foamy macrophages are seen in the small intestinal lamina propria. These are indistinguishable from Whipple's disease; however, an acid fast stain will show numerous acid fast organisms in the case of MAC.

○ **How does MAC cause peritonitis?**

Liquefaction necrosis. An abdominal lymph node may necrose and result in peritonitis.

○ **Describe a rational stepwise approach to the evaluation of chronic diarrhea in patients with AIDS.**

Careful attention should be directed toward a complete history and physical examinations including the HAART medications that the patient is taking. If one of the medications is a potential offender, consider discontinuation of the drug and observe for resolution. Diagnostically, multiple stool samples should be obtained. If nondiagnostic and CD4 count is <200 cells/mm³, consider sigmoidoscopy (or colonoscopy with biopsies of the terminal ileum) and/or upper endoscopy with small bowel biopsy and aspirate. These tests may provide a diagnosis in an additional 50% of cases.

○ **Which of the HAART medications cause diarrhea as a side effect?**

As a class, diarrhea is most commonly seen with protease inhibitors, prominent among which are nelfinavir (up to 50%), and up to 20% of those taking lopinavir/ritonavir and fosamprenavir/ritonavir. The mechanism of diarrhea is unclear. Additionally diarrhea has also been described with the nucleoside analogue reverse transcriptase inhibitor (RTI) didanosine, stavudine, and abacavir.

○ **What is the HIV/AIDS wasting syndrome?**

The involuntary loss of greater than 10% body weight from baseline over 12 months or 5% over 6 months with no identifiable infectious or neoplastic cause.

○ **What is the most significant cause of weight loss in AIDS patients without gastrointestinal symptoms?**

Decreased caloric intake. Stable weights are often punctuated by episodic short-term weight loss when patients develop opportunistic infections. Small intestinal malabsorption has been shown to commonly occur in these patients as well. In addition, altered energy expenditure and adrenal insufficiency may contribute.

○ **All patients with HIV disease should have what vitamin level checked because of a high prevalence of deficiency?**

Vitamin B_{12}. A landmark paper on the subject found a 15% prevalence of vitamin B_{12} deficiency in an unselected group of patients with AIDS and 7% prevalence in asymptomatic HIV infection. In AIDS patients with chronic diarrhea, the prevalence of B_{12} deficiency may be as high as 39%.

○ **What mechanisms are responsible for the development of vitamin B_{12} deficiency in HIV-infected patients?**

The most important mechanism is ileal absorptive dysfunction. Additional factors include achlorhydria (causing decreased liberation of food-bound cobalamin), decreased intrinsic factor secretion, bacterial or parasitic overgrowth in the small bowel, and pancreatic insufficiency.

○ **What is the most common cause of pancreatitis in patients with HIV/AIDS?**

Drug-induced. Common offending agents include pentamidine (inhaled and parenteral), didanosine (ddI), zalcitabine (ddC), and occasionally trimethoprim-sulfamethoxazole. Less commonly, infections involving the pancreas with organisms such as CMV, *Cryptosporidium*, and MAC can also cause pancreatitis.

○ **True/False: Pancreatic toxicity from pentamidine causes hypo- and hyperglycemia.**

True. Direct toxicity to the pancreatic islet cells causes insulin release and low blood sugar levels. Hyperglycemia occurs later as insulin deficiency worsens.

○ **Anorectal carcinomas are associated with what infections in homosexual patients with HIV infection?**

Human papillomavirus types 16 and 18. A CD4 count <500 is an independent risk factor. Cytological specimens of the anal canal are increasingly being used for screening and have been shown to have a high predictive value for dysplasia. Quadrivalent HPV vaccine against 6, 11, 16, and 18 has been approved by the FDA for immunization in males 9–26 years age to prevent anal cancer based on a randomized trial that included men who have sex with men, ages 16–26.

○ **What are the most common causes of gastrointestinal bleeding in an AIDS patient?**

The most common cause of upper GI bleeding is peptic ulcer disease. Lower GI bleeding is most commonly due to CMV colitis.

○ **What is the most common cause of drug-induced hepatomegaly and abnormal liver tests with AIDS?**

Medications, particularly sulfonamides and protease inhibitors.

○ **An HIV patient on abacavir as part of the HAART therapy presents with fever, rash, and abdominal pain. What is the most likely diagnosis?**

This is a hypersensitivity reaction to abacavir, described in 3%–8% of the patients taking the medication. This can be fatal and is more common in Caucasians and strongly associated with human leukocyte antigen (HLA)-B5701 haplotype.

○ **What is the meaning of the term "lactic acidosis syndrome" in patients on HAART therapy?**

This is a syndrome caused by nucleoside RTIs, most commonly stavudine, didanosine, and zidovudine. Progressive microvesicular steatosis occurs secondary to mitochondrial toxicity induced by these drugs. Clinical features include fatigue, abdominal pain, nausea or muscle aches, and hepatomegaly on physical examination along with abnormal liver enzyme tests. Metabolic acidosis and elevated arterial lactic acid levels greater than or equal to 5 mEq/L generally occur after 6 months of therapy and require discontinuance of the offending agent.

○ **What potential metabolic disorder is associated with HAART therapy?**

A lipodystrophy syndrome has been described consisting of peripheral fat loss (face, buttocks, and limbs) with central fat accumulation, gynecomastia, and hypertrophy of dosicervical fat pad (buffalo hump). This may also be associated with hypertriglyceridemia, insulin resistance, impaired glucose tolerance, lactic acidemia, and hepatic dysfunction. This may be due to toxic effects of protease inhibitors, particularly ritonavir, along with nucleoside RTI and nonnucleoside RTI.

○ **What are the antiretroviral medications associated with abnormal liver tests?**

- Raised aspartate aminotransferase (AST)/alanine aminotransferase (ALT):
  o Nucleoside RTI—stavudine, didanosine, abacavir
  o Nucleotide RTI—adefovir
  o Nonnucleoside RTI—nevirapine, delaviridine, efavirenz
  o Protease inhibitors—tipranavir, lopinavir/ritonavir
- Indirect hyperbilirubinemia (clinically benign)
  o Protease inhibitors—atazanavir, indinavir

○   **What risk factors for hepatotoxicity are associated with HAART therapy?**

Up to 10% of patients receiving HAART therapy will develop Grade 3 or 4 hepatotoxicity.
- Use of ritonavir
- Increase in CD4 cell count >50 cells/mm^3 during treatment
- Stage F3 and F4 fibrosis at the time of treatment
- Baseline elevation in serum aminotransferases
- Hepatitis C virus coinfection

○   **What is the most common hepatic pathogen in AIDS?**

MAC. The hallmark of this infection is poorly formed granulomas with acid fast staining organisms located within foamy macrophages.

○   **True/False:** *Pneumocystis jiroveci* **can infect the liver in AIDS?**

True. Isolated cases of *P. jiroveci* hepatitis have been described in patients on inhaled pentamidine, which fails to protect extrapulmonary sites from the pathogen.

○   **What tumor seen in HIV infection is made up of spindle cells and originates from lymphatic endothelial cells?**

Kaposi's sarcoma (KS). In the alimentary tract, KS typically occurs as purplish, bulky gingival or palatal lesions, or gastrointestinal lesions. The vast majority are asymptomatic. Rarely, gastrointestinal KS can cause weight loss, abdominal pain, nausea and vomiting, upper or lower gastrointestinal bleeding, malabsorption, intestinal obstruction, and/or diarrhea. Treatment is reserved for symptomatic cases, mainly by instituting HAART. Advanced lesions can additionally be treated with liposomal doxorubicin or daunorubicin.

○   **What percentage of patients with cutaneous KS have gastrointestinal or hepatic involvement?**

33%. These are usually asymptomatic. In the pre-HAART era, the gastrointestinal tract was involved in approximately 40% of patients with KS at initial diagnosis and in up to 80% at autopsy. Involvement can occur in the absence of cutaneous disease.

○   **A 43-year-old HIV-infected man complains of abdominal pain. He has fever, lymphadenopathy, skin angiomas, hepatomegaly, and lytic bone lesions. What is the most likely diagnosis?**

Bacillary peliosis hepatis. Caused by *Bartonella henselae*, this infection causes dilated vascular lakes and blood filled spaces within the liver. It is the fourth leading cause of abnormal liver tests and hepatomegaly in AIDS patients. It is treated with erythromycin or doxycycline.

○   **What are the six most common causes of abnormal liver tests and hepatomegaly in patients with AIDS?**

Drug-induced, mycobacterial infection, CMV, *Cryptosporidium*, hepatitis C, and lymphoma.

○   **What is AIDS cholangiopathy?**

This syndrome resembles sclerosing cholangitis and papillary stenosis. Patients present with upper abdominal pain, diarrhea, and, less commonly, fever and jaundice. Labs reveal elevated serum alkaline phosphatase levels. Occasionally, transaminase elevations are also seen. This syndrome usually results from infection with *Cryptosporidium*. Other potential causative organisms include CMV and microsporidiosis. Rarely, this may be caused by MAC, *Isospora belli*, and *Cyclospora cayetanensis*.

○ **True/False: The diagnosis of AIDS cholangiopathy is usually made by endoscopic retrograde cholangiopancreatography (ERCP).**

True. ERCP most commonly demonstrates a combination of papillary stenosis and sclerosing cholangitis. Therapy is endoscopic sphincterotomy in the setting of stenosis with or without stenting of bile duct strictures. The role of magnetic resonance cholangiopancreatography (MRCP) for diagnosing AIDS cholangiopathy has not been fully evaluated. Ultrasound is often used as an initial diagnostic study and appears to have a high specificity for the condition.

○ **How does the pattern of liver enzyme elevation assist in the diagnosis of HIV/AIDS-related disease?**

The elevation of aminotransferases is nonspecific. The pattern and extent is not useful to correlate with a specific diagnosis. However, an impressive rise in the alkaline phosphatase without extra- or intrahepatic obstruction is strongly suggestive of infection with MAC.

○ **True/False: HIV increases the risk of sexual transmission of the hepatitis C (HCV) virus.**

True. HIV also increases the vertical transmission of HCV from mother to child.

○ **What factors predict fibrosis and progression to cirrhosis in patients with hepatitis C who are also coinfected with HIV?**

Older age at infection, higher ALT levels, higher levels of inflammatory activity, alcohol consumption of more than 50 g/d, and a CD4 count <500.

○ **What is the most common cause of ascites in patients with AIDS?**

Lymphoma. Other causes include tuberculosis, atypical mycobacterial infections, disseminated fungal infections, disseminated *Pneumocystis*, and non-AIDS-related causes.

○ **True/False: Primary gastrointestinal fungal diseases are common in patients with HIV/AIDS.**

False. Fungal infections typically occur as part of a disseminated infection causing chronic fever, anorexia, nausea, vomiting, hepatomegaly, and abnormal liver tests. Histoplasmosis and coccidiomycosis are among the more common infections seen.

○ **A 37-year-old man with AIDS presents with severe anorectal pain associated with defecation. What is the most likely cause?**

Ulceration of the anal canal, usually associated with HCV or CMV infection. Benign anorectal causes of anorectal pain including anal fissures and thrombosed hemorrhoids should be considered. The possibility of anal carcinoma should be considered.

○ **What is the relationship between inflammatory bowel disease and AIDS?**

An idiopathic colitis resembling ulcerative colitis that responds to steroid therapy has been described in patients with AIDS.

• • • SUGGESTED READINGS • • •

Wilcox CM, Saag MS. Gastrointestinal complications of HIV infection: changing priorities in the HAART era. *Gut.* 2008;57(6): 861-870.

Panel on Antiretroviral Guidelines for Adults and Adolescents. Guidelines for the use of antiretroviral agents in HIV-1-infected adults and adolescents. Department of Health and Human Services. January 10, 2011;1-166. Available at http://www.aidsinfo.nih.gov/ ContentFiles/AdultandAdolescentGL.pdf. Accessed July 27, 2011.

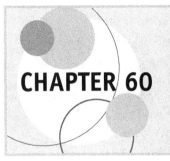

CHAPTER 60

Gastrointestinal and Hepatobiliary Disorders in Pregnancy

Erika Boroff, MD and Elizabeth Carey, MD

○ **True/False: Dietary micronutrient supplementation is a more important determinant of birth weight than overall calorie intake during pregnancy.**

False. Calorie intake is the most important determinant of birth weight. Micronutrients do not significantly affect birth weight or duration of pregnancy in well-nourished women in developed countries. However, a multivitamin supplement is recommended for pregnant patients who do not consume a varied diet.

Table 60-1. Recommended Daily Allowances for Nonpregnant and Pregnant Women

Nutrient	Nonpregnant	Pregnant
Calories (kcal)	2200	2500
Protein (g)	50 (0.8 g/kg/d)	60 (1.1 g/kg/d)
Calcium (mg)	800	1000 (age >19) 1300 (age 14–18)
Vitamin A (μg retinol equivalents)	800	800
Vitamin D (iu)	200	600
Thiamine (mg)	1.2	1.5
Riboflavin (mg)	1.3	1.6
Pyridoxine (mg)	1.6	2.2
Niacin (mg niacin equivalents)	15	17
Vitamin B_{12} (μg)	2.0	2.2
Folate (mg)	0.18	0.4–0.8
Vitamin C (mg)	60	70
Selenium (μg)	55	65
Iron (mg)	15	30

○ **What are the excess energy requirements (kcal/day) during pregnancy and lactation?**

Pregnancy increases energy requirements by 300 kcal/day during the second and third trimesters. Lactation increases energy requirements by 500 kcal/day.

○ **True/False: Activity of inflammatory bowel disease at conception affects the likelihood of disease flare during pregnancy.**

True. When conception occurs during a period of remission, one-third of patients will relapse during their pregnancy. When conception occurs during a period of active disease however, two-thirds of patients will experience persistently active disease, and of these, two-thirds will note disease progression. There does not appear to be increased risk of flare during the postpartum period if stable patients are continued on medical therapy.

○ **What are the risks to the pregnancy when inflammatory bowel disease is active at the time of conception?**

Increased risk of preterm birth (odds ratio [OR] 1.87, 95% confidence interval [CI] 1.52 to 2.31) and low birth weight (OR 2.1; 95% CI 1.38 to 3.19). The risk is higher for infants born to mothers with severe colitis during the pregnancy.

There is no clear evidence for an increased risk of congenital abnormalities or stillbirth; however, if surgery is required to treat refractory disease or fulminant colitis, fetal mortality is high (18%–40%).

○ **True/False: Spontaneous vaginal delivery should be avoided in all pregnant women with inflammatory bowel disease (IBD).**

False. In general, the decision to have a C-section should be based purely on obstetrical factors, with two exceptions: 1) the presence of active perianal disease at the time of delivery, and 2) the presence of an ileal pouch anal anastomosis (IPAA). Although the presence of an IPAA does not mandate a C-section, pouch function may deteriorate during pregnancy, particularly in the third trimester, and there is a theoretical concern that if there is damage to the anal sphincter during vaginal delivery, this can negatively impact pouch function over subsequent years. The patient should discuss with her obstetrician and her surgeon the risks to pouch function over the long term, before deciding on the planned mode of delivery.

○ **True/False: Inflammatory bowel disease has no effect on fertility.**

False. The effect of IBD on fertility depends on the activity of the disease at the time of attempted conception. Women with quiescent Crohn's disease (CD) and ulcerative colitis (UC) have similar fertility rates to that of the general population. In contrast, active CD is associated with reduced fertility. In addition, abdominal or pelvic surgery for CD and colectomy with IPAA for UC are associated with a reduction in fertility (threefold decrease for IPAA).

○ **True/False: All IBD medications should be stopped in those trying to conceive and those who become pregnant.**

False. Most IBD medications are considered low risk during pregnancy and lactation, with the exception of methotrexate and thalidomide which are teratogenic. Low-risk medications should be continued throughout the pregnancy, as discontinuation of such medications at conception may precipitate a disease flare, which is associated with poorer pregnancy outcomes. General consensus for anti-TNF therapy is that they should be continued through conception and the first and second trimesters of pregnancy. If a patient is in remission, consider discontinuing the medication in the latter half of the third trimester, unless the patient is being treated with certolizumab, in which case, the medication can be continued until delivery.

Table 60-2. Medications Used in the Treatment of Inflammatory Bowel Disease

Drug	FDA Pregnancy Category	Comments	Breastfeeding
Sulfasalazine	B	Take sulfasalazine with 2mg folic acid daily to offset its anti-folate effects.	Yes
Mesalamine	B		Yes
Balsalazide	B		Yes
Olsalazine	C		Yes
Metronidazole	B	Avoid in 1st trimester due to slight increase in cleft lip.	No
Ciprofloxacin	C	May damage joints, limited human data. Short courses for pouchitis considered, but generally avoided.	No
Levofloxacin	C		No
Amoxicillin-clavulanate	B	Safer alternative for pouchitis.	Yes
Corticosteroids: Budesonide	C	First trimester exposure associated with low risk of oral clefts. Budesonide retrospective study showed no negative outcomes. Enters breast milk.	
Immunomodulator: Azathioprine	D	Teratogenicity in animal studies, but no consistent malformation in humans. Usually continued in pregnancy to prevent flare.	Yes
6-Mercaptopurine	D		Yes
Methotrexate	X	Teratogenic. Have patient wait 6 months after discontinuing drug to conceive.	No
Thalidomide	X	Teratogenic.	No
Cyclosporine	C	Cyclosporine has been used successfully to delay colectomy for fulminate UC until post-partum.	No
Tacrolimus	C		No
Biologics: Infliximab	B	Infliximab does not cross placenta in 1st trimester. No test available to detect Adalimumab in the newborn to insure clearing, and so live vaccines (rotovirus) are avoided.	Yes
Adalimumab	B		Yes
Certolizumab	B		Yes

○ **What is the most common cause of upper gastrointestinal bleeding during pregnancy?**

Mallory–Weiss tear, followed by erosive esophagitis.

○ **What is the most frequent cause of an acute abdomen in pregnancy?**

Appendicitis, followed by cholecystitis and intestinal obstruction. Appendicitis occurs in roughly 1 of every 766 pregnancies. Perforated appendicitis increases fetal mortality compared with cases of uncomplicated appendicitis (6%–37%). Symptoms may be atypical as the appendix is displaced out of the pelvis by the gravid uterus, and abdominal distention may delay peritoneal irritation and peritoneal signs.

○ **What is the differential diagnosis of acute onset abdominal pain in pregnancy?**

Gastrointestinal, genitourinary, and gynecologic disorders including appendicitis, cholelithiasis, pancreatitis, small-bowel obstruction, infectious disease, inflammatory bowel disease, nephrolithiasis, urinary tract infection, ectopic pregnancy, ovarian torsion, and ovarian vein thrombosis.

○ **Describe the clinical presentations of gallstone disease during pregnancy.**

Most patients with symptomatic gallstones will report biliary-like abdominal pain. Although nausea and vomiting are common in pregnancy, abdominal pain should trigger further evaluation. The presence of fever, leukocytosis, and an ill appearing patient are suggestive of acute cholecystitis. A positive sonographic Murphy's sign carries a positive predictive value of 92%.

○ **During which trimester of pregnancy is pancreatitis most likely to occur?**

Third trimester, with increasing incidence with gestational age. Gallstone pancreatitis is the most common cause (66% of cases), and carries a better prognosis than alcoholic or hypertriglyceridemic pancreatitis. In pancreatitis, preterm delivery is increased (18%–32%) but maternal and fetal mortality is low (less than 1% and 4%, respectively).

○ **What potential causes of pancreatitis may be exacerbated during pregnancy?**

Gallstones, hypertriglyceridemia, and hypercalcemia due to hyperparathyroidism which may first become manifest during pregnancy.

○ **What features distinguish hyperemesis gravidarum from uncomplicated nausea and vomiting of pregnancy?**

Nausea and vomiting are common in early pregnancy (incidence of 50%), usually peaking at 9-week gestation. The majority of cases (91%) resolve by 20-week gestation. Outcomes are favorable as infants born to mothers who lost weight early in pregnancy have lower birth weights, but the rate of miscarriage is lower than that of women without nausea and vomiting.

Hyperemesis gravidarum occurs in 0.3%–1% of pregnancies, and is characterized by persistent vomiting associated with weight loss of over 5%, ketonuria, hypokalemia, and dehydration. Potential complications of hyperemesis gravidarum include peripheral neuropathy due to deficiency of vitamin B6 or B12, and Wernicke's encephalopathy due to deficiency of vitamin B1 (thiamine). With appropriate treatment, there is no increased risk of pregnancy loss, low birth weight, or congenital malformation compared with the general population.

○ **What conditions are associated with an increased incidence of hyperemesis gravidarum?**

Multiple pregnancies and hydatidiform mole.

○ **What is the significance of new onset nausea and vomiting in the third trimester of pregnancy?**

Nausea and vomiting with onset after 8-week gestation are rare in pregnancy and suggest a more serious condition than uncomplicated nausea and vomiting of pregnancy.

○ **Describe laboratory changes in pregnancy that may render the diagnosis of illness more difficult.**

Mild leukocytosis is normal in pregnancy. Hemodilution decreases measured hemoglobin, hematocrit, and albumin levels. Iron deficiency may occur in the absence of GI bleeding. Alkaline phosphatase rises (2–4 times normal) due to production of this enzyme by the placenta. Serum alanine aminotranserferase (ALT) and serum aspartate aminotransferase (AST) remain within normal limits. Serum bilirubin levels remain normal. Prothrombin time is unchanged.

○ **Describe the normal physiologic changes in GI motility during pregnancy.**

Lower esophageal sphincter tone is reduced. Nonpropulsive esophageal motor activity is increased, while esophageal contraction wave amplitude and velocity is decreased. Transit through the stomach, small bowel, and colon is prolonged. Intervals between the interdigestive phase III complexes of the migrating motor complex are prolonged. Gallbladder contractility is reduced with slowed gallbladder emptying. Intraabdominal pressure is increased due to gravid uterus.

○ **What medications used for gastroesophageal reflux disease (GERD) are safe for use in pregnancy?**

All proton pump inhibitors (PPIs) are FDA category B except omeprazole (category C). Meta-analyses and case control studies have not demonstrated a significant increase in spontaneous abortion, preterm delivery, or congenital birth defects in humans exposed to PPIs. Published guidelines suggest PPIs as first-line therapy for GERD in pregnancy. H$_2$ blockers are less effective than PPIs in managing symptoms of reflux in pregnancy but are safe (all are category B). Other medications for GERD that are safe in pregnancy include antacids and sucralfate.

○ **What imaging modality is recommended to evaluate acute right lower quadrant pain in pregnancy?**

MRI without gadolinium is the imaging test of choice. MRI without contrast has been determined to be safe in pregnancy. Gadolinium-based contrast is pregnancy category C and should not be used routinely. MRI has a high sensitivity (98%–100%) for diagnosing appendicitis, and a high negative predictive value (94%–100%) to rule out the diagnosis throughout pregnancy. CT should be avoided in pregnancy, except in instances where ultrasound (US) is indeterminate and MRI is not feasible. In comparison, US is safe for use in pregnancy and is accurate in the evaluation of the appendix in the first and second trimesters; however, US is technically difficult in the third trimester due to displacement of the appendix by the gravid uterus.

○ **What imaging modalities can be considered in the evaluation of suspected biliary pathology in pregnancy?**

Magnetic resonance cholangiopancreatography (MRCP) is recommended in pregnant patients with suspected biliary pathology. US has a sensitivity of 95% for detection of cholelithiasis but is limited in the evaluation of the common bile duct (CBD) and the pancreas. In cases where US identifies biliary dilation or there is a suspicion of CBD stones, MRCP has an accuracy of 100% in determining the cause and location of biliary obstruction, and can evaluate pancreatic disease as well. Patients with choledocholithiasis may then be referred for urgent endoscopic retrograde cholangiopancreatography (ERCP), with shielding of the uterus and minimizing fluoroscopy time to limit fetal radiation exposure.

○ **What liver diseases are unique to pregnancy?**

- Hyperemesis gravidarum (HG): first trimester—intractable nausea and vomiting with transaminase elevation (50%).
- Intrahepatic cholestasis of pregnancy (ICP): second or third trimester—pruritus (severe) with transaminase elevation and elevated serum bile acids (pathognomonic). Jaundice is uncommon (10%–25%) and should trigger evaluation for biliary obstruction.
- Preeclampsia: second or third trimester—hypertension, right upper quadrant (RUQ) pain, and transaminase elevation.
- HELLP syndrome (Hemolysis, Elevated Liver tests, and Low Platelet count syndrome): second trimester or third trimester—hypertension, RUQ pain (65%–90%), nausea and vomiting (35%–50%), a flu-like illness (90%), and headache (30%). Labs typically reveal proteinuria (86%), transaminase elevation (10–20 times normal), mild bilirubin elevation, hemolysis, and thrombocytopenia. Severe cases may present with disseminated intravascular coagulation (DIC).
- Acute fatty liver of pregnancy (AFLP): second or third trimester—1–2 weeks of anorexia followed by nausea and vomiting, headache, and RUQ pain. Patients may present with fulminant hepatic failure with encephalopathy.

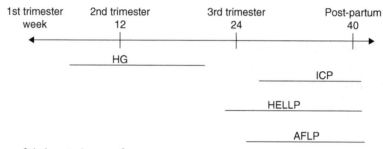

Figure 60-1. Onset of cholestatic diseases of pregnancy.

○ **True/False: The definitive treatment of ICP, HELLP, and AFLP is early delivery.**

True. Corticosteroids may improve maternal and fetal outcomes in HELLP.

○ **List the criteria for diagnosing HELLP syndrome.**

- Hemolysis (abnormal blood smear, elevated LDH, increased indirect bilirubin, low haptoglobin)
- AST > 70 IU/L
- Platelet count < 100,000

○ **What distinguishes AFLP from HELLP syndrome?**

Patients with AFLP may present with fulminant liver failure and encephalopathy. Jaundice is also a more common feature in AFLP.

○ **What common immunosuppressant used in liver transplant recipients is pregnancy category D?**

Most immunosuppression (tacrolimus, cyclosporine, and steroids) should be continued during pregnancy; however, mycophenolate mofetil is associated with an increased risk of birth defects and should be discontinued before a woman attempts to conceive. It is recommended a woman wait at least 1 year after transplant before attempting conception.

○ **What poses the greatest risk to the cirrhotic patient who is pregnant?**

Portal hypertension with variceal bleeding. Over 25% of women with portal hypertension will have a variceal bleed during pregnancy, and 70% if varices are detected prior to conception. Maternal mortality due to a variceal bleed is high, between 20% and 50%. Onset is usually in the third trimester, when blood volume is greatest. Treatment is the same as with nonpregnant patients. For women with known portal hypertension, endoscopy should be performed early in the second trimester. Beta-blocker prophylaxis should be offered if varices are found.

○ **True/False: Most cirrhotic women are anovulatory and infertile.**

True.

○ **Describe the clinical presentation of a ruptured splenic artery aneurysm.**

Rupture of a splenic artery aneurysm complicates up to 2.5% of pregnancies in cirrhotic women and is associated with a high mortality. Typical clinical presentation includes acute onset of abdominal pain, pulsatile mass in the left upper quadrant, and presence of an abdominal bruit.

○ **True/False: Endoscopic procedures are safe during pregnancy.**

True. Endoscopy is safe in pregnancy and can be performed with or without conventional sedation and analgesia.

○ **What interventions are utilized to reduce vertical transmission of hepatitis B virus (HBV) infection?**

Infants of mothers with HBV should receive HBV vaccination and hepatitis immunoglobulin within 12 hours of birth to prevent vertical transmission during labor and delivery. Completion of HBV vaccination should occur according to the standard schedule. Antiviral treatment such as lamivudine (FDA pregnancy category C), tenofovir (pregnancy category B), and hepatitis B immunoglobulin have each been used successfully in the third trimester to reduce vertical transmission of HBV.

○ **True/False: Antiviral treatment is recommended for pregnant patients with chronic hepatitis C (HCV) and high viral loads.**

False. Ribavirin is teratogenic and should not be used during pregnancy. Chemoprophylaxis of pregnant women with HCV to reduce the risk of vertical transmission is not recommended at this time. Vertical transmission of HCV is not as efficient as with HBV, occurring in only 4%–6% of pregnancies.

○ **True/False: Budd–Chiari syndrome (BCS) in pregnancy usually occurs during the second trimester.**

False. BCS presents with acute onset of RUQ pain, hepatomegaly, and ascites, usually in the third trimester (elevated estrogen levels and decrease in serum antithrombin III late in pregnancy promote thombogenesis).

○ **What is the most morbid form of acute viral hepatitis in pregnancy?**

Acute hepatitis E virus (HEV) infection is particularly virulent in pregnant patients and can present with fulminant hepatic failure in the third trimester. Mortality is high, 15%–25%. Cases are found primarily in Southeast Asia, Northern Africa, and Mexico, although less virulent strains have been identified in North America.

○ **What other virus can cause fulminant liver failure during the third trimester of pregnancy?**

Herpes simplex virus (HSV). Typical oral or genital lesions are present in only the minority of cases (30%). Fever and upper respiratory symptoms may be present. Bilirubin level may be normal or near normal at initial presentation. Diagnosis can be made by detection of viremia if no vesicular lesions are present. Treatment with antivirals may reduce mortality.

● ● ● **SUGGESTED READINGS** ● ● ●

Carey E, Hay J. Pregnancy and liver disease. In: Talley N, Lindor K, Vargas H, eds. *Practical Gastroenterology and Hepatology: Liver and Biliary Disease*. Hoboken, NJ: Wiley-Blackwell; 2010:152-163.

Niebyl JR. Clinical practice. Nausea and vomiting in pregnancy. *N Engl J Med*. 2010;363:1544-1550.

Parangi S, Levine D, Henry A, et al. Surgical gastrointestinal disorders during pregnancy. *Am J Surg*. 2007;193:223-232.

van der Woude CJ, Kolacek S, Dotan I, et al. European evidenced-based consensus on reproduction in inflammatory bowel disease. *J Crohns Colitis*. 2010;4:493-510.

CHAPTER 61 Gastrointestinal and Liver Radiology

Andrew D. Hardie, MD, Matthew Stephenson, MD, and David G. Koch, MD

○ **What are the primary diagnostic considerations for this liver lesion as seen on magnetic resonance imaging (MRI)?**

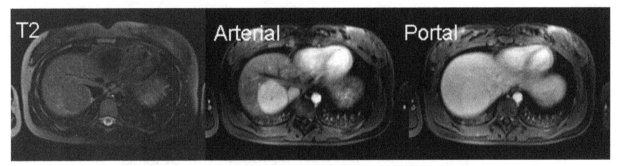

Figure 61-1

Focal nodular hyperplasia (FNH) or hepatic adenoma. FNH is usually seen as a multilobulated mass, which must be uniformly hypervascular/hyperenhancing to the liver on imaging during the "arterial phase" of contrast administration but isovascular/isoenhancing during the "portal venous phase." FNH also often, but not always, has a central scar, which is T2 bright and enhances progressively following contrast administration. In contrast, hepatic adenoma is often round or oval with smooth margins. It also often has arterial enhancement but can have a variable postcontrast appearance (often slightly hypoenhancing on later phases of contrast).

○ **True/False: The availability of biliary specific MRI contrast agents has effectively made nuclear imaging studies such as the sulfur colloid scan obsolete for the differentiation of FNH from hepatic adenoma.**

True. The availability of biliary specific contrast agents for MRI has markedly improved the ability to differentiate these lesions, as FNH will take up the agent while adenoma will not.

○   **How would the bowel gas pattern in the figure shown be characterized?**

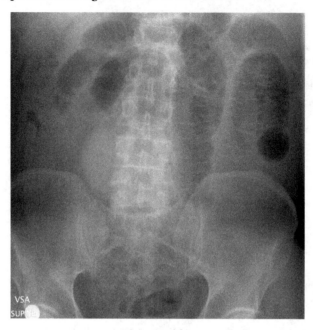

Figure 61-2

The pattern is typical of a small bowel obstruction (SBO). Key elements are dilation of the proximal small bowel to greater than 3 cm with relative decompression of distal small and large bowel. Adhesions related to prior intraabdominal surgery or intraabdominal infection are the most common cause of an SBO.

○   **In this patient with known cirrhosis, what is the likely etiology of the lesion depicted in figure below?**

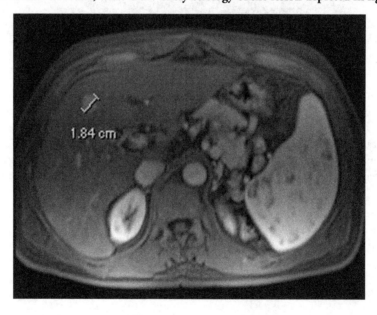

Figure 61-3

Hepatocellular carcinoma (HCC). This solid liver lesion has the typical arterial phase enhancement compared with the liver. Note the presence of collateral vessels near the lesser curve of the stomach and splenomegaly indicating portal hypertension.

○ **What is the most likely diagnosis depicted in this abdominal radiograph? What would be an appropriate intervention?**

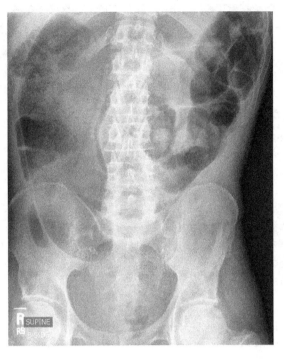

Figure 61-4

The markedly dilated sigmoid colon with a "coffee bean" configuration is typical of sigmoid volvulus. Attempts to reduce the volvulus with either water soluble enema or flexible sigmoidoscopy are appropriate in the absence of free intraperitoneal air.

○ **What is the likely etiology of this liver lesion in a patient presenting with recent onset of left lower quadrant pain and fever?**

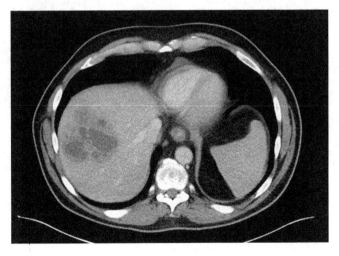

Figure 61-5

This is a typical appearance of hepatic abscesses. Note the poorly defined collection in the right lobe of the liver with an enhancing *internal* wall surrounded by low density edema. In this case, the etiology was related to sigmoid diverticulitis.

○ **What is the most likely etiology of this pancreatic cystic mass?**

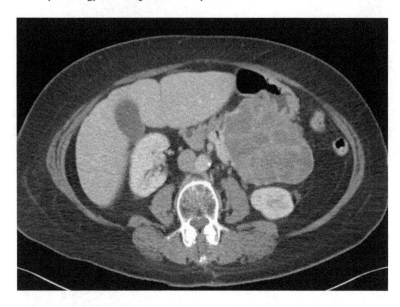

Figure 61-6

This is a typical appearance of serous cystadenoma with features consisting of a large cystic mass with multilobulated contours. Endoscopic ultrasound with fine needle aspiration (FNA) of the cyst fluid may be confirmatory.

○ **What is the most likely cause of the abnormal appearance of the small bowel in this 26-year-old patient with chronic intermittent abdominal pain and weight loss? What type of radiologic study was performed?**

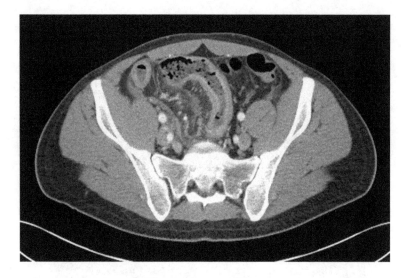

Figure 61-7

Crohn's disease. This is a computed tomography (CT) enterography study performed using a *negative* oral contrast agent in the *arterial phase* of intravenous (IV) contrast. This technique is necessary in order to visualize the mural enhancement of the bowel wall, which is present due to active inflammation.

○ **True/False: The finding in the figure would fall within the Milan criteria for HCC.**

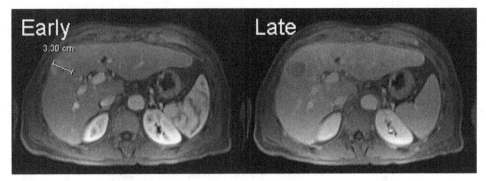

Figure 61-8

True. The 3.3-cm lesion in the left hepatic lobe has a typical imaging appearance of HCC on MRI (arterial phase enhancement and "wash out" of contrast on delayed imaging). For a single tumor, the Milan criteria require that the lesion be less than 5 cm. The Milan criteria are used to assess postoperative survival in patients undergoing liver transplantation for HCC. They are also the basis for applying model for end-stage liver disease (MELD) exception points to patients being placed on the transplant waiting list.

○ **What is the relevant finding shown in this abdominal radiograph from a patient presenting with an acute abdomen? What is the presumed etiology?**

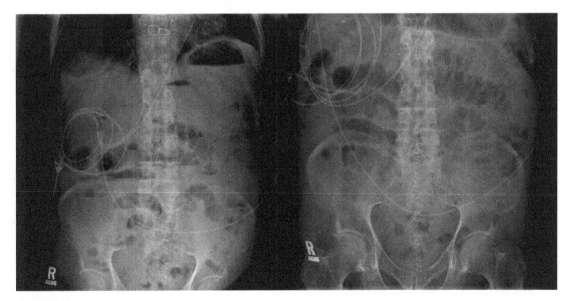

Figure 61-9

There is "pneumatosis" or air within the wall of the small bowel in the left upper quadrant. Given the location and appearance of the pneumatosis combined with the clinical presentation, bowel ischemia with impending infarction is the most likely diagnosis.

○ **What is the finding shown on this endoscopic retrograde cholangiopancreatography (ERCP) done on a patient with abdominal pain and fever 3 days after laparoscopic cholecystectomy for gallstones?**

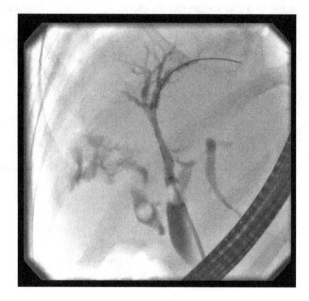

Figure 61-10

This balloon occlusion cholangiogram demonstrates a round filling defect in the cystic duct (cholelithiasis) as well as contrast extravasation from the cystic duct stump.

○ **What is the differential diagnosis of the finding on this CT of the abdomen?**

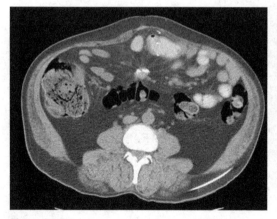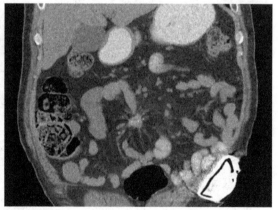

Figure 61-11

Carcinoid tumor versus sclerosing mesenteritis. There is a partially calcified mass in the small bowel mesentery with stellate (star-like) borders. This is a case of carcinoid tumor and this lesion actually represents the first site of spread of carcinoid tumor of the small bowel to mesenteric nodes. The primary tumor is usually in the small bowel lumen but is rarely identified by imaging. Sclerosing mesenteritis is a poorly understood inflammatory condition of the mesentery that can have a virtually identical appearance as carcinoid.

○ **What is the abnormal finding of the liver shown in the figure in this patient with chronically elevated aminotransferase levels taking a statin-based medication for hyperlipidemia?**

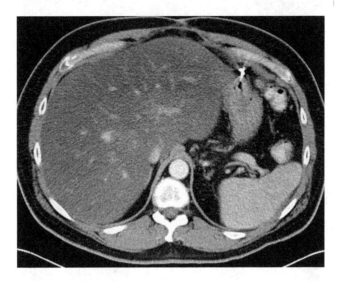

Figure 61-12

Hepatic steatosis. The liver is abnormally low in density on contrast-enhanced CT in comparison with the spleen. The normal liver should be similar in density to the spleen on both noncontrast and contrast-enhanced CT. Density on CT is measured in Hounsfield units (HU).

○ **What laboratory abnormalities would be expected for the patient with acute abdominal pain and the CT findings shown?**

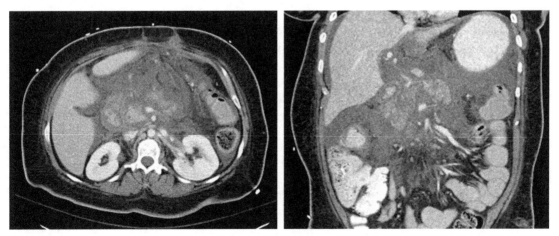

Figure 61-13

Elevated amylase and lipase. This is a typical CT appearance of acute pancreatitis, with edema of the pancreas and retroperitoneum. Furthermore, the lack of enhancement of portions of the pancreatic parenchyma indicates the presence of pancreatic necrosis.

○   **What is the finding shown in the figure from a patient following colonoscopy?**

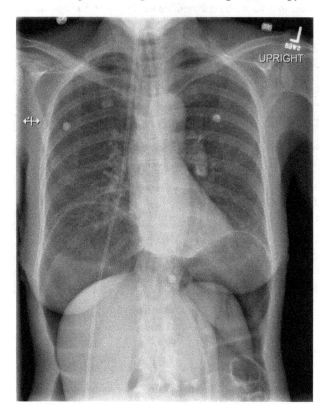

Figure 61-14

Free intraperitoneal air. The patient likely has a perforated colon. Prompt surgical consultation is indicated.

○   **What is the difference between T1 weighting and T2 weighting in MRI?**

Images in MRI are possible because of the inherent differences in resonance frequencies of protons (hydrogen nuclei) in tissues under the influence of a powerful magnet. By emitting radiofrequency pulses, which excite the protons, numerous types of images can be created based on the variable relaxation of the excited protons. The degree to which a series of radiofrequency pulses (sequence) highlights the proton relaxation in the longitudinal plane (T1) or transverse plane (T2) determines whether the image is predominantly T1 or T2 weighted. Fluid in pure T1 weighted images is dark, but is bright on pure T2 weighted images. Fat is bright on both T1 and T2 weighted images, although fat saturation techniques are often employed on either. Most organs have characteristic intermediate signal characteristics on both sequences.

○   **True/False: IV contrast for CT is contraindicated in patients with acute or chronic renal failure.**

True, usually. CT contrast agents contain high quantities of iodine, which can precipitate worsening renal failure in patients with already compromised renal function. However, in patients with end-stage renal disease (ESRD) on chronic dialysis, IV contrast can be used as long as there is no chance for recovery of renal function.

○ **What is the radiological sign depicted in the colon on this abdominal radiograph? What is a typical etiology for the finding on this CT of the abdomen?**

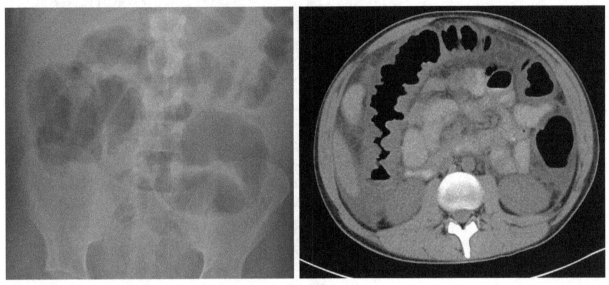

Figure 61-15

Thumbprinting. The haustral folds in the colon (particularly transverse) are markedly thickened in this patient with colitis, becoming as wide as a thumb. The CT demonstrates the same finding in better detail. Especially in an inpatient setting, *Clostridium difficile* is a common etiology.

○ **What is the radiological sign depicted on this CT of the abdomen in a patient with jaundice? What are the potential etiologies?**

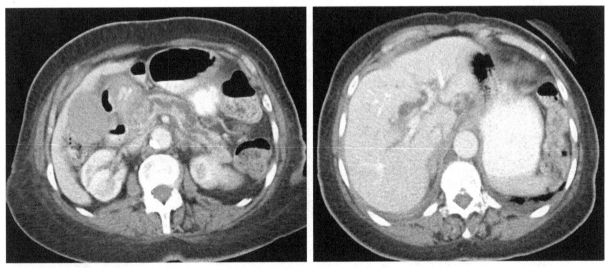

Figure 61-16

Double duct sign. The pancreatic duct is abnormally dilated as is the common bile duct. This indicates an obstruction in the pancreatic head or ampullary region where the ducts converge. Etiologies include adenocarcinoma of the pancreas or cholangiocarcinoma of the distal common bile duct, obstructing stone(s) near the ampulla, or an ampullary adenoma/adenocarcinoma.

○ **What is the liver lesion depicted on this CT of the abdomen?**

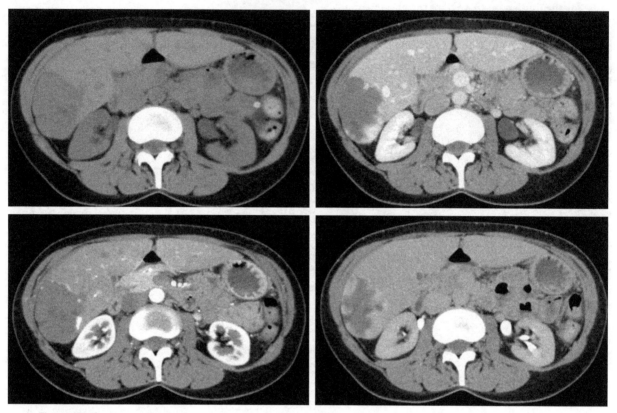

Figure 61-17

Hemangioma (aka, cavernous hemangioma). This benign neoplasm of capillary origin appears near fluid density prior to contrast. Following contrast, there is a typical "peripheral discontinuous nodular" enhancement pattern. Also, note how the enhancing portions of the lesion match the contrast level in the aorta at all times.

○ **What is the likely etiology of this patient's liver dysfunction based on this MRI?**

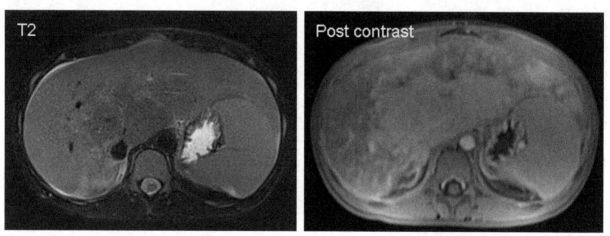

Figure 61-18

Budd–Chiari syndrome. There is abnormal signal and enhancement of the liver parenchyma that is confined to the periphery, while the liver parenchyma surrounding the inferior vena cava (IVC) and caudate lobe enhances normally. This phenomenon is due to the fact that the latter mentioned portions of the liver can drain through the IVC and not the hepatic veins, which are obstructed.

○   **Based on the findings in this figure, what is the likely etiology of jaundice in this patient?**

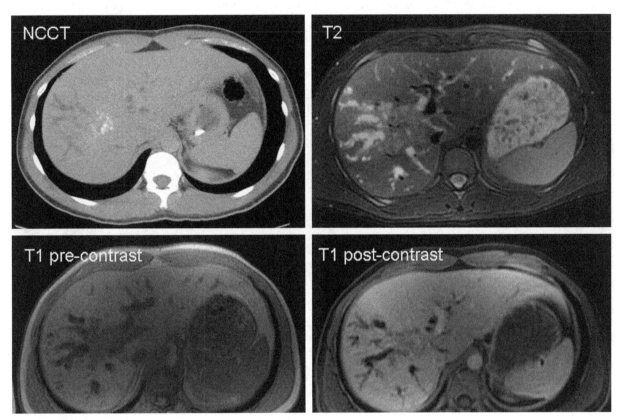

Figure 61-19

Cholangiocarcinoma. There is severe biliary obstruction of the right and left hepatic lobe biliary system from an ill-defined mass. Other findings suggestive of cholangiocarcinoma are punctate calcifications on noncontrast CT and an infiltrative appearance on MRI. When occurring at the confluence of the right and left hepatic ducts, this type of tumor is referred to as a Klatskin tumor.

○   **True/False: IV contrast agents for MRI are safe in patients with renal failure.**

False. Gadolinium (a rare earth metal) is used to achieve contrast in MRI studies. In patients with normal renal function, it is rapidly cleared and poses no health risks; however, in patients with severely compromised renal function, gadolinium has been discovered to deposit in tissues and lead to a condition called nephrogenic systemic fibrosis (NSF), which can be debilitating or even fatal. Gadolinium use is absolutely contraindicated in patients with ESRD.

○ **When might MRI be preferred to CT for evaluating a pancreatic mass?**

In general, MRI better visualizes fluid containing ductal structures and better characterizes cystic lesions than CT. Hence, MRI is the test of choice for evaluating intraductal papillary mucinous neoplasm (IPMN), which arises from the pancreatic duct. It also is more often definitive for differentiating pseudocysts, serous cystadenomas, and mucinous cystadenomas/carcinomas than CT. However, CT can often more easily discern abnormalities that require fine detail, such as the local spread of pancreatic adenocarcinomas into the retroperitoneal fat and around vascular structures. However, even in this case, MRI can be superior to CT at definitely characterizing liver lesions, adrenal nodules, and lymphadenopathy, which may be essential in deciding final treatment options.

○ **What is the likely etiology of the mass lesions in the liver seen in this patient with recent onset of constipation?**

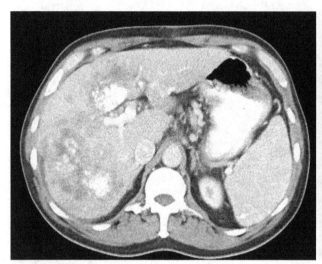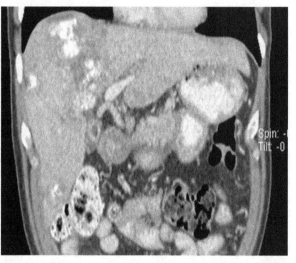

Figure 61-20

Metastatic disease from colorectal cancer. Although uncommon, colorectal metastases can have internal calcifications as is evident on this abdominal CT scan. Other adenocarcinomas, such as gastric carcinoma, can also calcify, but are less common.

○ **What are the inherent advantages and disadvantages of small bowel follow-thru, CT enterography, and MR enterography?**

Small bowel follow-thru:

Advantages: readily accessible, cheap, ability to see functional aspect of bowel

Disadvantages: long examination time (3 hours), high radiation (particularly for young patients needing serial imaging), variable interpretations, no ability to see extraluminal complications

CT enterography:

Advantages: accessible (can be performed on most CT scanners), rapid to perform (seconds), usually a consistent technique, moderately expensive, identifies extraluminal complications, anatomy recognizable to clinicians

Disadvantages: high radiation (particularly for young patients needing serial imaging), no functional information as it is only a single "snapshot," difficult to characterize bowel disease as acute or chronic inflammation and therefore may not be clear how to best treat

MR enterography:

Advantages: no radiation, combines functional and anatomic information as well as allowing for rapidly advancing newer MRI techniques, probably the best method to characterize bowel disease in order to decide how best to treat

Disadvantages: less accessible, takes 30–40 minutes to perform, not always a consistent technique, expensive, less recognizable to clinicians

○ **True/False: Based on the Milan criteria, a patient with three HCC tumors is potentially eligible for transplantation.**

True. For patients with more than one tumor: a) there can be no more than three lesions, b) the largest tumor must be less than 3 cm in size, and c) the aggregate of the tumor sizes must be less than 6 cm. If all three criteria are met, then the patient would have acceptable survival with liver transplantation and may be eligible for MELD exception points when being placed on the transplant waiting list.

○ **True/False: CT is the preferred choice for visualizing and diagnosing esophageal diseases.**

False. Despite advances in CT and MRI technology, esophageal pathology is still best imaged by fluoroscopy. Not only does fluoroscopy allow for functional assessment of esophageal motility and strictures, it is much more sensitive to mucosal abnormalities than any other radiologic study.

○ **What is the significance of pancreatic necrosis as described on CT or MRI?**

Depending on the size and location of the area of necrosis, its presence is associated with increased morbidity and mortality and often leads to eventual formation of pseudocysts and disruptions of the pancreatic duct. Pancreatic duct disruptions can cause fluid collections, which are unable to be resolved by catheter drainage and occasionally lead to pancreatico-pleural fistulae.

○ **What are the reasons to consider CT (aka, "virtual") colonography among the choices for colon cancer screening?**

In experienced hands, CT colonography (CTC) has a sensitivity approaching that of traditional optical colonoscopy for polyps greater than 1 cm in size; the lesions that are at greatest risk for progressing to cancer. As sedation is not required, CTC may be preferred for some patients. Although still requiring evacuation of feces and rectal air insufflation, some patients prefer CTC due to a lower risk of complications; hence, they may be more likely to get screened.

○ **True/False: CTC obviates the need for conventional colonoscopy.**

False. The main disadvantage of CTC is that it does not allow lesions identified to be biopsied or removed, which still requires conventional optical colonoscopy.

● ● ● SUGGESTED READINGS ● ● ●

Ros PR, Koenraad JM, Pelsser V, Lee S. *CT and MRI of the Abdomen and Pelvis: A Teaching File.* 2nd ed. Philadelphia, PA: Lippincott Williams and Wilkins; 2007.

Johnson CD, Schmit GD. *Mayo Clinic Gastrointestinal Imaging Review.* Rochester, MN: Mayo Clinic Scientific Press; 2005.

Halpert RD. *Case Review Series: Gastrointestinal Imaging.* Philadelphia, PA: Mosby/Elsevier; 2007.

CHAPTER 62

Gastrointestinal and Pancreaticobiliary Endoscopy

Ivana Dzeletovic, MD and Rahul Pannala, MD

○ **Describe approaches to palliation of jaundice due to malignant biliary obstruction.**

Obstructive jaundice secondary to inoperable malignant biliary strictures can be palliated with endoscopic stent placement (self-expanding metal stents [SEMS] or plastic stents). Percutaneous transhepatic biliary drainage (PTBD) and surgical bypass are alternatives to endoscopic stenting.

○ **Describe complications associated with biliary stents.**

Stent occlusion from debris or tumor ingrowth, cholangitis, stent migration, and cystic duct obstruction leading to cholecystitis (typically with fully covered SEMS).

○ **What is Bouveret's syndrome?**

It refers to gastric outlet obstruction caused by duodenal impaction by a large gallstone, which passes into the duodenal bulb via a cholecystogastric or cholecystoduodenal fistula. First-line treatment is endoscopic retrieval with or without mechanical lithotripsy.

○ **True/False: Hot biopsy removal of diminutive polyps and treatment of angiectasia in the right colon is associated with a high incidence of bleeding.**

True. Alternative means of polyp removal and lesion treatment are available and recommended instead of hot biopsy for lesions in the right colon.

○ **Describe qualities of an optimal colonoscopy bowel preparation.**

Convenient, safe, tolerable, and effective.

○ **True/False: Serious electrolyte and renal complications have been reported in patients with certain risk factors (eg, heart failure, renal failure, liver failure) receiving oral sodium phosphate products for their colonoscopy bowel preparation.**

True. As a result, the Food and Drug Administration (FDA) has required manufacturers of oral sodium phosphate products to include a black box warning regarding potential complications.

○ **A 27-year-old man presents with vague epigastric discomfort and fatigue, and is noted to have conjunctival icterus. He denies any other gastrointestinal complaints. Liver tests demonstrate a cholestatic picture. An abdominal ultrasound is normal. An endoscopic retrograde cholangiopancreatography (ERCP) is subsequently done demonstrating the following. What is the diagnosis? What other noninvasive test could have been used to make the diagnosis? What other endoscopic test should be considered in this patient?**

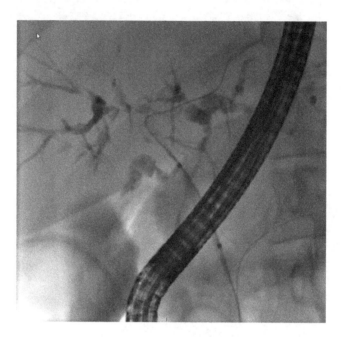

Figure 62-1

Primary sclerosing cholangitis (PSC), note the extensive stricturing of the intrahepatic ducts. Magnetic resonance cholangiopancreatography (MRCP). Colonoscopy should be considered to evaluate for underlying inflammatory bowel disease.

○ **What are the established risk factors for cholangiocarcinoma?**

PSC, Caroli's disease, choledochal cysts, infection with hepatobiliary flukes, hepatolithiasis, and toxins (Thorotrast).

○ **What imaging modalities are used to diagnose choledocholithiasis?**

The initial study of choice is transabdominal ultrasound (TUS) because it is noninvasive, cheap, and readily available. However, its sensitivity is only 40%, mostly due to poor visibility of the distal common bile duct (CBD). Endosopic ultrasound (EUS) and MRCP have excellent sensitivity and specificity; EUS is more sensitive for sludge and stones <6 mm. The use of EUS or MRCP in patients with low to intermediate pretest probability of choledocholithiasis guides patient selection for ERCP. While ERCP has sensitivity of >90% and specificity of 100%, it is rarely used for diagnosis of choledocholithiasis due to its invasiveness and potential risks.

○ **What clinical factors are highly predictive of the presence of a retained CBD stone?**

Clear presence of a CBD stone on transabdominal US, ascending cholangitis, and total bilirubin greater than 4. A strong suspicion of retained CBD stone occurs with a dilated CBD to more than 6 mm or a serum bilirubin between 1.8 to 4 mg/dL, while a moderate suspicion occurs with elevated transaminases, age >55, and gallstone pancreatitis.

○ **What are the criteria for the diagnosis of type I sphincter of Oddi dysfunction?**

- Abdominal pain associated with abnormal alanine aminotransferase (ALT) and aspartate aminotransferase (AST) more than two times upper limit of normal on at least two occasions
- Dilated CBD >10 mm on US or 12 mm on ERCP
- Delayed drainage of contrast from the CBD after >45 minutes in the supine position

○ **What is Mirrizi's syndrome?**

It is a rare complication in which a stone impacted in the neck of the gallbladder or cystic duct extrinsically compresses the CBD with resulting proximal biliary obstruction.

○ **What is recurrent pyogenic cholangitis (RPC)?**

It is a syndrome characterized by recurrent bacterial cholangitis, intrahepatic stones, and biliary strictures that is usually seen in young patients of South East Asian descent. Cholangiocarcinoma and secondary biliary cirrhosis are long-term complications.

○ **What are the sites of a postcholecystectomy bile leak and what is the treatment of choice?**

Most likely sites are the cystic duct stump or a duct of Luschka. Treatment with ERCP and stent placement is successful in the majority of cases.

○ **What noninvasive test is most useful in detecting postcholecystectomy bile leaks?**

Hepatobiliary scintigraphy (hepatoiminodiacetic acid [HIDA] scan) is highly sensitive and specific.

○ **What are the indications for preoperative ERCP prior to laparoscopic cholecystectomy?**

Preoperative ERCP is indicated when there is concomitant cholangitis, persistent biliary pancreatitis, or in the setting of a large CBD stone (>1 cm) or multiple CBD stones.

○ **What are the most common complications of chronic pancreatitis?**

In addition to endocrine and exocrine insufficiency, chronic pancreatitis may be complicated by pseudocyst formation, biliary stricture due to CBD obstruction, gastric outlet obstruction, pancreatic ascites/pleural effusion, splenic vein thrombosis with isolated gastric varices, and splenic artery pseudoaneurysm formation.

○ **What is the role of endotherapy in patients with chronic pancreatitis?**

The role of pancreatic endotherapy in chronic pancreatitis is usually limited to symptomatic patients with a dominant pancreatic duct stricture or an obstructing stone in the head of the pancreas. Surgical drainage (Peustow procedure) or resection (Whipple operation) offers more definitive and longer-lasting pain relief in chronic pancreatitis. The use of EUS-guided celiac plexus block for the management of chronic pain is controversial given its generally poor efficacy.

○ **What are the indications for pancreatic pseudocyst drainage?**

The traditional teaching requiring intervention if the pseudocyst is larger than 6 cm or last longer than 6 weeks is no longer recommended. Currently, a more conservative approach is suggested with serial imaging (ultrasound or CT every 3–6 months) followed by pseudocyst drainage only if the patient is symptomatic (eg, abdominal pain, gastric outlet obstruction) or if the pseudocyst is infected. Drainage may be achieved by endoscopic or surgical cystgastrostomy or cystduodenostomy or percutaneously depending on communication of the cyst with the main pancreatic duct.

○ **What are the complications of endoscopic pseudocyst drainage?**

Bleeding, which can be severe enough to require surgical intervention in 5% of cases, retroperitoneal perforation, and infection. Failure to achieve resolution occurs in 10%–35% of cases and recurrence in 6%–18%. EUS-guided pseudocyst drainage decreases risk of bleeding associated with endoscopic drainage. Treatment of an associated pancreatic duct leak with pancreatic duct stent placement decreases the risk of recurrence.

○ **What are the risk factors for post-ERCP pancreatitis?**

Patient factors: young age, female gender, suspected sphincter of Oddi dysfunction, and history of recurrent pancreatitis.

Procedural factors: difficult cannulation, precut sphincterotomy, pancreatic contrast injection, and pancreatic duct sphincterotomy.

○ **What are the proven measures to decrease the risk of post-ERCP pancreatitis?**

In high-risk patients, placement of a temporary pancreatic duct stent at the time of ERCP significantly decreases the risk of pancreatitis. Several pharmacologic measures have been tried but have not proven to be beneficial.

○ **What are the potential complications of pancreatic duct stenting?**

Early complications: pancreatitis, pain, pancreatic duct rupture, bleeding, guidewire fracture requiring surgical removal, and acute cholangitis.

Late complications: development of pancreatic duct changes resembling chronic pancreatitis.

○ **What are the diagnostic criteria for autoimmune pancreatitis?**

HISORt criteria: **H**istology, characteristic **I**maging, **S**erology (elevated IgG4), other **O**rgan involvement (biliary strictures, parotid/lacrimal gland involvement, mediastinal lymphadenopathy, retroperitoneal fibrosis), **R**esponse to steroid **t**reatment.

○ **What are the two most common sites of heterotopic pancreas (ie, pancreatic rest)?**

Stomach (antrum) and duodenum.

○ **What is hereditary pancreatitis?**

It is a syndrome of recurrent acute pancreatitis. The most common cause is a mutation in the cationic trypsinogen gene (PRSS1) expressed in an autosomal dominant pattern. Patients with hereditary pancreatitis have a markedly higher lifetime risk of pancreatic cancer as compared to the general population.

○ **What is annular pancreas?**

It is a congenital anomaly in which a portion of the pancreas forms a thin band around the periampullary portion of the duodenum, leading to complete or partial duodenal obstruction. It is associated with trisomy 21, cardiac defects, intestinal malrotation, genitourinary anomalies, and tracheoesophageal fistula.

○ **When is cholecystectomy indicated for gallbladder polyps?**

Polyps that are 10–20 mm in size could be malignant (25%–77%). Laparoscopic cholecystectomy with removal of the entire connective tissue layer to expose the liver is recommended. Polyps larger than 20 mm are usually malignant and require preoperative staging with CT and EUS.

○ **Name five causes of secondary sclerosing cholangitis.**

Operative trauma and ischemia, chronic choledocholithiasis, cholangiocarcinoma, chronic pancreatitis, and toxins (absolute alcohol and formaldehyde).

○ **How frequently do patients with hepatic artery aneurysms present with jaundice?**

Hepatic artery aneurysms, which are situated close to the bile ducts, present with jaundice in 50% of cases. The classic triad of epigastric pain, hemobilia, and jaundice is present in 33% of cases.

○ **When should hemobilia be suspected?**

Hemobilia should be considered in patients with upper GI bleeding and a recent history of hepatic parenchymal or biliary tract injury, including percutaneous and transjugular liver biopsy, cholecystectomy, endoscopic biliary biopsies and stenting, transjugular intrahepatic portosystemic shunt (TIPS), angioembolization, and blunt abdominal trauma. Other causes include gallstones, cholecystitis, hepatic or bile duct tumors, and hepatic abscesses.

○ **What are the indications for EUS?**

Common indications for EUS include locoregional staging and tissue acquisition in luminal GI malignancies, pancreatico-biliary neoplasms, and subepithelial lesions. Other indications are evaluation for chronic pancreatitis, posterior mediastinal lesions, perianal disease, and therapeutic applications.

○ **Describe the characteristic five layer pattern of the GI tract as seen on EUS.**

1. Mucosal interface
2. Muscularis mucosa
3. Submucosa
4. Muscularis propria
5. Serosa/adventitia

○ **Describe the tumor classification of the TNM staging system for esophageal cancer.**

TX	Primary tumor cannot be assessed
T0	No evidence of primary tumor
Tis	High grade dysplasia
T1	Tumor invades lamina propria, muscularis mucosae or submucosa
T1a	Tumor invades lamina propria or muscularis mucosae
T1b	Tumor invades submucosa
T2	Tumor invades muscularis propria
T3	Tumor invades adventitia
T4	Tumor invades adjacent structures
T4a	Resectable tumor invading pleura, pericardium, or diaphragm
T4b	Unresectable tumor invading other adjacent structures, such as aorta, vertebral body, trachea, etc

○   **An EUS image of a distal esophageal exophytic mass is shown below. Using the TNM staging system, what is the T-stage?**

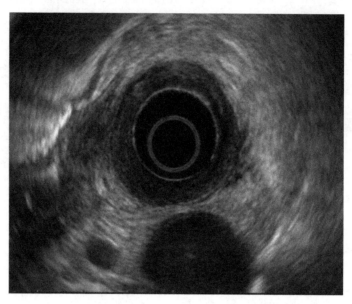

Figure 62-2

The image demonstrates a hypoechoic mass lesion involving the entire circumference of the esophagus leading to loss of the five layer architecture. In addition, there is extension beyond the muscularis propria at 4 o'clock and 9 o'clock positions suggesting a T3 tumor.

○   **A 67-year-old woman presents with painless jaundice and without other systemic complaints. CT scan demonstrates a possible mass in the head of the pancreas. EUS demonstrates the following image. What is the next diagnostic test of choice?**

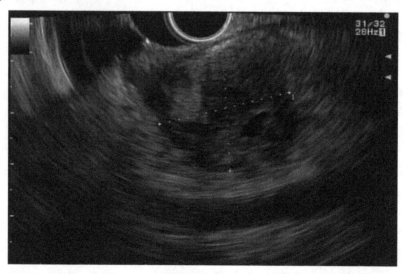

Figure 62-3

Note the hypoechoic mass in the head of the pancreas. Tissue diagnosis may be established through EUS-guided fine needle aspiration (FNA).

○   **What is the layer of origin of the mass noted in the following EUS image? What is the most likely diagnosis?**

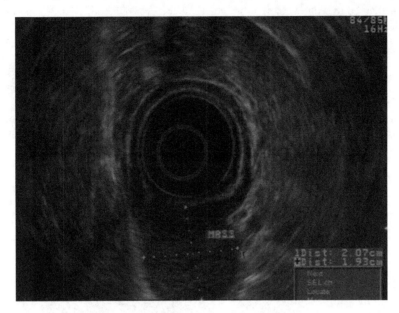

Figure 62-4

Fourth layer (muscularis propria). Gastrointestinal stromal tumors (GISTs) typically arise from the fourth layer (muscularis propria) and are most commonly seen in the stomach. On EUS, they are usually hypoechoic, homogeneous lesions with well-defined margins. Spindle cell neoplasms (leiomyoma and neuroma) have a similar appearance. FNA or tru-cut biopsy with immunohistochemistry is helpful in distinguishing between these lesions.

○   **What are the EUS characteristics of GISTs that predict malignant transformation?**

Size >4 cm, irregular margins, cystic spaces, and echogenic foci.

○   **What is the characteristic immunohistochemical staining pattern for GISTs?**

GISTs characteristically exhibit positive staining for cKIT/CD117 (tyrosine kinase), CD34, and DOG1. Staining for smooth muscle actin (SMA) is negative, a feature that helps to differentiate them from leiomyomas.

○   **What is the characteristic EUS appearance of a lipoma?**

Lipomas usually arise from the third layer (submucosa), appear hyperechoic (bright) and homogeneous on EUS, and have regular margins. A positive pillow-sign on routine endoscopy is highly suggestive of a lipoma.

○   **What is the reported risk of pancreatitis after EUS-FNA of pancreas?**

1%–2%.

○   **What are EUS characteristics that suggest malignant transformation in pancreatic cysts?**

Increase in cyst size over time, thick wall, mural nodularity, or the presence of a solid component within the cyst.

○   **What is the most appropriate maneuver when a "white out" or "red out" occurs during colonoscopy?**

Withdraw the colonoscope until the lumen comes into view.

○ **How is cyst fluid analysis helpful in the evaluation of pancreatic cystic lesions?**

EUS-FNA is usually used to acquire cyst fluid for chemical and cytological analysis. An elevated carcinoembryonic antigen (CEA) level (>200 mg/dL) is more indicative of a mucinous cyst. Elevated cyst fluid amylase level is suggestive of a pseudocyst. Cytology can help in the evaluation of dysplasia within the cyst but sensitivity is limited. EUS-FNA of the cyst wall can also be helpful in evaluating suspected malignancy.

○ **How is EUS helpful in the staging of rectal cancer?**

EUS is indicated for locoregional staging of rectal cancer and for selection of patients who would benefit from neoadjuvant treatment (ie, patients with T3 or higher stage and those with nodal involvement [N1 or higher]). Both EUS and MRI are helpful in defining the extent of invasion into adjacent structures.

○ **An otherwise healthy 73-year-old man presents for open-access colonoscopy due to the recent development of bright red blood per rectum. A rectal lesion shown in the figure is found. What is the likely diagnosis? Subsequent EUS of the lesion is done and demonstrates the finding shown in the figure below. What is the T-stage of the tumor?**

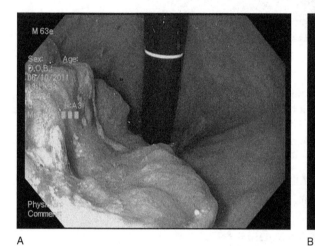
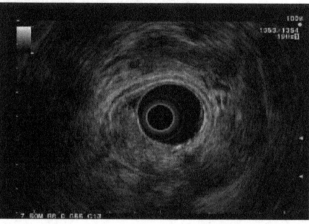

A   B

Figure 62-5 For Figure 62-5A, see also color plate.

The endoscopic image shows a lesion highly suspicious for malignancy, which was subsequently proven following biopsies. The EUS image shows an eccentric mass lesion with involvement of the muscularis propria consistent with a T2 lesion. (see Figure 62-5A)

○ **What are the durations of actions of antiplatelet agents and anticoagulants?**

Aspirin	10 days
Clopidogrel	3–7 days
Warfarin	3–5 days
Low molecular weight heparin	12–24 hours
Unfractionated heparin	4–6 hours

○   **True/False: You should stop warfarin for low-risk endoscopic procedures.**

False. Low-risk procedures include diagnostic endoscopy including biopsy, ERCP without sphincterotomy, EUS without FNA, diagnostic balloon-assisted enteroscopy, capsule endoscopy, and enteral stent deployment without dilation.

○   **What are the high-risk conditions associated with thromboembolic complications that require bridging therapy?**

Atrial fibrillation associated with valvular heart disease, prosthetic valves, active congestive heart failure, left ventricular ejection fraction <35%, history of a thromboembolic event, hypertension, diabetes, age >75 years, mechanical valve in the mitral valve position, mechanical valve in any position with history of thromboembolic event, recently placed coronary stent (<1 year), and acute coronary syndrome.

○   **What are low-risk conditions that do not require bridging therapy?**

Uncomplicated or paroxysmal atrial fibrillation, bioprosthetic valve, mechanical valve in the aortic position, and deep vein thrombosis.

○   **Name the high-risk procedures that require stopping both antiplatelet and anticoagulation therapy?**

Polypectomy, biliary or pancreatic sphincterotomy, pneumatic or bougie dilation, percutaneous endoscopic gastrostomy placement, therapeutic balloon-assisted enteroscopy, EUS with FNA, tumor ablation by any technique, cystogastrostomy, and treatment of varices.

○   **Which endoscopic procedures require antibiotic prophylaxis?**

ERCP with anticipated incomplete drainage of bile duct obstruction, ERCP for sterile pancreatic fluid collection (pseudocyst, necrosis), which communicates with pancreatic duct, transmural drainage of sterile pancreatic fluid collection, EUS-FNA for cystic lesions along GI tract or in the pancreas, PEG tube placement, cirrhosis with acute GI bleed.

○   **What is the rebleed rate of peptic ulcers with 1) active bleeding, 2) nonbleeding visible vessel, 3) adherent clot, and 4) pigmented spot?**

55%–90%, 40%–50%, 10%–36%, and 7%–10%, respectively.

○   **What medications are preferred for procedural sedation during pregnancy?**

Meperidine (category B) alone is preferred but midazolam (category D) can be used as needed. Propofol (category B) can be used for deep sedation.

○   **What medication is preferred for procedural sedation during breastfeeding?**

Fentanyl has the lowest breast milk concentrations of the medications typically used. Infants should not be breastfed for at least 4 hours after maternal midazolam or propofol administration.

○   **What are the indications for diagnostic balloon-assisted enteroscopy?**

Evaluation of obscure GI bleed, suspected nonsteroidal anti-inflammatory drug (NSAID)-induced injury, suspected or established small bowel Crohn's disease, refractory celiac disease, evaluation and tattooing of small bowel malignancies or other abnormal findings on imaging studies, detection of polyps in patients with polyposis syndromes, assistance with difficult and/or previously incomplete colonoscopies, and examination of the excluded stomach in patients who have undergone Roux-en-Y gastric bypass.

○ **What are the therapeutic applications of balloon-assisted enteroscopy?**

Treatment of GI bleeding, small bowel polypectomy, stricture dilation, stenting of small bowel obstructions, foreign body retrieval, endoscopic mucosal resection (EMR), and placement of direct percutaneous jejunostomy.

○ **What are potential complications of balloon-assisted enteroscopy?**

Pancreatitis, perforation, bleeding, and aspiration pneumonia. The overall complication rate is 1.2%–1.6%.

○ **True/False: Moderate sedation (conscious sedation) refers to drug-induced depression of consciousness during which patients 1) cannot be easily aroused but respond purposefully following repeated or painful stimulation, 2) may have impaired ability to independently maintain ventilatory function, and 3) may require assistance in maintaining a patent airway.**

False. The preceding is correct for deep sedation not moderate sedation, which is defined as a drug-induced depression of consciousness during which patients 1) respond purposefully to verbal commands, either alone or accompanied by light tactile stimulation, 2) do not require interventions to maintain a patent airway, and 3) maintain adequate spontaneous ventilation.

○ **True/False: Capnography is recommended for all patients undergoing moderate (conscious) sedation.**

False. Capnography is a noninvasive technique that measures carbon dioxide in exhaled breath and is more sensitive than direct visual observation or pulse oximetry for detecting hypoventilation. The American Society of Anesthesiologists (ASA) currently recommends that capnography be considered for patients receiving deep sedation and for patients whose ventilation cannot be observed directly during moderate sedation. It is not yet recommended for routine use during endoscopy.

○ **True/False: The patency capsule is used to assure small bowel patency before video capsule endoscopy (VCE) and can also be used as a diagnostic test for suspected small bowel strictures that cannot be identified by standard radiographic means.**

True. The patency capsule does not have any image acquisition capability.

○ **True/False: Incomplete transit of the VCE capsule during its recording time occurs in approximately 33% of procedures**

False. It occurs in < 20% and is of no clinical consequence, other than resulting in an incomplete examination of the small bowel.

○ **Topical anesthetics for upper endoscopy should be avoided in patients with glucose-6-phosphate-dehydrogenase (G6PD) deficiency.**

True. Topical anesthetics have been associated with methemoglobinemia in these patients.

○ **True/False: Bougie esophageal dilation and pneumatic balloon dilation are equally effective in the treatment of achalasia.**

False. The more forceful pneumatic dilation is necessary.

○ **True/False: The endpoint of an esophageal dilation should be a lumen diameter of 13 mm.**

False. Although there is no consensus, an endpoint of 18 mm is often chosen for most benign causes of esophageal strictures as it usually allows ingestion of a regular diet. Certainly, in some complex strictures (eg, radiation, caustic), a lesser diameter may be more appropriate.

○ **What is the rule of 3's?**

The rule of 3's pertains to esophageal dilation using bougie dilators whereby, once mild resistance is felt, continued dilation should only continue to a maximum of three additional dilator sizes (ie, 3 mm increase in diameter) during a single session.

○ **What are some quality indicators for the performance of colonoscopy?**

Cecal intubation rate, polyp and adenoma detection rates, photodocumentation of the cecum, documentation of the quality of the bowel preparation, retroflexion in the rectum, and complication rate.

○ **True/False: Carbon dioxide (CO_2) insufflation in deeply and moderately sedated patients during colonoscopy has been clearly shown to be superior to conventional air insufflation with regards to patient satisfaction.**

False. A recent study reported that CO_2 insufflation had no impact on patients' satisfaction with the procedure or on their attitude to voluntary colorectal cancer screening; however, it was associated with significantly diminished abdominal pain after the procedure.

○ **True/False: EMR is a suitable endoscopic alternative to surgical resection of mucosal and submucosal neoplastic lesions and intramucosal (T1) cancers.**

True.

○ **True/False: Puckering or nonlifting of the lesion during injection of saline for a saline-assisted polypectomy suggests invasion of the muscularis propria.**

True. Submucosal injection may decrease the incidence of perforation during saline-assisted polypectomy and EMR.

○ **True/False: Complications with India ink injection, used for lesion localization, are common and may be related to the wide variety of organic and inorganic compounds contained in the ink solution such as carriers, stabilizers, binders, and fungicides.**

False. Complications with India ink are rare, although the second part of the sentence is correct.

● ● ● SUGGESTED READINGS ● ● ●

ASGE Practice Guideline on the management of low-molecular weight heparin and nonaspirin antiplatelet agents for endoscopic procedures. *Gastrointest Endosc.* 2005;61:189-194.

Cotton PB, Williams CB, Hawes RH, Saunders BP. *Practical gastrointestinal endoscopy: The fundamentals.* 6th ed. Hoboken, NJ: Wiley-Blackwell; 2008.

Baron TH, Kozarek RA, Carr-Locke D, eds. *ERCP.* 1st ed. Philadelphia, PA: WB Saunders Co; 2007.

CPSIA information can be obtained
at www.ICGtesting.com
Printed in the USA
BVHW010733070819
555146BV00028B/61/P